A–Z Guide to
Drug-Herb-Vitamin
Interactions

A–Z Guide to Drug-Herb-Vitamin Interactions

REVISED AND UPDATED 2ND EDITION

Improve Your Health and Avoid Side Effects When Using
Common Medications and Natural Supplements Together

Alan R. Gaby, M.D., Chief Science Editor

Forrest Batz, Pharm.D.

Rick Chester, R.Ph., N.D., Dipl.Ac.

George Constantine, R.Ph., Ph.D.

With contributions by

Steve Austin, N.D.
Eric Yarnell, N.D.
Donald J. Brown, N.D.
Jeremy Appleton, N.D.

Schuyler W. Lininger, Healthnotes Publisher

 THREE RIVERS PRESS · NEW YORK

healthnotes®

Copyright © 2006 by Healthnotes, Inc.

Published in the United States by Three Rivers Press, an imprint of the Crown Publishing Group, a division of Random House, Inc., New York.
www.crownpublishing.com

THREE RIVERS PRESS and the Tugboat design are registered trademarks of Random House, Inc.

Library of Congress Cataloging-in-Publication Data

A–Z guide to drug-herb-vitamin interactions : improve your health and avoid side effects when using common medications and natural supplements together / edited by Alan R. Gaby; with contributions by Steve Austin . . . [et al.].—Rev. and expanded 2nd ed.
Includes index.
1. Drug-herb interactions.   2. Drug-nutrient interactions.   I. Gaby, Alan.
RM666.H33A16 2006
615'.7045—dc22
2005022327

ISBN-13: 978-0-307-33664-4
ISBN-10: 0-307-33664-6

Printed in the United States of America

Design by Cynthia Dunne

10 9 8 7 6

Second Edition

For my wife, Beth, who has shared my journey
in pursuing the truth regarding natural medicine. —*ARG*

For the Healthnotes team. —*SWL*

Acknowledgments

This book is the result of the work of many dedicated healthcare professionals who believe in the power of evidence-based natural medicine. They receive well-deserved credit on the title page, but special recognition goes to Chief Science Editor Alan R. Gaby, M.D. His hard work, sense of humor, and dedication to excellence and quality are an inspiration to all of us.

The "hidden" work is done by the hardworking, talented, and dedicated members of the Product Development and Marketing teams at Healthnotes, Inc. Although many people were involved, Jenefer Angell, Loren Jenkins, Kurt Kremer, and Jeannette Shupp deserve special mention for their efforts on this book.

Thanks are also due our publisher, Three Rivers Press. Our editor, Kathryn McHugh, has been a strong advocate for this new and greatly expanded edition. Her efforts are really appreciated.

Finally, thanks to our families, friends, and customers who continue to strongly support our company and our work.

—Dr. Skye Lininger, Healthnotes Publisher

Contents

Interactions by Herb or Vitamin

Herbs

Foreword

As PEOPLE INCREASINGLY explore their power to improve their own lives and an aging baby boomer population reaches out for alternatives to traditional therapies, attention has turned to integrative medicine. At the same time, the rising cost of healthcare has encouraged consumers to take more responsibility for their own physical well-being, from prevention to treatment. In particular, the emergence of new public health issues, such as the epidemic increases in childhood obesity and diabetes, urges us to find complementary and alternative solutions to these problems.

When one is taking a more active role in self-care, the importance of education cannot be overstated, particularly as it relates to the different forms of nutritional supplements, the potencies of different extracts, and how specific intake amounts may benefit particular health concerns. The *A–Z Guide to Drug-Herb-Vitamin Interactions* gives people a quick, easy tool to become informed about the effects of drugs and natural treatments.

This book lists both over-the-counter and prescription medications. It breaks compound substances into their component parts while making the information easily accessible by listing both brand and generic names. Not only are the drug interactions with dietary supplements addressed, but also interactions with herbs, foods, and alcohol are discussed. Interactions—both positive and negative—include nutrient depletions, side-effect risk reduction, potential adverse reactions, reduced drug absorption and bioavailability, and supportive interactions.

The *A–Z Guide to Drug-Herb-Vitamin Interactions* is the only comprehensive book to take into consideration that drug depletions can be a severe problem and that we sometimes need to replace what medications take out of our system to put our bodies back in balance.

Consumers need objective, reliable sources of health information. Accessible science, such as readers will find here, helps them come to safe conclusions about healthcare and natural treatments. The *A–Z Guide to Drug-Herb-Vitamin Interactions* is grounded in the mission of providing comprehensive, scientifically based information from leading natural medicine experts, empowering individuals to make informed decisions about their health. As a physician, I can't emphasize strongly enough how important it is to review the supplements you're considering with your physician, especially any potential interactions you've uncovered in this very useful guide.

— *Dr. Bob Arnot, NBC news correspondent, expert health and fitness author and columnist*

Preface

RECENT TIMES HAVE seen an explosion of interest in natural medicine, and sales of nutritional supplements and herbal remedies continue to grow each year. One factor helping to drive this change has been the growing recognition that natural medicine can often promote healing in a way that is safer, less expensive, and more effective than conventional medical practices. Another important force in the move toward natural medicine is growing discomfort with the largely symptom-suppressive approach to healthcare. Individuals are becoming increasingly concerned about both the safety and effectiveness of pharmaceutical drugs, and questions are even being asked about the scrupulousness and integrity of the companies that make them.

More and more, people are feeling motivated to take their health issues into their own hands and are finding that natural medicine often provides them with the tools to do so. However, while the use of pharmaceutical drugs can be fraught with hazards, there is no doubt that these agents can bring profound benefits to some, and indeed may even save lives. And while natural remedies such as nutritional supplements and medicinal herbs are broadly safe, they also have the potential for harm—particularly when taken in conjunction wth conventional drugs. Natural remedies can, for instance, reduce or increase the effects of prescription or over-the-counter medication. Also, some drugs can deplete the body of nutrients, which can have adverse effects on health.

With increasing numbers of individuals using natural medicines alongside conventional drugs, it is now critically important that individuals have access to reliable and trustworthy information about any hazards that may ensue. To this end, the *A–Z Guide to Drug-Herb-Vitamin Interactions* is a truly comprehensive and reliable guide. It details some 18,000 drug-nutrient-herb interactions and provides critical information people need if they are to use natural remedies in a way that is truly educated and safe. To my mind, the *A–Z Guide to Drug-Herb-Vitamin Interactions* is a must for anyone seeking to use remedies of all kinds in a way that minimizes risk and maximizes benefit.

—Dr. John Briffa, leading British natural medicine
specialist, award-winning journalist,
author, and columnist

Introduction

OVER THE LAST several decades, use of vitamins, minerals, and herbs to treat a wide range of health concerns has become so widespread that many remedies are familiar to the general public and have been adopted as part of many individuals' regular self-care practices. However, while people have come to enjoy and trust the benefits of natural medicine, the incorrect perception that a natural substance is always healthful and safe persists, so many users of vitamins and herbs take prescription and nonprescription medicines along with supplements, unaware of possible interactions. Though relatively rare and less frequent than negative reactions to over-the-counter and prescription medications, those cases in which an herb or supplement causes a negative reaction become highly publicized by the media, which then warns people against the substance in question, rather than educating them about specific risks and safe usage. Furthermore, while people interested in natural remedies often don't know to ask their healthcare providers about interactions, those who do may find that many practitioners don't know how to access reliable information.

Fortunately, the gap between natural and Western medicine is rapidly closing, evidenced by the explosion of research on natural treatments in recent years. As more doctors recognize the efficacy of natural protocols there has also been more interest in combining them with conventional treatments. Despite this increased attention, however, safety information on the interactions between drugs, herbs, and vitamins is as difficult to find as it was when we published the first edition of the best-selling *A–Z Guide to Drug-Herb-Vitamin Interactions*. So we are happy now to publish this updated version, with a new format that makes it even easier to use.

The Healthnotes medical writing team—the group that created the Healthnotes electronic knowledgebase and our original book, *The Natural Pharmacy*—has compiled safety and interaction information from over 25,000 scientific articles pulled from more than 600 journals, to give you the essential information you need to determine whether you should take a vitamin or herb with your medicine. This revised edition of the *A–Z Guide to Drug-Herb-Vitamin Interactions* is much expanded, with coverage of almost 200 additional drugs, including 31 new combination drugs. It also provides 167 new drug-nutrient interaction articles. In addition, every article has been updated with the latest scientific research. We have added an informative new article, "What Are Depletions and Interactions?" and articles on new, high-profile drugs.

Otherwise, this edition shares the same characteristics as the original:

- All statements that might be controversial have been documented with references from the scientific literature.

- Thousands of citations are referenced and available online, so the serious reader can retrieve the article and review the material we relied on.

- In addition, we have tried to use primarily human studies, although in the area of drug-nutrient and drug-herb interactions, animal or test tube trials are in some cases the only resources available.

- Our expert scientific and evidence-based medical team consists of medical doctors, pharmacists, naturopaths, and doctors of chiropractic. All of our key contributors have actually been in practice with real patients and are also trained to recognize the difference between reliable and questionable scientific evidence.

In short, we have done our best to create the most useful, authoritative, and balanced book available on this topic—a place you can turn to for answers. For more information on using vitamins and herbs to treat health conditions, see our companion volume, *The Natural Pharmacy*.

All of the Healthnotes team joins me in wishing you good health.

—Alan R. Gaby, M.D., Chief Medical Editor,
Healthnotes, Inc.

How to Use This Book

The *A–Z Guide to Drug-Herb-Vitamin Interactions* reviews more than 18,000 known major interactions between pharmaceutical medicines and food, nutrients, and herbs, such as iron deficiency triggered by long-term use of aspirin, or inhibition of vitamin K caused by antibiotics. This handy reference book gives you information about how some herbs or nutritional supplements help drugs work better, which drugs deplete your body of crucial nutrients, which drugs and supplements should never be taken together, and which drug side effects can be reduced by taking the right nutritional supplement or herb.

Note that in this book the words *drug, medicine,* and *medication* are used interchangeably.

Important Features

- **Generic Drugs**—All the prescription and over-the-counter medications covered in the *A–Z Guide to Drug-Herb-Vitamin Interactions* are listed alphabetically in the table of contents by generic name (the active ingredient).

- **Brand-Name Drugs**—Generic drugs are often packaged and branded by different companies. For example, the generic drug ibuprofen is sold under several brand names, such as Advil, Motrin, and Nuprin. Brand names can be found in the index and are listed under the generic name in each entry.

- **Combination Drugs**—Some drugs are combinations of other drugs. In the Drug Interactions section, an entry on a combination drug will have the text "Contains the following ingredients," listing each component with page numbers directing you to that

ingredient's interactions entry. Generic combination drugs are listed in the table of contents; brand-name combination drugs are listed in the index.

- **Drug Interactions by Herb or Vitamin**—This section allows you to look up a vitamin or herb to see what drugs it interacts with, positively or negatively. This book sometimes refers to vitamins and minerals as "nutritional supplements."

- **Summary of Interactions Table**—The summary table rates each nutrient with which the drug reacts and provides a quick reference. See the next section, **"What Are Depletions and Interactions?"** (page xxvii), for a full description of the summary table, a topic overview, and answers to some frequently asked questions.

- **Cross References**—For easy navigation, drug names, herbs, and vitamins are bolded and followed by a page number that will take you to information on that topic, much the way hyperlinks work online. If a drug topic mentions vitamin C, for example, then "vitamin C" will appear in bold type, followed by a page number that takes you to the entry on vitamin C.

- **Use the Table of Contents and Index**—The table of contents lists generic drugs, vitamins, and herbs by their common names. Try the index for alternate names, drug brand names, and for botanical names of herbs.

- **Find References**—We have tried not to make any statements without referring to scientific documentation. We rely most heavily on human studies published in major medical and scientific journals, which can be found using reference numbers. If you or your doctor wants to see the original study, the full references for each entry can be easily accessed online at www.healthnotes.com/a-zguide.

What Is *Not* Covered in This Book

Please be aware that you will not find the following in the *A–Z Guide to Drug-Herb-Vitamin Interactions*:

- **Other Types of Interactions**—The following types of interactions are not discussed:

    - Side effects that may be caused by a drug only (see your prescription or OTC drug package insert for this information)

    - Interactions between two or more drugs

    - Interactions between alcohol and specific nutrients

    - Interactions between drugs and water (for example, drugs inducing dehydration)

- **Every Possible Drug-Herb-Vitamin Interaction**—Although this book is extensive, it includes only documented drug-nutrient or drug-herb interactions. In other words, a drug not included in the book may still have drug-food, drug-nutrient, or drug-herb interactions that have not yet been identified or written about. For these reasons, it is not sufficient to rely solely on the information presented here.

- **Information That Replaces Medical Advice**—It is always wise for people seeking information about interactions between a prescription drug and food, specific nutrients, or herbs to talk with their pharmacist, prescribing physician, or other healthcare professional. In addition, the information in this book is not intended to replace information supplied by a doctor or pharmacist; neither is it intended to replace package inserts or other printed material that may be available for or accompany a particular drug.

What Are Depletions and Interactions?

Body chemistry

Your body functions because millions of chemical reactions are constantly going on inside you. Everything that you eat and drink influences those reactions, including foods, beverages, and drugs.

Using drugs to treat illness

Drugs are manufactured to help correct the body's chemistry when irregularities are caused by illness or genetic makeup.

When the body isn't working properly, drugs can often replace a chemical that is missing, block an unwanted reaction, or enhance a desired reaction. In the process, a drug may also cause the body to lose or need more of important nutrients, such as potassium, sodium, calcium, or some vitamins.

Sometimes, taking an herb or nutrient with a drug can cause an unhealthy or harmful reaction. Other times, an herb or nutrient might actually improve the action of a drug. Some herbs or nutrients, when taken at the same time as a drug, might reduce the amount of medication absorbed into the body, reducing its effectiveness. (This can often be avoided by taking the drug and the herb or nutrient at different times.)

Side effects

All drugs have the potential to cause unwanted symptoms, or side effects. Some herbs or nutrients, when taken with a drug, might help to prevent the side effects or make them less severe.

Depletions

Depletion happens when a drug causes the body to lose a nutrient. The drug might also interfere with the nutrient's absorption.

A good example of a drug that depletes nutrients from the body is the diuretic furosemide. Furosemide causes the body to lose potassium, so people taking furosemide might need to supplement with potassium to avoid unwanted problems such as muscle cramps, fatigue, or heart rhythm disturbances.

Interactions

Interactions happen when a nutrient affects the way a drug works, or when a drug affects the way a nutrient works. Interactions can be beneficial or harmful.

An example of a good interaction might be when a person taking the drug fluoxetine (Prozac) also takes the nutrient folic acid. This combination might increase the drug's effectiveness.

An example of a bad result of an interaction might be a person taking the herb St. John's wort while taking the drug digoxin (Lanoxin). In this situation, the herb might reduce the absorption of the drug, which would result in lower-than-necessary blood levels of the drug.

Reading the Summary Tables

For your safety, the *A–Z Guide to Drug-Herb-Vitamin Interactions* provides depletion and interaction information for drugs, nutritional supplements, herbs, and foods. All medications are indexed alphabetically by both their generic and brand names.

Within each drug entry you will find a summary listing the interacting supplements, herbs, and foods in one or more of the following six categories:

May be beneficial

✓ *Depletion or interference*—The medication may deplete or interfere with the absorption or function of the nutrient. Taking these nutrients may help replenish them.

✓ *Side effect reduction/prevention*—Taking these supplements may help reduce the likelihood and/or severity of a potential side effect caused by the medication.

✓ *Supportive interaction*—Taking these supplements may support or otherwise help your medication work better.

Avoid

⊘ *Adverse interaction*—Avoid these supplements when taking this medication because taking them together may cause undesirable or dangerous results.

⊘ *Reduced drug absorption/bioavailability*—Avoid these supplements when taking this medication since the supplement may decrease the absorption and/or activity of the medication in the body.

Explanation required

ⓘ *Other*—Before taking any of these supplements or eating any of these foods with your medication, read the drug article in full for details.

An asterisk (*) next to an item in the Summary Table indicates that the interaction is supported only by weak, fragmentary, and/or contradictory information.

Frequently Asked Questions

Why do you sometimes list a supplement as both beneficial and something to avoid for the same drug?

When a medication depletes the body of a nutrient, it may be beneficial to take more of that nutrient to compensate; however, it might also be necessary to avoid taking the nutritional supplement at the same time of day as the drug because taking them together might reduce drug absorption.

For example, calcium is listed both as beneficial and as something to avoid when taking thyroid medication. Taking extra calcium might be necessary to replace the calcium that is depleted by thyroid hormone, but it should not be taken at the same time of day as thyroid hormone because calcium might reduce absorption of the drug.

How do I know if my drug is causing a depletion or interaction?

Usually a person does not know that a drug is depleting a nutrient until the body shows symptoms of deficiency. In some cases, your healthcare provider might run blood tests to check whether nutrient levels are low. For example, individuals taking the diuretic furosemide should have potassium blood levels monitored regularly to detect depletion.

You might notice a bad interaction if your drug stops working as effectively or if you develop unwanted symptoms when you begin taking a new nutrient or add a new food to your diet. Similarly, you might notice a beneficial interaction if your drug starts working better after adding a new food or nutrient.

As natural substances, are herbs and vitamins safer than drugs?

Herbs and vitamins are not necessarily safer just because they are natural. Though herbs and vitamins are generally safer than drugs, some might produce unwanted side effects when a person takes too much. And if you are taking medications, you should always check with your doctor or pharmacist before taking new herbs or nutritional supplements.

When nutrients are depleted, are supplements the only way to replace them?

Though supplements are more commonly used than foods to replace depleted nutrients, certain foods may also work. For example, people who need to replace potassium might choose to eat bananas or other fruit rather than take supplements.

Interactions by Drug

Some interactions may increase the need for the drug (✓), other interactions may be negative (⊘) and indicate the drug should not be taken without first speaking with your physician or pharmacist. Others may require further explanation (ⓘ). Refer to the individual drug entry for specific details about an interaction.

ACCURETIC

Contains the following ingredients:
Hydrochlorothiazide
Quinapril (page 226)

ACEBUTOLOL

Common names: Sectral

Combination drug: Secradex

Acebutolol is used to treat high blood pressure and certain forms of heart arrhythmia, and is in a family of drugs known as **beta-adrenergic blockers** (page 37).

Summary of Interactions for Acebutolol

In some cases, an herb or supplement may appear in more than one category, which may seem contradictory. For clarification, read the full article for details about the summarized interactions.

⊘ Avoid: Reduced drug absorption bioavailability	Food
⊘ Avoid: Adverse interaction	High-potassium foods* Pleurisy root* Potassium supplements*
Depletion or interference	None known
Side effect reduction/prevention	None known
Supportive interaction	None known

Interactions with Dietary Supplements

Potassium

Some beta-adrenergic blockers (called "nonselective" beta blockers) decrease the uptake of potassium from the blood into the cells,[1] leading to excess potassium in the blood, a potentially dangerous condition known as hyperkalemia.[2] People taking beta-blockers should therefore avoid taking potassium supplements, or eating large quantities of fruit (e.g., bananas), unless directed to do so by their doctor.

Interactions with Herbs

Pleurisy root

As pleurisy root and other plants in the *Aesclepius* genus contain cardiac glycosides, it is best to avoid use of pleurisy root with heart medications such as beta-blockers.[3]

Interaction with Foods and Other Compounds

Taking acebutolol with food slows the rate of absorption and reduces the maximum blood levels of the drug, though overall absorption is not affected.[4] However, the blood level of an active breakdown product of acebutolol is reduced.[5] Though the activity of acebutolol is affected by food, people taking the drug on a daily basis are not likely to experience a reduction in the effectiveness of the drug if it is taken with a meal.

ACETAMINOPHEN

Common names: 222 AF, Abenol, Acetab, Acet, Alisphene Forte, Alvedon, Anadin Paracetamol, APAP, Apo-Acetaminophen, Artritol, Atasol, Boots Children's Pain Relief Syrup, Boots Cold Relief Hot

Acetaminophen

Blackcurrant, Boots Cold Relief Hot Lemon, Boots Infant Pain Relief, Calpol 6 Plus, Calpol Infant, Calpol Pediatric, Calpol, Cephanol, Children's Acetaminophen, Children's Feverhalt, Cupanol Over 6, Cupanol Under 6, Disprol, Dom-Acetaminophen, Fanalgic, Fennings Children's Cooling Powders, Hill's Balsam Flu Strength Hot Lemon Powders, Infadrops, Lem-Plus Powders, Medinol, Novogesic, Pain Aid Free, Paldesic, Panaleve 6+, Panaleve Junior, Pandol, Panodol Baby and Infant, Paracetamol, Paracets, Paraclear, Paramin, Pediatrix, PMS Acetaminophen, Resolve, Robigesic Elixir, Rounox, Salzone, Tantaphen, Tempra, Tixymol, Tramil 500, Trianon, Tylenol, WestCan Extra Strength Acetaminophen, WestCan Regular Strength Acetaminophen

Combination drugs: Alka-Seltzer Plus, Co-Proxamol, Coalgesic, Darvocet N, Distalgesic, Endocet, Excedrin PM, Fioricet, Lortab, Midrin, Nyquil, Nyquil Hot Therapy Powder, Percocet, Phrenilin, Propacet 100, Roxicet, Theraflu, Tylenol Allergy Sinus, Tylenol Cold, Tylenol Flu NightTime Maximum Strength Powder, Tylenol Multi-Symptom Hot Medication, Tylenol PM, Tylenol Sinus, Tylenol with Codeine, Vicodin, Wygesic

Acetaminophen is used to reduce pain and fever. Unlike NSAIDs (**nonsteroidal anti-inflammatory drugs**) (page 193), it lacks anti-inflammatory activity. Acetaminophen is available by itself or in nonprescription and prescription-only combination products used to relieve pain and the symptoms associated with colds and flu.

Summary of Interactions for Acetaminophen

In some cases, an herb or supplement may appear in more than one category, which may seem contradictory. For clarification, read the full article for details about the summarized interactions.

✓ May be Beneficial: Side effect reduction/prevention	Milk thistle* N-acetyl cysteine
✓ May be Beneficial: Supportive interaction	Vitamin C*
⊘ Avoid: Reduced drug absorption/ bioavailability	Hibiscus
ⓘ Check: Other	Schisandra
Depletion or interference	None known
Adverse interaction	None known

Interactions with Dietary Supplements

N-acetyl cysteine (NAC)

Hospitals use oral and intravenous N-acetyl cysteine (NAC) to treat liver damage induced by acetaminophen overdose poisoning.[1] NAC is often administered intravenously by emergency room doctors. Oral NAC appears to be effective for acetaminophen toxicity.

An uncontrolled trial compared intravenous NAC with oral NAC in children with acetaminophen poisoning and found that both methods were equally effective in reversing acetaminophen-induced liver toxicity.[2] However, acetaminophen toxicity is a potential medical emergency, and should only be managed by qualified healthcare professionals.

Vitamin C

Taking 3 grams vitamin C with acetaminophen has been shown to prolong the amount of time acetaminophen stays in the body.[3] This theoretically might allow people to use less acetaminophen, thereby reducing the risk of side effects. Consult with a doctor about this potential before reducing the amount of acetaminophen.

Interactions with Herbs

Hibiscus

One small study found that hibiscus could decrease levels of acetaminophen if the drug was taken after the tea was consumed though it was not entirely clear if the decreases were clinically significant.[4]

Milk thistle (Silybum marianum)

Silymarin is a collection of complex flavonoids found in milk thistle that has been shown to elevate liver glutathione levels in rats.[5] Acetaminophen can cause liver damage, which is believed to involve glutathione depletion.[6] In one study involving rats, silymarin protected against acetaminophen-induced glutathione depletion.[7] While studies to confirm this action in humans have not been conducted, some doctors recommend silymarin supplementation with 200 mg milk thistle extract, containing 70–80% silymarin, three times per day for people taking acetaminophen in large amounts for more than one year and/or with other risk factors for liver problems.

Schisandra (Schisandra chinensis)

Gomisin A is a constituent found in the Chinese herb schisandra. In a study of rats given liver-damaging amounts of acetaminophen, gomisin A appeared to protect against some liver damage but did not prevent glutathione depletion[8] (unlike milk thistle, as reported above). Studies have not yet confirmed this action in humans.

Interactions with Foods and Other Compounds

Food

Food, especially foods high in pectin (including jellies), carbohydrates, and large amounts of cruciferous vegetables (broccoli, Brussels sprouts, cabbage, and others) can interfere with acetaminophen absorption.[9] It is unclear how much effect this interaction has on acetaminophen activity.

Alcohol
Moderate to high amounts of acetaminophen have caused liver damage in people with alcoholism.[10] To prevent problems, people taking acetaminophen should avoid alcohol.

ACEZIDE

Contains the following ingredients:
    Captopril (page 47)
    Hydrochlorothiazide

ACTONORM GEL

Contains the following ingredients:
    Aluminium
    Dimethicone
    Magnesium
    Peppermint oil

ACYCLOVIR ORAL

Common names: Virovir, Zovirax Oral

Acyclovir is an antiviral drug used to treat shingles, genital herpes, and chickenpox.

Summary of Interactions for Oral Acyclovir
In some cases, an herb or supplement may appear in more than one category, which may seem contradictory. For clarification, read the full article for details about the summarized interactions.

✓	May be Beneficial: Supportive interaction	Citrus root bark* Flavonoids* *Geum japonicum** *Rhus javanica** *Syzygium aromaticum** *Terminalia chebula** *Tripterygium wilfordii**

Depletion or interference	None known
Side effect reduction/prevention	None known
Reduced drug absorption/bioavailability	None known
Adverse interaction	None known

Interactions with Dietary Supplements
Flavonoids
The flavonoids quercetin, quercitrin, and apigenin enhanced the antiviral activity of acyclovir in test tube studies.[1] Controlled research is needed to determine whether taking quercetin or other flavonoid supplements would increase the effectiveness of acyclovir in humans.

Interactions with Herbs
Citrus species
The alkaloid citrusinine-1 from the root bark of citrus plants has been shown to enhance the antiviral activity of acyclovir.[2] Further research is needed to determine whether taking citrus root bark would increase the effectiveness of acyclovir in humans.

Tripterygium wilfordii
Test tube studies show that triptofordin C-2 increases the antiviral activity of acyclovir against the herpes virus.[3] Controlled human research is needed to determine whether taking tripterygium would increase the effectiveness of acyclovir in humans.

Other herbs
Animal studies have shown that other herbs, including *Geum japonicum*, *Rhus javanica*, *Syzygium aromaticum*, and *Terminalia chebula* enhance the antiviral activity of acyclovir.[4] Controlled human studies are needed to determine whether taking these herbs would increase the effectiveness of acyclovir in humans.

ACYCLOVIR TOPICAL

Common names: Aciclovir Topical, Boots Avert, Herpetad, Soothelip, Viralief, Virasorb, Zovirax Topical

Acyclovir is an antiviral drug applied to the skin to treat the first outbreaks of genital herpes as well as herpes infections in people with poor immune systems. Topical application of acyclovir speeds up the healing process and the duration of pain.

Summary of Interactions for Topical Acyclovir

In some cases, an herb or supplement may appear in more than one category, which may seem contradictory. For clarification, read the full article for details about the summarized interactions.

Depletion or interference	None known
Side effect reduction/prevention	None known
Supportive interaction	None known
Reduced drug absorption/bioavailability	None known
Adverse interaction	None known

ADAPALENE

Common names: Differin

Adapalene is a vitamin A–related drug that is applied to the skin to treat acne.

Summary of Interactions for Adapalene

In some cases, an herb or supplement may appear in more than one category, which may seem contradictory. For clarification, read the full article for details about the summarized interactions.

Depletion or interference	None known
Side effect reduction/prevention	None known
Supportive interaction	None known
Reduced drug absorption/bioavailability	None known
Adverse interaction	None known

Interaction with Foods and Other Compounds

Topical application of adapalene may cause skin irritation in some individuals. This irritation can be worsened when alcohol, astringents, spices, and lime are also applied to the area.[1] Sensitive individuals should use caution when using adapalene and other topical compounds.

ADCORTYL WITH GRANEODIN

Contains the following ingredients:
Gramicidin
Neomycin (page 187)
Triamcinolone

ADGYN COMBI

Contains the following ingredients:
Estradiol (page 108)
Norethisterone

ADVANCED FORMULA DI-GEL TABLETS

Contains the following ingredients:
Calcium carbonate
Magnesium hydroxide (page 166)
Simethicone (page 239)

ALBUTEROL

Common names: Aerolin, Airomir, Albuterol Inhaled, Alti-Salbutamol Sulfate, Asmasal, Asmavent, Gen-Salbutamol, Novo-Salmol, Nu-Salbutamol, PMS-Salbutamol, Proventil, Rho-Salbutamol, Salbutamol, Salmol, Ventodisks, Ventolin, Volmax

Combination drug: Combivent

Albuterol is a short-acting, beta-adrenergic bronchodilator drug used for relief and prevention of bronchospasm. It is also used to prevent exercise-induced bronchospasm. While albuterol is available in tablet form, it is most commonly used by oral inhalation into the lungs.

Summary of Interactions for Albuterol

In some cases, an herb or supplement may appear in more than one category, which may seem contradictory. For clarification, read the full article for details about the summarized interactions.

✓ May be Beneficial: Depletion or interference	Calcium* Magnesium* Phosphate* Potassium*
✓ May be Beneficial: Supportive interaction	Coleus*
ⓘ Check: Other	Digitalis
Side effect reduction/prevention	None known
Reduced drug absorption/bioavailability	None known
Adverse interaction	None known

Interactions with Dietary Supplements

Minerals

Therapeutic amounts of intravenous salbutamol (albuterol) in four healthy people were associated with decreased plasma levels of calcium, magnesium, phosphate, and potassium.[1] Decreased potassium levels have been reported with oral,[2] intramuscular, and subcutaneous albuterol administration.[3] How frequently this effect occurs is not known; whether these changes are preventable through diet or supplementation is also unknown.

Interactions with Herbs

Digitalis (Digitalis lanata, Digitalis purpurea)

Digitalis refers to a family of plants (commonly called foxglove) that contain digitalis glycosides, chemicals with actions and toxicities similar to the prescription drug **digoxin** (page 90).

In a small study of salbutamol (albuterol) in people receiving digoxin, albuterol was associated with decreased serum digoxin levels.[4] No interactions between albuterol and digitalis have been reported. Until more is known, albuterol and digitalis-containing products should be used only under the direct supervision of a doctor trained in their use.

Coleus

A test tube study demonstrated that the bronchodilating effects of salbutamol (albuterol) were significantly increased by the addition of forskolin, the active component of the herb *Coleus forskohlii*.[5] The results of this preliminary research suggest that the combination of forskolin and beta-agonists such as albuterol might provide an alternative to raising the doses of the beta-agonist drugs as they lose effectiveness. Until more is known, coleus should not be combined with albuterol without the supervision of a doctor.

Interactions with Foods and Other Compounds

Food

Albuterol may be taken with food to prevent stomach upset.[6]

ALDACTAZIDE

Contains the following ingredients:
    Hydrochlorothiazide
    Spironolactone (page 243)

ALDOCLOR

Contains the following ingredients:
    Chlorothiazide
    Methyldopa (page 174)

ALDORIL

Contains the following ingredients:
    Hydrochlorothiazide
    Methyldopa (page 174)

ALENDRONATE

Common names: Alendronic Acid, Biophosphonates, Fosamax

Alendronate is a member of the bisphosphonate family of drugs used to treat/prevent osteoporosis. It is also used to treat some bone diseases and some cases of cancer that have spread to bones.

Summary of Interactions for Alendronate

In some cases, an herb or supplement may appear in more than one category, which may seem contradictory. For clarification, read the full article for details about the summarized interactions.

ⓘ Check: Other	Calcium Magnesium
Depletion or interference	None known
Side effect reduction/prevention	None known
Supportive interaction	None known
Reduced drug absorption/bioavailability	None known
Adverse interaction	None known

Interactions with Dietary Supplements

Calcium

Calcium supplements may interfere with alendronate absorption.[1] However, one researcher suggested that addition of large amounts of supplemental calcium to alendronate therapy in patients with bone metastases (with evidence of osteomalacia) related to prostate cancer might improve the clinical outcome.[2] Moreover, both calcium and alendronate are commonly used in the treatment of osteoporosis in the same people. To prevent potential interactions, alendronate should be taken two hours before or after calcium supplements.

Magnesium
Absorption of tiludronate, a drug related to alendronate, is reduced when taken with **magnesium** (page 308) and/or **aluminum** (page 10)-containing antacids.[3] This interaction has not yet been reported with alendronate. Until more is known, alendronate should be taken two hours before or after magnesium and/or aluminum-containing **antacids** (page 18).

Interactions with Foods and Other Compounds
Food
Food, coffee, and orange juice significantly reduce absorption of alendronate.[4]

Alendronate should be taken with a large glass of plain water, upon arising in the morning, and 30 minutes or more before any food, beverages, supplements, or other medications.[5] People taking alendronate should remain upright (do not lie down) for 30 minutes after taking the drug.[6]

ALFUZOSIN

Common names: UroXatral

Alfuzosin is used to treat the signs and symptoms of benign prostatic hyperplasia, also known as BPH. There are currently no reported nutrient or herb interactions involving alfuzosin.

ALKA-SELTZER

Contains the following ingredients:
Aspirin (page 26)
Citric acid
Sodium bicarbonate (page 240)

ALKA-SELTZER PLUS

Contains the following ingredients:
Acetaminophen (page 3)
Pseudoephedrine
Chlorpheniramine (page 59)

ALLEGRA-D

Contains the following ingredients:
Fexofenadine (page 115)
Pseudoephedrine

ALLOPURINOL

Common names: Apo-Allopurinol, Caplenal, Cosuric, Lopurim, Rimapurinol, Xanthomax, Zyloprim, Zyloric

Allopurinol is a xanthine oxidase inhibitor used to prevent gout and to lower blood levels of uric acid in certain people taking drugs for cancer.

Summary of Interactions for Allopurinol
In some cases, an herb or supplement may appear in more than one category, which may seem contradictory. For clarification, read the full article for details about the summarized interactions.

✓ May be Beneficial: Supportive interaction	L-tryptophan
ⓘ Check: Other	L-carnitine Vitamin D
Depletion or interference	None known
Side effect reduction/prevention	None known
Reduced drug absorption/bioavailability	None known
Adverse interaction	None known

Interactions with Dietary Supplements
Vitamin D
Individuals with gout have low blood concentration of the active form of vitamin D (1,25 dihydroxycholecalciferol), and allopurinol corrects this problem.[1]

L-carnitine
People who have Duchenne muscular dystrophy have low levels of L-carnitine in their muscles. Allopurinol restores L-carnitine to normal levels, resulting in improved muscle strength.[2] Whether L-carnitine supplementation might improve this effect of allopurinol has not been investigated.

L-tryptophan
In a preliminary study, seven of eight individuals with severe mental depression showed improvement when they took L-tryptophan and allopurinol;[3] of these

seven, five experienced full remission. Controlled research is necessary to determine whether this combination might be more effective for severe depression than standard treatment.

Interactions with Foods and Other Compounds

Food
Allopurinol may be taken with food to prevent stomach upset.[4]

Protein
Compared with people on high-protein diets, people on low-protein diets excrete less allopurinol, resulting in a threefold increase in the time it takes for the drug to be removed from the body.[5] Vegetarians and those who eat low-protein diets (20 grams of protein a day or less) should discuss this possible interaction with their healthcare practitioner before taking allopurinol.

Alcohol
According to animal research, alcohol reduces the activity of antioxidant systems involving vitamin E, vitamin C, and selenium, leading to tissue damage in the cerebellum; however, allopurinol reverses this effect.[6] Drinking alcoholic beverages also increases the removal of allopurinol from the body, thereby reducing the effectiveness of the drug.[7] Therefore, people taking allopurinol should avoid alcohol.

ALPHADERM

Contains the following ingredients:
   Hydrocortisone
   Urea

ALPRAZOLAM

Common names: Xanax

Alprazolam is used to treat anxiety and panic disorder, and is in a family of drugs known as **benzodiazepines** (page 36).

Summary of Interactions for Alprazolam
In some cases, an herb or supplement may appear in more than one category, which may seem contradictory. For clarification, read the full article for details about the summarized interactions.

🚫 Avoid: Adverse interaction	Alcohol Kava*
Depletion or interference	None known
Side effect reduction/prevention	None known
Supportive interaction	None known
Reduced drug absorption/bioavailability	None known

Interactions with Dietary Supplements

Vinpocetine
In a preliminary trial, an extract of periwinkle called vinpocetine was shown to produce minor improvements in short-term memory among people taking flunitrazepam, a benzodiazepine.[1] Further study is needed to determine if vinpocetine would be a helpful adjunct to use of benzodiazepines, or alprazolam specifically.

Interaction with Herbs

Kava (Piper methysticum)
Kava is an herb used to treat anxiety disorder. One individual who took alprazolam and kava together, along with two other medications (**cimetidine** [page 61] and **terazosin** [page 253]) was hospitalized in a lethargic and disoriented condition.[2] Further research is needed to determine whether the combination of kava and alprazolam produces an adverse interaction. However, individuals should not take alprazolam and kava together unless supervised by a doctor.

Interaction with Foods and other Compounds

Alcohol
Drinking alcoholic beverages while taking alprazolam may increase side effects such as drowsiness, confusion, and dizziness.[3] Consequently, people taking alprazolam should avoid drinking alcohol, especially when they must stay alert.

ALTACITE

Contains the following ingredients:
   Aluminium
   Magnesium

ALUDROX TABLETS

Contains the following ingredients:
   Aluminium
   Magnesium

Aludrox Tablets

Aluminum Hydroxide

ALUMINUM HYDROXIDE

Common names: Actal, Algedrate, Alu-Cap, Alu-Tab, Aludrox Liquid, Aludrox, Alugel, Amphojel, Basaljel, Di-Gel, Metapharma Aluminum Hydroxide Gel, Riopan

Combination drugs: Co-Magaldrox, Maalox Plus, Maalox, Mucaine, Mylanta, Tempo Tablets

Aluminum hydroxide acts as an **antacid** (page 18) and is most commonly used in the treatment of heartburn, gastritis, and peptic ulcer. This drug is also sometimes used to reduce absorption of phosphorus for people with kidney failure.

Aluminum hydroxide is found in a variety of **antacids** (page 18). People should read the ingredient label for over-the-counter (OTC) drugs carefully before purchase to know exactly what they contain.

Summary of Interactions for Aluminum Hydroxide

In some cases, an herb or supplement may appear in more than one category, which may seem contradictory. For clarification, read the full article for details about the summarized interactions.

✓ May be Beneficial: Depletion or interference	Calcium Folic acid Phosphorus
✓ May be Beneficial: Supportive interaction	Alginates
⊘ Avoid: Adverse interaction	Citrate
Side effect reduction/prevention	None known
Reduced drug absorption/bioavailability	None known

Interactions with Dietary Supplements

Alginates

A thick gel derived from algae has been used together with aluminum antacids to treat heartburn. Together, alginate gel and antacid were more effective at relieving symptoms[1] and improving healing.[2] Alginate is believed to work by physically blocking stomach acid from touching the esophagus. According to these studies, two tablets containing 200 mg alginic acid should be chewed before each meal and at bedtime.

Calcium

Aluminum hydroxide may increase urinary and stool loss of calcium.[3] Also, aluminum is a toxic mineral, and a limited amount of aluminum absorption from aluminum-containing antacids does occur.[4] As a result,

most doctors do not recommend routine use of aluminum-containing **antacids** (page 18).[5] Other types of antacids containing calcium or **magnesium** (page 166) instead of aluminum are available.

Citrate

Several studies have shown that combination of citrate, either as calcium citrate supplements or from orange and lemon juice, with aluminum-containing antacids increases aluminum levels in the body.[6, 7, 8] Calcium in forms other than calcium citrate has been shown to not increase aluminum absorption.[9] Drinking 7–10 ounces of orange juice provides sufficient citrate to be problematic.[10, 11] Intake of 950 mg calcium citrate greatly elevates aluminum absorption.[12] People with renal failure may be at particular risk of kidney damage due to elevated aluminum levels if they combine aluminum hydroxide with citrate.[13]

Folic acid

Folic acid is needed by the body to utilize vitamin B_{12}. Antacids,[14] including aluminum hydroxide, inhibit folic acid absorption. People taking antacids are advised to supplement with folic acid.

Phosphorus

Depletion of phosphorus may occur as a result of taking aluminum hydroxide. For those with kidney failure, reducing phosphorus absorption is the purpose of taking the drug, as excessive phosphorus levels can result from kidney failure. However, when people with normal kidney function take aluminum hydroxide for extended periods of time, it is possible to deplete phosphorus to unnaturally low levels.

AMANTADINE

Common names: Endantadine, Gen-Amantadine, Symadine, Symmetrel

Amantadine is used to treat influenza, Parkinson's disease, side effects caused by certain drugs, and tiredness associated with multiple sclerosis. It may be classified either as an **antiviral** (page 26) or an antiparkinson drug.

Summary of Interactions for Amantadine

In some cases, an herb or supplement may appear in more than one category, which may seem contradictory. For clarification, read the full article for details about the summarized interactions.

Depletion or interference	None known
Side effect reduction/prevention	None known
Supportive interaction	None known
Reduced drug absorption/bioavailability	None known
Adverse interaction	None known

Interactions with Foods and Other Compounds

Alcohol

Drinking alcoholic beverages while taking amantadine may enhance side effects of the drug, such as dizziness, confusion, and light-headedness.[1] Therefore, combining alcohol and amantadine should be avoided.

AMILORIDE

Common names: Amilamount, Amilospare, Midamor

Combination drugs: Kalten, Moducren, Moduretic

Amiloride is a potassium-sparing (prevents excess loss of potassium) **diuretic** (page 94) drug. Diuretics increase urinary water loss from the body and are used to treat high blood pressure, congestive heart failure, and some kidney or liver conditions.

Summary of Interactions for Amiloride

In some cases, an herb or supplement may appear in more than one category, which may seem contradictory. For clarification, read the full article for details about the summarized interactions.

⃠ Avoid: Adverse interaction	Magnesium* Potassium
ⓘ Check: Other	Sodium
Depletion or interference	None known
Side effect reduction/prevention	None known
Supportive interaction	None known
Reduced drug absorption/bioavailability	None known

Interactions with Dietary Supplements

Folic acid

One study showed that people taking diuretics for more than six months had dramatically lower blood levels of folic acid and higher levels of homocysteine compared with individuals not taking diuretics.[1] Homocysteine, a toxic amino acid by-product, has been associated with atherosclerosis. Until further information is available, people taking diuretics for longer than six months should probably supplement with folic acid.

Magnesium

Preliminary research in animals suggests that amiloride may reduce the urinary excretion of magnesium.[2] It is unknown if this same effect would occur in humans. Nevertheless, persons taking more than 300 mg of magnesium per day and amiloride should consult with a doctor, as this combination may lead to potentially dangerous elevations in levels of magnesium in the body. The combination of amiloride and hydrochlorothiazide would likely eliminate this problem, as hydrochlorothiazide may deplete magnesium.

Potassium

As a potassium-sparing drug, amiloride reduces urinary loss of potassium.[3] This can cause potassium levels to build up in the body. People taking this drug should avoid use of potassium chloride–containing products, such as Morton Salt Substitute, No Salt, Lite Salt, and others. Even eating several pieces of fruit per day can sometimes cause problems for people taking potassium-sparing diuretics, due to the high potassium content of fruit.

Sodium

Diuretics, including amiloride, cause increased loss of sodium in urine. By removing sodium from the body, diuretics cause water to leave the body as well. This reduction of water in the body is the purpose of taking amiloride. Therefore, there is usually no reason to replace lost sodium, although strict limitation of salt intake in combination with the action of diuretics can sometimes cause excessive sodium depletion. On the other hand, people who restrict sodium intake and in the process reduce blood pressure may need to have the dose of their diuretics lowered.

AMINOGLYCOSIDE ANTIBIOTICS

Aminoglycosides are **antibiotics** (page 19) that are often administered into veins or muscle to treat serious bacterial infections. Some aminoglycosides are also used orally to treat intestinal infections or topically to treat eye infections.

There are interactions that are common to **antibacterial drugs** (page 19) in general and interactions involving a specific aminoglycoside. For the latter interactions, refer to the highlighted drugs listed below.

- Amikacin (Amikin)
- **Gentamicin** (page 129) (Garamycin)
- Kanamycin (Kantrex)
- **Neomycin** (page 187) (Mycifradin)
- Netilmicin (Netromycin)
- Paromomycin (Humatin)
- Streptomycin
- **Tobramycin** (page 264) (TOBI Solution, TobraDex, Nebcin)

Summary of Interactions for Aminoglycoside Antibiotics

In some cases, an herb or supplement may appear in more than one category, which may seem contradictory. For clarification, read the full article for details about the summarized interactions.

✓	May be Beneficial: Depletion or interference	Vitamin K*
✓	May be Beneficial: Side effect reduction/prevention	Bifidobacterium longum* Lactobacillus acidophilus* Lactobacillus casei* Saccharomyces boulardii* Saccharomyces cerevisiae* Vitamin K*
✓	May be Beneficial: Supportive interaction	Saccharomyces boulardii*
	Reduced drug absorption/bioavailability	None known
	Adverse interaction	None known

Interactions common to many, if not all, Aminoglycoside Antibiotics are described in this article. Interactions reported for only one or several drugs in this class may not be listed in this article. Some drugs listed in this article are linked to articles specific to that respective drug; please refer to those individual drug articles. The information in this article may not necessarily apply to drugs in this class for which no separate article exists. If you are taking an Aminoglycoside Antibiotic for which no separate article exists, talk with your doctor or pharmacist.

Interactions with Dietary Supplements
Probiotics

A common side effect of antibiotics is diarrhea, which may be caused by the elimination of beneficial bacteria normally found in the colon. Controlled studies have shown that taking probiotic microorganisms—such as

Lactobacillus casei, Lactobacillus acidophilus, Bifidobacterium longum, or *Saccharomyces boulardii*—helps prevent antibiotic-induced diarrhea.[1]

The diarrhea experienced by some people who take antibiotics also might be due to an overgrowth of the bacterium *Clostridium difficile,* which causes a disease known as pseudomembranous colitis. Controlled studies have shown that supplementation with harmless yeast—such as *Saccharomyces boulardii*[2] or *Saccharomyces cerevisiae* (baker's or brewer's yeast)[3]—helps prevent recurrence of this infection. In one study, taking 500 mg of *Saccharomyces boulardii* twice daily enhanced the effectiveness of the antibiotic vancomycin in preventing recurrent clostridium infection.[4] Therefore, people taking antibiotics who later develop diarrhea might benefit from supplementing with saccharomyces organisms.

Treatment with antibiotics also commonly leads to an overgrowth of yeast *(Candida albicans)* in the vagina (candida vaginitis) and the intestines (sometimes referred to as "dysbiosis"). Controlled studies have shown that *Lactobacillus acidophilus* might prevent candida vaginitis.[5]

Vitamin K

Several cases of excessive bleeding have been reported in people who take antibiotics.[6, 7, 8, 9] This side effect may be the result of reduced vitamin K activity and/or reduced vitamin K production by bacteria in the colon. One study showed that people who had taken broad-spectrum antibiotics had lower liver concentrations of vitamin K_2 (menaquinone), though vitamin K_1 (phylloquinone) levels remained normal.[10] Several antibiotics appear to exert a strong effect on vitamin K activity, while others may not have any effect. Therefore, one should refer to a specific antibiotic for information on whether it interacts with vitamin K. Doctors of natural medicine sometimes recommend vitamin K supplementation to people taking antibiotics. Additional research is needed to determine whether the amount of vitamin K_1 found in some multivitamins is sufficient to prevent antibiotic-induced bleeding. Moreover, most multivitamins do not contain vitamin K.

AMIODARONE

Common names: Amidox, Cordarone X, Cordarone, Pacerone

Amiodarone is a drug occasionally used to treat life-threatening arrhythmias of the heart.

Summary of Interactions for Amiodarone

In some cases, an herb or supplement may appear in more than one category, which may seem contradictory. For clarification, read the full article for details about the summarized interactions.

✓ May be Beneficial: Side effect reduction/prevention	Vitamin E
⊘ Avoid: Adverse interaction	Grapefruit juice
Depletion or interference	None known
Supportive interaction	None known
Reduced drug absorption/bioavailability	None known

Interactions with Dietary Supplements

Vitamin E

Test tube research on human lung tissue suggests that vitamin E might reduce lung toxicity caused by amiodarone.[1] More research is needed to further investigate this possibility.

Interactions with Foods and Other Compounds

Grapefruit juice

In one controlled study, drinking grapefruit juice while taking amiodarone dramatically increased blood levels of the drug.[2] Consequently, people taking amiodarone should avoid drinking grapefruit juice (and eating grapefruit) to prevent potentially serious side effects.

AMI-TEX LA

Contains the following ingredients:
Guaifenesin (page 133)
Phenylpropanolamine (page 218)

AMLODIPINE

Common names: Istin, Norvasc

Combination drug: Lotrel

Amlodipine is a calcium channel blocker used to treat angina and high blood pressure.

Summary of Interactions for Amlodipine

In some cases, an herb or supplement may appear in more than one category, which may seem contradictory. For clarification, read the full article for details about the summarized interactions.

⊘ Avoid: Adverse interaction	Pleurisy root*
ⓘ Check: Other	DHEA Grapefruit juice
Depletion or interference	None known
Side effect reduction/prevention	None known
Supportive interaction	None known
Reduced drug absorption/bioavailability	None known

Interactions with Dietary Supplements

Dehydroepiandrosterone (DHEA)

Amlodipine has been shown to raise blood levels of DHEA-sulfate in insulin-resistant, obese men with high blood pressure.[1]

Interactions with Herbs

Pleurisy root

As pleurisy root and other plants in the *Aesclepius* genus contain cardiac glycosides, it is best to avoid use of pleurisy root with heart medications such as calcium channel blockers.[2]

Interactions with Foods and Other Compounds

Grapefruit juice

Ingestion of grapefruit juice has been shown to increase the absorption of **felodipine** (page 113) (a drug similar in structure and action to that of amlodipine) and to increase the adverse effects of the medication in patients with hypertension. Until more is known, it seems that grapefruit juice should not be ingested by people taking amlodipine or similar drugs.[3] The same effects might be seen from eating grapefruit as from drinking its juice.

Food

Amlodipine may be taken with or without food.[4]

AMOXICILLIN

Common names: Almodan, Amix, Amoram, Amoxil, Amoxycillin, Apo-Amoxil, Galenamox, Novamoxin, Nu-Amoxil, Polymox, Rimox-allin, Trimox, Wymox

Combination drug: Augmentin

Amoxicillin is a member of the penicillin family of **antibiotics** (page 19). Amoxicillin is used to treat bacterial infections, including infections of the middle ear. The combination of amoxicillin/clavulanate (Augmentin) is an extended-spectrum antibiotic used to treat bacterial infections resistant to amoxicillin alone.

Summary of Interactions for Amoxicillin

In some cases, an herb or supplement may appear in more than one category, which may seem contradictory. For clarification, read the full article for details about the summarized interactions.

✓ May be Beneficial: Depletion or interference	Vitamin K*
✓ May be Beneficial: Side effect reduction/prevention	*Bifidobacterium longum* * *Lactobacillus acidophilus* * *Lactobacillus casei* * Probiotics *Saccharomyces boulardii* * *Saccharomyces cerevisiae* * Vitamin K*
✓ May be Beneficial: Supportive interaction	Bromelain *Saccharomyces boulardii* *
Reduced drug absorption/bioavailability	None known
Adverse interaction	None known

Interactions with Dietary Supplements

Bromelain

When taken with amoxicillin, bromelain was shown to increase absorption of amoxicillin in humans.[1] When 80 mg of bromelain was taken together with amoxicillin and **tetracycline** (page 253), blood levels of both drugs increased, though how bromelain acts on drug metabolism remains unknown.[2] An older report found bromelain also increased the actions of other antibiotics, including penicillin, chloramphenicol, and **erythromycin** (page 106), in treating a variety of infections. In that trial, 22 out of 23 people who had previously not responded to these antibiotics did so after adding bromelain taken four times per day.[3]

Doctors will sometimes prescribe enough bromelain to equal 2,400 gelatin dissolving units (listed as GDU on labels) per day. This amount would equal approximately 3,600 MCU (milk clotting units), another common measure of bromelain activity.

Probiotics

A common side effect of antibiotics is diarrhea, which may be caused by the elimination of beneficial bacteria normally found in the colon. A nonpathogenic yeast known as *Saccharomyces boulardii* has been shown in two double-blind studies to decrease frequency of diar-

rhea in people taking amoxicillin as well as other penicillin-type drugs compared to placebo.[4, 5] There were overall few people in these studies using amoxicillin specifically, so there is no definitive proof that *Saccharomyces boulardii* will be beneficial for everyone when it is combined with amoxicillin. The studies used 1 gram of *Saccharmoyces boulardii* per day.

A separate double-blind study found that taking a combination of *Lactobacillus acidophilus* and *Lactobacillus bulgaricus,* two normal gut bacteria, with amoxicillin did not protect children from developing diarrhea.[6] The authors of the study point out some problems such as the parents' inability to consistently define diarrhea. However, at this time, it is unknown if lactobacillus products will reduce diarrhea due to amoxicillin.

Controlled studies have shown that taking other probiotic microorganisms—such as *Lactobacillus casei* or *Bifidobacterium longum*—also helps prevent antibiotic-induced diarrhea.[7]

The diarrhea experienced by some people who take antibiotics also might be due to an overgrowth of the bacterium *Clostridium difficile*, which causes a disease known as pseudomembranous colitis. Controlled studies have shown that supplementation with harmless yeast—such as *Saccharomyces boulardii*[8] or *Saccharomyces cerevisiae* (baker's or brewer's yeast)[9]—helps prevent recurrence of this infection. In one study, taking 500 mg of *Saccharomyces boulardii* twice daily enhanced the effectiveness of the antibiotic vancomycin in preventing recurrent clostridium infection.[10] Therefore, people taking antibiotics who later develop diarrhea might benefit from supplementing with saccharomyces organisms.

Treatment with antibiotics also commonly leads to an overgrowth of yeast *(Candida albicans)* in the vagina (candida vaginitis) and the intestines (sometimes referred to as "dysbiosis"). Controlled studies have shown that *Lactobacillus acidophilus* might prevent candida vaginitis.[11]

Vitamin K

Several cases of excessive bleeding have been reported in people who take antibiotics.[12, 13, 14, 15] This side effect may be the result of reduced vitamin K activity and/or reduced vitamin K production by bacteria in the colon. One study showed that people who had taken broad-spectrum antibiotics had lower liver concentrations of vitamin K_2 (menaquinone), though vitamin K_1 (phylloquinone) levels remained normal.[16] Several antibiotics appear to exert a strong effect on vitamin K activity, while others may not have any effect. Therefore, one should refer to a specific antibiotic for information on whether it interacts with vitamin K. Doctors of natural medicine sometimes recommend vitamin K supplementation to people taking antibiotics. Additional research is needed to determine whether the amount of vitamin K_1 found in some multivitamins is sufficient to prevent antibiotic-induced bleeding. Moreover, most multivitamins do not contain vitamin K.

AMPHOTERICIN B

Common names: Fungilin, Fungizone

Amphotericin B is an antifungal drug. Topically, it is used to treat skin yeast infections. Intravenously, it is used to treat a variety of life-threatening fungal infections.

Summary of Interactions for Amphotericin B

In some cases, an herb or supplement may appear in more than one category, which may seem contradictory. For clarification, read the full article for details about the summarized interactions.

✓ May be Beneficial: Depletion or interference	Magnesium*
Side effect reduction/prevention	None known
Supportive interaction	None known
Reduced drug absorption/bioavailability	None known
Adverse interaction	None known

Interactions with Dietary Supplements
Magnesium
Amphotericin B has been reported to increase urinary excretion of magnesium.[1] It remains unclear whether it is important for people taking this drug to supplement magnesium.

AMPICILLIN

Common names: Amficot, Apo-Ampi, Novo-Ampicillin, Nu-Ampi, Omnipen, Penbritin, Principen, Rimacillin, Totacillin, Vidopen

Ampicillin is used to treat diseases caused by bacterial infections; it is a type of **antibiotic** (page 19) called an aminopenicillin.

Summary of Interactions for Ampicillin

In some cases, an herb or supplement may appear in more than one category, which may seem contradictory. For clarification, read the full article for details about the summarized interactions.

✓ May be Beneficial: Depletion or interference	Vitamin C* Vitamin K*
✓ May be Beneficial: Side effect reduction/prevention	*Bifidobacterium longum* *Lactobacillus acidophilus* *Lactobacillus casei* Probiotics* *Saccharomyces boulardii* *Saccharomyces cerevisiae* Vitamin K*
✓ May be Beneficial: Supportive interaction	*Saccharomyces boulardii*
🚫 Avoid: Reduced drug absorption/ bioavailability	Khat
Adverse interaction	None known

Interactions with Dietary Supplements
Vitamin C
Test tube studies show that ampicillin significantly reduces the amount of vitamin C in the blood.[1] Controlled research is needed to determine whether individuals might benefit from supplementing vitamin C while taking ampicillin.

Probiotics
A common side effect of antibiotics is diarrhea, which may be caused by the elimination of beneficial bacteria normally found in the colon. Controlled studies have shown that taking probiotic microorganisms—such as *Lactobacillus casei, Lactobacillus acidophilus, Bifidobacterium longum,* or *Saccharomyces boulardii*—helps prevent antibiotic-induced diarrhea.[2]

The diarrhea experienced by some people who take antibiotics also might be due to an overgrowth of the bacterium *Clostridium difficile,* which causes a disease known as pseudomembranous colitis. Controlled studies have shown that supplementation with harmless yeast—such as *Saccharomyces boulardii*[3] or *Saccharomyces cerevisiae* (baker's or brewer's yeast)[4]—helps prevent recurrence of this infection. In one study, taking 500 mg of *Saccharomyces boulardii* twice daily enhanced the effectiveness of the antibiotic vancomycin in preventing recurrent clostridium infection.[5] Therefore, people taking antibiotics who later develop diarrhea might benefit from supplementing with saccharomyces organisms.

Treatment with antibiotics also commonly leads to an overgrowth of yeast *(Candida albicans)* in the vagina (candida vaginitis) and the intestines (sometimes referred to as "dysbiosis"). Controlled studies have shown that *Lactobacillus acidophilus* might prevent candida vaginitis.[6]

Vitamin K

Several cases of excessive bleeding have been reported in people who take antibiotics.[7, 8, 9, 10] This side effect may be the result of reduced vitamin K activity and/or reduced vitamin K production by bacteria in the colon. One study showed that people who had taken broad-spectrum antibiotics had lower liver concentrations of vitamin K_2 (menaquinone), though vitamin K_1 (phylloquinone) levels remained normal.[11] Several antibiotics appear to exert a strong effect on vitamin K activity, while others may not have any effect. Therefore, one should refer to a specific antibiotic for information on whether it interacts with vitamin K. Doctors of natural medicine sometimes recommend vitamin K supplementation to people taking antibiotics. Additional research is needed to determine whether the amount of vitamin K_1 found in some multivitamins is sufficient to prevent antibiotic-induced bleeding. Moreover, most multivitamins do not contain vitamin K.

Interactions with Herbs

Khat (Catha edulis)

Khat is an herb found in East Africa and Yemen that has recently been imported into the United States. Studies have shown that chewing khat significantly reduces the absorption of ampicillin,[12] which might reduce the effectiveness of the **antibiotic** (page 19). Therefore, people taking ampicillin should avoid herbal products that contain khat.

Interactions with Foods and Other Compounds

Food

Taking ampicillin with food reduces the amount of drug that is absorbed regardless of the type of meal eaten.[13] Therefore, ampicillin should be taken an hour before or two hours after a meal.

Carbohydrates

Normally, bacteria in the intestines help break down indigestible carbohydrates into useable forms. Ampicillin

blocks this process, which may result in increased undigested carbohydrates in the intestine, increased water in the stool, and diarrhea.[14] Consequently, people taking ampicillin might experience fewer episodes of diarrhea if they eat a diet low in indigestible carbohydrate during the treatment period. Consult a health practitioner to learn about sources of indigestible carbohydrate.

Dietary Fiber

Controlled studies with **amoxicillin** (page 13), an **antibiotic** (page 19) similar to ampicillin, have shown that a diet low in fiber (7 g/day) increases the absorption of the drug when compared to a high-fiber diet (36 g/day).[15] However, further research is needed to determine whether different amounts of dietary fiber exert the same effect on ampicillin. Until more information is available, people taking ampicillin might benefit more from eating a low-fiber diet during the treatment period.

Alcohol

Normally, the body converts alcohol to acetaldehyde, which test tube studies show blocks the action of ampicillin.[16] Whether drinking alcoholic beverages affects the activity of ampicillin in the body is unknown; therefore, until more information is available, people taking ampicillin should avoid alcohol.

ANACIN

Contains the following ingredients:
   Aspirin (page 26)
   Caffeine (page 44)

ANASTROZOLE

Common names: Arimidex

Anastrozole is used to treat advanced breast cancer in postmenopausal women who have not responded to the drug **tamoxifen** (page 251). At the time of this writing, no evidence of nutrient or herb interactions involving anastrozole was found in the medical literature.

Summary of Interactions for Anastrozole

In some cases, an herb or supplement may appear in more than one category, which may seem contradictory. For clarification, read the full article for details about the summarized interactions.

Depletion or interference	None known
Side effect reduction/prevention	None known
Supportive interaction	None known
Reduced drug absorption/bioavailability	None known
Adverse interaction	None known

ANDREWS ANTACID

Contains the following ingredients:
    Calcium
    Magnesium

ANGIOTENSIN II RECEPTOR BLOCKERS

Common names: Eprosartan, Micardis, Telmisartan, Teveten

Angiotensin II receptor blockers are used—either alone or in combination with other drugs—to treat high blood pressure.

For interactions involving specific medications, refer to the highlighted drugs listed below.
- **Candesartan** (page 47) (Atacand)
- **Irbesartan** (page 146) (Avapro)
- **Losartan** (page 162) (Cozaar)
- Telmisartan (Micardis)
- **Valsartan** (page 278) (Diovan)

> For interactions involving a specific Angiotensin II Receptor Blocker, see the individual drug article. For interactions involving an Angiotensin II Receptor Blocker for which no separate article exists, talk to your doctor or pharmacist.

ANGIOTENSIN-CONVERTING ENZYME (ACE) INHIBITORS

Common names: ACE Inhibitors, Aceon, Cilazapril, Coversyl, Fosinopril, Gopten, Imidapril, Mavik, Monopril, Odrik, Perindopril, Staril, Tanatril, Trandolapril, Vascace

Angiotensin-converting enzyme (ACE) inhibitors constitute a family of drugs used to treat high blood pres-

sure and heart failure, as well as to improve survival following a heart attack. ACE inhibitors are also used to slow the progression of kidney disease in people with diabetes.

Interactions that are common to all ACE inhibitors are described below. For interactions involving specific ACE inhibitors, refer to the highlighted drugs listed below.
- **Benazepril** (page 34) (Lotensin)
- **Captopril** (page 47) (Capoten)
- **Enalapril** (page 103) (Vasotec)
- Fosinopril (Monopril)
- **Lisinopril** (page 156) (Prinivil, Zestril)
- **Moexipril** (page 182) (Univasc)
- Perindopril (Aceon)
- **Quinapril** (page 226) (Accupril)
- **Ramipril** (page 229) (Altace)
- Trandolapril (Mavik)

Summary of Interactions for ACE Inhibitors

In some cases, an herb or supplement may appear in more than one category, which may seem contradictory. For clarification, read the full article for details about the summarized interactions.

✓	May be Beneficial: Side effect reduction/prevention	Iron
⊘	Avoid: Adverse interaction	High-potassium foods Potassium supplements Salt substitutes
	Depletion or interference	None known
	Supportive interaction	None known
	Reduced drug absorption/bioavailability	None known

Interactions common to many, if not all, ACE Inhibitors are described in this article. Interactions reported for only one or several drugs in this class may not be listed in this article. Some drugs listed in this article are linked to articles specific to that respective drug; please refer to those individual drug articles. The information in this article may not necessarily apply to drugs in this class for which no separate article exists. If you are taking an ACE Inhibitor for which no separate article exists, talk with your doctor or pharmacist.

Interactions with Dietary Supplements
Potassium

An uncommon yet potentially serious side effect of taking ACE inhibitors is increased blood potassium levels.[1, 2, 3] Taking potassium supplements,[4] potassium-containing salt substitutes (No Salt, Morton Salt

Angiotensin-Converting Enzyme

Substitute, and others),[5, 6, 7] or large amounts of high-potassium foods at the same time as ACE inhibitors could cause life-threatening problems.[8] Therefore, individuals should consult their healthcare practitioner before supplementing additional potassium and should have their blood levels of potassium checked periodically while taking ACE inhibitors.

Iron
In a double-blind study of patients who had developed a cough attributed to an ACE inhibitor, supplementation with iron (in the form of 256 mg of ferrous sulfate per day) for four weeks reduced the severity of the cough by a statistically significant 45%, compared with a non-significant 8% improvement in the placebo group.[9]

ANTACIDS/ACID BLOCKERS

Common names: Esomeprazole, Nexium

Antacids/acid blockers are a family of drugs that includes antacids, which help prevent damage to tissue by neutralizing stomach acid, and histamine-2 blockers (H2-blockers) and proton pump inhibitors that reduce acid production.

For interactions involving specific antacids and acid blocker drugs, refer to the highlighted medications listed below.

Antacids
- Aluminum and magnesium hydroxide (Maalox, Mylanta)
- Aluminum carbonate gel (Basajel)
- **Aluminum hydroxide** (page 10) (Amphojel, AlternaGEL)
- Calcium carbonate (Tums, Titralac, Calcium Rich Rolaids)
- **Magnesium hydroxide** (page 166) (Phillips' Milk of Magnesia)
- **Sodium bicarbonate** (page 240)

H2-Blockers
- **Cimetidine** (page 61) (Tagamet, Tagamet HB)
- **Famotidine** (page 112) (Pepcid, Pepcid AC)
- **Nizatidine** (page 192) (Axid)
- **Ranitidine** (page 230) (Zantac)

Proton Pump Inhibitors
- **Lansoprazole** (page 153) (Prevacid)
- **Omeprazole** (page 197) (Prilosec)
- Pantoprazole (Protonix)
- Rabeprazole (Aciphex)

For interactions involving a specific Antacid/Acid Blocker, see the individual drug article. For interactions involving an Antacid/Acid Blocker for which no separate article exists, talk to your doctor or pharmacist.

ANTHELMINTICS

Common names: Albendazole, Albenza, Antiminth, Biltricide, Diethylcarbamazine, Hetrazan, Ivermectin, Mebendazole, Mintezol, Oxamniquine, Pin-Rid, Praziquantel, Pyrantel, Stromectol, Thiabendazole, Vansil, Vermox

Anthelmintic drugs are used to kill parasites, including roundworms, whipworms, hookworms, pinworms, trichinella (trichinosis), and other less common organisms.
- Albendazole (Albenza)
- Diethylcarbamazine (Hetrazan)
- Ivermectin (Stromectol)
- Mebendazole (Vermox)
- Oxamniquine (Vansil)
- Praziquantel (Biltricide)
- Pyrantel (Antiminth, Pin-Rid)
- Thiabendazole (Mintezol)

For interactions involving a specific Anthelmintic, see the individual drug article. For interactions involving an Anthelmintic for which no separate article exists, talk to your doctor or pharmacist.

ANTHRALIN

Common names: Anthraderm, Anthraforte, Anthranol, Anthrascalp, Dithranol, Drithocreme, Micanol Cream, Psorin Ointment

Anthralin is a drug applied only to affected skin areas to treat psoriasis.

Summary of Interactions for Anthralin
In some cases, an herb or supplement may appear in more than one category, which may seem contradictory. For clarification, read the full article for details about the summarized interactions.

✓	May be Beneficial: Side effect reduction/prevention	Vitamin E (topical)
	Depletion or interference	None known
	Supportive interaction	None known
	Reduced drug absorption/bioavailability	None known
	Adverse interaction	None known

Interactions with Dietary Supplements

Vitamin E

Anthralin can cause inflammation of the skin. A preliminary study found that topical use of vitamin E was able to protect against this side effect.[1] This report used a tocopherol form of the vitamin rather than tocopheryl. This makes sense, as there is no conclusive proof that the tocopheryl forms (which require an enzyme to split vitamin E from the fatty acid to which it is attached) have any activity on the skin.

ANTI-INFECTIVE AGENTS

Anti-infective agents are used to treat disorders caused by bacteria, viruses, protozoa, worms, fungi, and yeast.

Please refer to the specific anti-infective agent categories below for information regarding drug interactions.

- **Anthelmintics** (page 18) (Worms)
- **Antibiotics** (page 19) (Bacteria)
- **Antifungal** (page 25) (Fungi and Yeast)
- **Antimalarial** (page 25) (Malaria)
- **Anti-Protozoal** (page 19) (Protozoa)
- **Antitubercular** (page 25) (Tuberculosis)
- **Antiviral** (page 26) (Virus)

For interactions involving a specific Anti-Infective Agent, see the individual drug article. For interactions involving an Anti-Infective Agent for which no separate article exists, talk to your doctor or pharmacist.

ANTI-PROTOZOAL DRUGS

Anti-protozoal drugs, including amebicides, are used to kill parasites that infect the intestines, the male and female reproductive tract, or the entire body. Anti-protozoals treat diseases such as intestinal amebiasis (amebic dysentery), trichomosiasis, malaria, toxoplasmosis, cryptosporidiosis, pneumocystis carinii pneumonia, and giardiasis.

For interactions involving a specific anti-protozoal drug, refer to the highlighted medication listed below.

- Atovaquone (Mepron)
- Chloroquine (Aralen)
- Eflornithine (Ornidyl)
- Iodoquinol (Yodoxin)
- **Metronidazole** (page 177) (Flagyl, Protostat)
- Paromomycin (Humatin)
- Pentamidine (Pentam, NebuPent)

For interactions involving a specific Anti-Protozoal Drug, see the individual drug article. For interactions involving an Anti-Protozoal Drug for which no separate article exists, talk to your doctor or pharmacist.

ANTIBIOTICS

Common names: Bacitracin, Caci-IM, Chloramphenicol, Chlormycetin, Colistimethate, ColyMycin, Furazolidone, Furoxone, Lincocin, Lincomycin, Linezolid, Vancocin, Vancomycin, Zyvox

Antibiotics are used to either kill or slow down the growth of bacteria and are divided into the categories listed below.

Interactions common to most, if not all, antibiotics are described in this article. For interactions involving a specific antibiotic refer to the highlighted drugs listed below.

Aminoglycosides (page 11)
- Amikacin (Amikin)
- **Gentamicin** (page 129) (Garamycin)
- Kanamycin (Kantrex)
- **Neomycin** (page 187) (Mycifradin)
- Netilmicin (Netromycin)
- Paromomycin (Humatin)
- Streptomycin
- **Tobramycin** (page 264) (TOBI Solution, TobraDex, Nebcin)

Beta-lactam antibiotics
- Clavulanic acid
- **Cephalosporins** (page 52)
- Imipenem
- **Penicillins** (page 211)
- Sulbactam

Antibiotics

Cephalosporins *(page 52)*
- Aztreonam (Azactam for injection)
- Cefaclor (Ceclor)
- Cefadroxil (Duricef)
- Cefamandole (Mandol)
- Cefazolin (Ancef, Kefzol)
- Cefdinir (Omnicef)
- Cefepime (Maxipime)
- Cefixime (Suprax)
- Cefoperazone (Cefobid)
- Cefotaxime (Claforan)
- Cefotetan (Cefotan)
- Cefoxitin (Mefoxin)
- Cefpodoxime (Vantin)
- Cefprozil (Cefzil)
- Ceftazidime (Ceptaz, Fortaz, Tazicef, Tazidime)
- Ceftibuten (Cedax)
- Ceftizoxime (Cefizox)
- Ceftriaxone (Rocephin)
- Cefuroxime (Ceftin, Kefurox, Zinacef)
- Cephalexin (Keflex, Keftab)
- Cephapirin (Cefadyl)
- Cephradine (Anspor, Velocef)
- Imipenem and Cilastatin (Primaxin I.V.)
- **Loracarbef** (page 161) (Lorabid)
- Meropenem (Merrem I.V.)

Macrolides *(page 164)*
- **Azithromycin** (page 31) (Zithromax)
- **Clarithromycin** (page 68) (Biaxin)
- Dirithromycin (Dynabac)
- **Erythromycin** (page 106) oral (EES, EryPed, Ery-Tab, PCE Dispertab, Pediazole)
- Erythromycin topical (A/T/S, Akne-Mycin, Erygel, Erycette, Eryderm, Erygel)
- Troleandomycin (Tao)

Penicillins *(page 211)*
- **Amoxicillin** (page 13) (Amoxil, Trimox)
- Amoxicillin and Clavulanate (Augmentin)
- **Ampicillin** (page 15) (Principen, Totacillin)
- Ampicillin + sulbactam (Unisyn)
- Bacampicillin (Spectrobid)
- Carbenicillin (Geocillin)
- Cloxacillin (Cloxapen)
- **Dicloxacillin** (page 88) (Dynapen, Dycill)
- Mezlocillin (Mezlin)
- Nafcillin (Unipen)
- Oxacillin (Bactocill)
- Penicillin G (Bicillin C-R, Bicillin L-A, Pfizerpen)
- **Penicillin V** (page 210) (Beepen-VK, Veetids)

- Piperacillin (Pipracil)
- Piperacillin and Tazobactam (Zosyn)
- Ticarcillin (Ticar)
- Ticarcillin and Clavulantae (Timentin)

Quinolones *(page 228)*
- Cinoxacin (Cinobac)
- **Ciprofloxacin** (page 62) (Cipro)
- Enoxacin (Penetrex)
- Gatifloxacin (Tequin)
- **Levofloxacin** (page 155) (Levaquin)
- Lomefloxacin (Maxaquin)
- Moxifloxacin (Avelox)
- Nalidixic acid (NegGram)
- Norfloxacin (Noroxin)
- **Ofloxacin** (page 195) (Floxin)
- Sparfloxacin (Zagam)
- Trovafloxacin and Alatrofloxacin (Trovan)

Sulfonamides *(page 248)*
- Silver sulfadiazine (Silvadene, SSD)
- Sodium sulfacetamide (AK-Sulf, Bleph-10, Sodium Sulamyd)
- **Sulfamethoxazole** (page 245) (Gantanol)
- Sulfanilamide (AVC)
- **Sulfasalazine** (page 246) (Azulfidine)
- Sulfisoxazole (Gantrisin)
- **Trimethoprim/Sulfamethoxazole** (page 273) (Bactrim, Cotrim, Septra, Sulfatrim Pediatric)
- Triple Sulfa (Sultrin Triple Sulfa)

Tetracyclines *(page 255)*
- Demeclocycline (Declomycin)
- **Doxycycline** (page 101) (Monodox, Periostat, Vibramycin, Vibra-Tabs)
- **Minocycline** (page 179) (Dynacin, Minocin, Vectrin)
- Oxytetracycline (Terramycin)
- **Tetracycline** (page 253) (Sumycin, Tetracyn)

Miscellaneous antibiotics
- Bacitracin (Caci-IM)
- Chloramphenicol (Chloromycetin)
- **Chlorhexidine** (page 58) (Peridex)
- Colistimethate (ColyMycin M)
- **Dapsone** (page 85)
- Furazolidone (Furoxone)
- Lincomycin (Lincocin)
- Linezolid (Zyvox)
- **Nitrofurantoin** (page 190) (Macrobid, Macrodantin)

- **Clindamycin Oral** (page 70) (Cleocin)
- **Clindamycin Topical** (page 71) (Cleocin T)
- **Trimethoprim** (page 271) (Proloprim, Trimpex)
- Vancomycin (Vancocin)

Summary of Interactions for Antibiotics

In some cases, an herb or supplement may appear in more than one category, which may seem contradictory. For clarification, read the full article for details about the summarized interactions.

✓ May be Beneficial: Depletion or interference	Vitamin K
✓ May be Beneficial: Side effect reduction/prevention	Bifidobacterium longum Lactobacillus acidophilus Lactobacillus casei Saccharomyces boulardii Saccharomyces cerevisiae Vitamin K
✓ May be Beneficial: Supportive interaction	Saccharomyces boulardii
Reduced drug absorption/bioavailability	None known
Adverse interaction	None known

Interactions common to many, if not all, Antibiotics are described in this article. Interactions reported for only one or several drugs in this class may not be listed in this article. Some drugs listed in this article are linked to articles specific to that respective drug; please refer to those individual drug articles. The information in this article may not necessarily apply to drugs in this class for which no separate article exists. If you are taking an Antibiotic for which no separate article exists, talk with your doctor or pharmacist.

Interactions with Dietary Supplements

Probiotics

A common side effect of antibiotics is diarrhea, which may be caused by the elimination of beneficial bacteria normally found in the colon. Controlled studies have shown that taking probiotic microorganisms—such as *Lactobacillus casei*, *Lactobacillus acidophilus*, *Bifidobacterium longum*, or *Saccharomyces boulardii*—helps prevent antibiotic-induced diarrhea.[1]

The diarrhea experienced by some people who take antibiotics also might be due to an overgrowth of the bacterium *Clostridium difficile*, which causes a disease known as pseudomembranous colitis. Controlled studies have shown that supplementation with harmless yeast—such as *Saccharomyces boulardii*[2] or *Saccharomyces cerevisiae* (baker's or brewer's yeast)[3]—helps prevent recurrence of this infection. In one study, taking 500 mg of *Saccharomyces boulardii* twice daily enhanced the effectiveness of the antibiotic vancomycin in preventing recurrent clostridium infection.[4] Therefore, people taking antibiotics who later develop diarrhea might benefit from supplementing with saccharomyces organisms.

Treatment with antibiotics also commonly leads to an overgrowth of yeast *(Candida albicans)* in the vagina (candida vaginitis) and the intestines (sometimes referred to as "dysbiosis"). Controlled studies have shown that *Lactobacillus acidophilus* might prevent candida vaginitis.[5]

Vitamin K

Several cases of excessive bleeding have been reported in people who take antibiotics.[6, 7, 8, 9] This side effect may be the result of reduced vitamin K activity and/or reduced vitamin K production by bacteria in the colon. One study showed that people who had taken broad-spectrum antibiotics had lower liver concentrations of vitamin K_2 (menaquinone), though vitamin K_1 (phylloquinone) levels remained normal.[10] Several antibiotics appear to exert a strong effect on vitamin K activity, while others may not have any effect. Therefore, one should refer to a specific antibiotic for information on whether it interacts with vitamin K. Doctors of natural medicine sometimes recommend vitamin K supplementation to people taking antibiotics. Aditional research is needed to determine whether the amount of vitamin K_1 found in some multivitamins is sufficient to prevent antibiotic-induced bleeding. Moreover, most multivitamins do not contain vitamin K.

ANTICONVULSANTS

Common names: Apo-Carbamazepine, Apo-Primidone, Carbamazepine, Carbatrol, Celontin, Dilantin, Epanutin, Epitol, Ethosuximide, Ethotoin, Felbamate, Felbatol, Fosphentyoin, Keppra, Lamictal, Lamotrigine, Levetiracetam, Mesantoin, Methsuximide, Milontin, Mysoline, Novo-Carbamaz, Nu-Carbamazepine, Oxcarbazepine, Peganone, Phenobarbital (Anticonvulsants), Phensuximide, Phenytoin, Primaclone, Primidone, Taro-Carbamazepine, Tegretol, Teril, Timonil, Topamax, Topiramate, Tridione, Trileptal, Trimethadione, Zarontin, Zonegran, Zonisamide

Anticonvulsants are a family of drugs that depress abnormal nerve activity in the brain, thereby blocking seizures. **Barbiturates** (page 34) and **benzodiazepines** (page 36) are commonly used to prevent and treat seizure disorders, as well as other conditions. Though some people are maintained on a single drug, most take two or more anticonvulsant medications to prevent seizures. Consequently, many studies report interactions that occur in individuals taking several anticonvulsants.

Interactions that occur with multiple drug therapy are described on this page. For interactions involving a specific anticonvulsant, refer to the highlighted drugs listed below.

Barbiturates
- Mephobarbital (Mebaral)
- Pentobarbital (Nembutal)
- **Phenobarbital** (page 215) (Luminol, Solfoton)

Benzodiazepines
- Chlorazepate (Tranxene)
- Clonazepam (Klonopin)
- Diazepam (Valium)

GABA Analogues
- **Gabapentin** (page 125) (Neurontin)
- Tiagabine (Gabitril)

Hydantoins
- Ethotoin (Peganone)
- Fosphentyoin (Mesantoin)
- Phenytoin (Dilantin)

Oxazolidinediones
- Trimethadione (Tridione)

Phenyltriazines
- Lamotrigine (Lamictal)

Succinimides
- Ethosuximide (Zarontin)
- Methsuximide (Celontin)
- Phensuximide (Milontin)

Miscellaneous
- Acetazolamide (Diamox)
- Carbamazepine (Carbatrol, Tegretol)
- Felbamate (Felbatol)
- Levetiracetam (Keppra)
- Oxcarbazepine (Trileptal)
- Primidone (Mysoline)
- Topiramate (Topamax)
- **Valproic acid** (page 275) (Depakene, Depakote)
- Zonisamide (Zonegran)

Summary of Interactions for Anticonvulsants

In some cases, an herb or supplement may appear in more than one category, which may seem contradictory.

For clarification, read the full article for details about the summarized interactions.

✓ May be Beneficial: Depletion or interference	Biotin Calcium Folic acid L-carnitine Vitamin A Vitamin B$_{12}$ Vitamin B$_6$ Vitamin D Vitamin K
✓ May be Beneficial: Side effect reduction/prevention	Folic acid L-carnitine Vitamin B$_{12}$ Vitamin D Vitamin K
✓ May be Beneficial: Supportive interaction	Folic acid
⊘ Avoid: Adverse interaction	Folic acid
Reduced drug absorption/bioavailability	None known

Interactions common to many, if not all, Anticonvulsants are described in this article. Interactions reported for only one or several drugs in this class may not be listed in this article. Some drugs listed in this article are linked to articles specific to that respective drug; please refer to those individual drug articles. The information in this article may not necessarily apply to drugs in this class for which no separate article exists. If you are taking an Anticonvulsant for which no separate article exists, talk with your doctor or pharmacist.

Interactions with Dietary Supplements

Biotin

Several controlled studies have shown that long-term anticonvulsant treatment decreases blood levels of biotin.[1, 2, 3, 4] In children, a deficiency of biotin can lead to withdrawn behavior and a delay in mental development. Adults with low biotin levels might experience a loss of appetite, feelings of discomfort or uneasiness, mental depression, or hallucinations. To avoid side effects, individuals taking anticonvulsants should supplement with biotin either alone or as part of a multivitamin.

Calcium

Individuals on long-term multiple anticonvulsant therapy may develop below-normal blood levels of calcium, which may be related to drug-induced vitamin D deficiency.[5] Two infants born to women taking high doses of phenytoin and **phenobarbital** (page 215) while pregnant developed jitteriness and tetany (a syndrome characterized by muscle twitches, cramps, and spasm) during the first two weeks of life.[6] Controlled research is needed to determine whether pregnant women who are taking anticonvulsant medications should supplement with additional amounts of calcium and vitamin D.

L-carnitine

Several controlled and preliminary studies showed that multiple drug therapy for seizures results in dramatic reductions in blood carnitine levels.[7, 8, 9] Further controlled research is needed to determine whether children taking anticonvulsants might benefit by supplementing with L-carnitine, since current studies yield conflicting results. For example, one controlled study indicated that children taking **valproic acid** (page 275) and carbamazepine received no benefit from supplementing with L-carnitine.[10] However, another small study revealed that children taking valproic acid experienced less fatigue and excessive sleepiness following L-carnitine supplementation.[11] Despite the lack of well-controlled studies, individuals who are taking anticonvulsants and experiencing side effects might benefit from supplementing with L-carnitine.

Folic acid

Several studies have shown that multiple anticonvulsant therapy reduces blood levels of folic acid and dramatically increases homocysteine levels.[12, 13, 14] Homocysteine, a potential marker for folic acid deficiency, is a compound used experimentally to induce seizures and is associated with atherosclerosis. Carbamazepine alone has also been shown to reduce blood levels of folic acid.[15]

One preliminary study showed that pregnant women who use anticonvulsant drugs without folic acid supplementation have an increased risk of having a child with birth defects, such as heart defects, cleft lip and palate, neural tube defects, and skeletal abnormalities. However, supplementation with folic acid greatly reduces the risk.[16] Consequently, some healthcare practitioners recommend that women taking multiple anticonvulsant drugs supplement with 5 mg of folic acid daily, for three months prior to conception and during the first trimester, to prevent folic acid deficiency–induced birth defects.[17] Other practitioners suggest that 1 mg or less of folic acid each day is sufficient to prevent deficiency during pregnancy.[18]

One well-controlled study showed that adding folic acid to multiple anticonvulsant therapy resulted in reduced seizure frequency.[19] In addition, three infants with seizures who were unresponsive to medication experienced immediate relief following supplementation with the active form of folic acid.[20]

Despite the apparent beneficial effects, some studies have indicated that as little as 0.8 mg of folic acid taken daily can increase the frequency and/or severity of seizures.[21, 22, 23, 24] However, a recent controlled study showed that both healthy and epileptic women taking less than 1 mg of folic acid per day had no increased risk for seizures.[25] Until more is known about the risks and benefits of folic acid, individuals taking multiple anticonvulsant drugs should consult with their healthcare practitioner before supplementing with folic acid. In addition, pregnant women or women who might become pregnant while taking anticonvulsant drugs should discuss folic acid supplementation with their practitioner.

Vitamin A

Anticonvulsant drugs can occasionally cause birth defects when taken by pregnant women, and their toxicity might be related to low blood levels of vitamin A. One controlled study showed that taking multiple anticonvulsant drugs results in dramatic changes in the way the body utilizes vitamin A.[26] Further controlled research is needed to determine whether supplemental vitamin A might prevent birth defects in children born to women on multiple anticonvulsant therapy. Other research suggests that ingestion of large amounts of vitamin A may promote the development of birth defects, although the studies are conflicting.

Vitamin B6

One controlled study revealed that taking anticonvulsant drugs dramatically reduces blood levels of vitamin B6.[27] A nutritional deficiency of vitamin B6 can lead to an increase in homocysteine blood levels, which has been associated with atherosclerosis. Vitamin B6 deficiency is also associated with symptoms such as dizziness, fatigue, mental depression, and seizures. On the other hand, supplementation with large amounts of vitamin B6 (80–200 mg per day) has been reported to reduce blood levels of some anticonvulsant drugs, which could theoretically trigger seizures. People taking multiple anticonvulsant drugs should discuss with their doctor whether supplementing with vitamin B6 is advisable.

Vitamin B12

Anemia is an uncommon side effect experienced by people taking anticonvulsant drugs. Though many researchers believe that low blood levels of folic acid are involved, the effects might be caused by a vitamin B12 deficiency. Deficiencies of folic acid and vitamin B12 can lead to nerve and mental problems. One study revealed that individuals on long-term anticonvulsant therapy, despite having no laboratory signs of anemia, had dramatically lower levels of vitamin B_{12} in their cerebrospinal fluid (the fluid that bathes the brain) when compared with people who were not taking seizure medications. Improvement in mental status and nerve function was observed in a majority of symptomatic individuals after taking 30 mcg of vitamin B_{12} daily for a few days.[28] Another study found that long-term anticonvulsant therapy had no effect on blood levels of vitamin B_{12}.[29] The results of these two studies indicate that people taking anticonvulsant drugs might experience side effects of vitamin B_{12} deficiency, and that the deficiency is not easily detected by the usual blood tests. Therefore, individuals taking anticonvulsant drugs for several months or years might prevent nerve and mental problems by supplementing with vitamin B_{12}.

Vitamin D

Though research results vary, long-term use of anticonvulsant drugs appears to interfere with vitamin D activity, which might lead to softening of bones (osteomalacia). One study showed that blood levels of vitamin D in males taking anticonvulsants were lower than those found in men who were not taking seizure medication.[30] In a controlled study, bone strength improved in children taking anticonvulsant drugs who were supplemented with the activated form of vitamin D and 500 mg per day of calcium for nine months.[31] Some research suggests that differences in exposure to sunlight—which normally increases blood levels of vitamin D—might explain why some studies have failed to find a beneficial effect of vitamin D supplementation. In one controlled study, blood vitamin D levels in children taking anticonvulsants were dramatically lower in winter months than in summer months.[32] Another study of 450 people in Florida taking anticonvulsants found that few had drug-induced bone disease.[33] Consequently, people taking anticonvulsant drugs who do not receive adequate sunlight should supplement with 400 IU of vitamin D each day to help prevent osteomalacia.

Vitamin E

Two studies showed that individuals taking phenytoin and **phenobarbital** (page 215) had lower blood vitamin E levels than those who received no treatment for seizures.[34, 35] Though the consequences of lower blood levels of vitamin E are unknown, people taking multiple anticonvulsant drugs should probably supplement with 100 to 200 IU of vitamin E daily to prevent a deficiency.

Vitamin K

Some studies have shown that babies born to women taking anticonvulsant drugs have low blood levels of vitamin K, which might cause bleeding in the infant.[36] Though some researchers recommend vitamin K supplementation prior to delivery,[37, 38] not all agree that supplementation for women taking anticonvulsant drugs is necessary.[39] Until more information is available, pregnant women or women who might become pregnant while taking anticonvulsant drugs should discuss vitamin K supplementation with their healthcare practitioner.

ANTIDEPRESSANTS

Antidepressants are a family of drugs primarily used to treat mental depression as well as chronic pain, childhood bed-wetting, anxiety, panic disorder, eating disorders, cigarette addiction, obsessive-compulsive disorder, obesity, social anxiety disorder, and premenstrual depression. Antidepressants are classified according to their action on brain chemicals or by their chemical structure and are divided into the following four categories:

Monoamine Oxidase Inhibitors (MAOIs)
- **Phenelzine** (page 214) (Nardil)
- Tranylcypromine (Parnate)

Tricyclic Antidepressants *(page 270)*
- Amitriptyline (Elavil)
- Amoxapine (Asendin)
- Clomipramine (Anafranil)
- Desipramine (Norpramin, Pertofrane)
- Doxepin (Adapin, Sinequan)
- Imipramine (Tofranil, Janimine)
- Nortriptyline (Aventyl, Pamelor)
- Protriptyline (Vivactil)
- Trimipramine (Surmontil)

Selective Serotonin Reuptake Inhibitors (SSRIs)
- **Citalopram** (page 68) (Celexa)
- **Fluoxetine** (page 120) (Prozac)
- **Fluvoxamine** (page 122) (Luvox)
- **Paroxetine** (page 208) (Paxil)
- **Sertraline** (page 237) (Zoloft)

Miscellaneous Antidepressants
- **Bupropion** (page 43) (Wellbutrin, Zyban)
- Maprotiline (Ludiomil)
- **Mirtazapine** (page 180) (Remeron)
- **Nefazodone** (page 187) (Serzone)

- **Trazodone** (page 267) (Desyrel)
- **Venlafaxine** (page 279) (Effexor)

> For interactions involving a specific Antidepressant, see the individual drug article. For interactions involving an Antidepressant for which no separate article exists, talk to your doctor or pharmacist.

ANTIFUNGAL AGENTS

Common names: Ancobon, Butoconazole, Clotrimazole, Femizol-M, Femstat, Flucytosine, Gyne-Lotrimin, Itraconazole, Lotrimin, Lotrisone, Miconazole, Monistat, Mycelex, Sporanox, Tioconazole, Vagistat

Antifungal drugs are used to kill fungi and yeast that cause infection in many areas of the body. They are used to treat common conditions, such as athlete's foot, ringworm, dandruff, and vaginitis, as well as serious infections that have spread throughout the body. Antifungal medication is often used in individuals with poorly functioning immune systems, as observed in people with AIDS, and in people who are taking drugs that suppress immune function.

For interactions involving a specific antifungal drug, refer to the highlighted medications listed below.

- **Amphotericin B** (page 15) (Amphocin, Fungizone)
- Butoconazole (Femstat)
- Clotrimazole (Mycelex, Gyne-Lotrimin, Lotrimin, Lotrisone)
- **Fluconazole** (page 116) (Diflucan)
- Flucytosine (Ancobon)
- **Griseofulvin** (page 133) (Fulvicin P/G, Grifulvin V, Gris-PEG)
- Itraconazole (Sporanox)
- **Ketoconazole** (page 149) (Nizoral)
- Miconazole (Femizol-M, Monistat)
- **Nystatin** (page 195) (Mycostatin)
- **Terbinafine** (page 253) (Lamisil)
- **Terconazole** (page 253) (Terazol)
- Tioconazole (Vagistat)

> For interactions involving a specific Antifungal Agent, see the individual drug article. For interactions involving an Antifungal Agent for which no separate article exists, talk to your doctor or pharmacist.

ANTIMALARIAL DRUGS

Antimalarials are **anti-protozoal** (page 19) drugs that are primarily used to treat malaria. Certain antimalarials are useful in treating other conditions as well, including quinine for leg cramps and hydroxychloroquine for severe cases of rheumatoid arthritis.

For interactions involving a specific antimalarial drug, refer to the medications listed below.

- Chloroquine (Aralen)
- Halofantrine (Halfan)
- **Hydroxychloroquine** (page 137) (Plaquenil)
- Mefloquine (Lariam)
- Primaquine
- Pyrimethamine (Daraprim)
- **Quinine Sulfate** (page 227) (Quinamm)
- Sulfadoxine and pyrimethamine (Fansidar)

> For interactions involving a specific Antimalarian Drug, see the individual drug article. For interactions involving an Antimalarial Drug for which no separate article exists, talk to your doctor or pharmacist.

ANTITUBERCULAR AGENTS

Antitubercular drugs are **antibiotics** (page 19) specifically used to prevent or treat tuberculosis. Most patients with tuberculosis take more than one antibiotic at a time due to the high number of drug-resistant strains of bacteria that cause the disease.

For interactions involving a specific antitubercular drug, refer to the highlighted medications listed below.

- Aminosalicylic acid (Paser)
- Capreomycin (Capastat)
- **Cycloserine** (page 82) (Seromycin)
- Ethambutol (Myambutol)
- Ethionamide (Trecator-SC)
- **Isoniazid** (page 146) (INH, Nydrazid, Laniazid)
- Isoniazid and rifampin (Rifamate)
- Isoniazid, rifampin, and pyrazinamide (Rifater)
- Pyrazinamide
- Rifabutin (Mycobutin)
- Rifampin (Rifadin, Rimactane)
- Rifapentine (Priftin)
- Streptomycin

For interactions involving a specific Antitubercular Agent, see the individual drug article. For interactions involving an Antitubercular Agent for which no separate article exists, talk to your doctor or pharmacist.

For interactions involving a specific Antiviral Drug, see the individual drug article. For interactions involving an Antiviral Drug for which no separate article exists, talk to your doctor or pharmacist.

ANTIVIRAL DRUGS

Antiviral drugs are used to treat diseases caused by viruses, such as AIDS, genital herpes, influenza, chickenpox, shingles, and cold sores.

For interactions involving a specific antiviral drug, refer to the highlighted medications listed below.

Reverse Transcriptase Inhibitors, AIDS Therapy
- Abacavir (Ziagen)
- Delavirdine (Rescriptor)
- **Didanosine** (page 90) (Videx)
- Efavirenz (Sustiva)
- **Lamivudine** (page 153) (Epivir, Epivir-HBV)
- Nevirapine (Viramune)
- **Stavudine** (page 244) (Zerit)
- Zalcitabine (Hivid)
- Zidovudine (Retrovir)
- Zidovudine and Lamivudine (Combivir)

Protease Inhibitors, AIDS Therapy
- Amprenavir (Agenerase)
- **Indinavir** (page 141) (Crixivan)
- Nelfinavir (Viracept)
- Ritonavir (Norvir)
- Saquinavir (Fortovase, Invirase)

Herpes Therapy
- **Acyclovir oral** (page 5) (Zovirax)
- Cidofovir (Vistide for Injection)
- Famciclovir (Famvir)
- Gancyclovir (Cytovene)
- **Valacyclovir** (page 275) (Valtrex)

Miscellaneous Antiviral
- **Amantadine** (page 10) (Symmetrel)
- **Interferon** (page 144) (Alferon N Injection, Infergen, Intron A for Injection)
- Oseltamivir (Tamiflu)
- Palivizumab (Synagis)
- Ribavirin (Virazole)
- Ribavirin and Interferon (Rebetron)
- Rimantadine (Flumadine)
- Zanamivir (Relenza)

APPEDRINE

Contains the following ingredients:
Multiple vitamins and minerals
Phenylpropanolamine (page 218)

APRESAZIDE

Contains the following ingredients:
Hydralazine (page 136)
Hydrochlorothiazide

ARTHROTEC

Contains the following ingredients:
Diclofenac (page 87)
Misoprostol (page 180)

ASILONE ANTACID LIQUID

Contains the following ingredients:
Aluminium
Dimethicone
Magnesium

ASPIRIN

Common names: Acetylsalicylic Acid, Angettes 75, Apo-ASA, ASA, Asaphen, Aspro Clear, Aspro, Beecham Aspirin, Beecham's Powder Tablets, Boots Back Pain Relief, Caprin, Entrophen, Fynnon Calcium Aspirin, Maximum Strength Aspro Clear, MSD Enteric Coated ASA, Novasen, Nu-Seals Aspirin

Combination drugs: Alka-Seltzer, Anacin, Darvon Compound, Empirin with Codeine, Fiorinal, Imazin XL Forte, Imazin XL, Percodan, Roxiprin, Soma Compound, Soma Compound with Codeine

Aspirin is a drug that reduces swelling, pain, and fever. In recent years, long-term low-dose aspirin has been recommended to reduce the risk of heart attacks and strokes. In the future aspirin may be recommended to reduce the risk of some cancers. Reye's syndrome, a rare but serious illness affecting children and teenagers, has been associated with aspirin use. To prevent Reye's syndrome, people should consult their doctor and/ or pharmacist before giving aspirin, aspirin-containing products, or herbs containing salicylates to children and teenagers.

Summary of Interactions for Aspirin

In some cases, an herb or supplement may appear in more than one category, which may seem contradictory. For clarification, read the full article for details about the summarized interactions.

✓ May be Beneficial: Depletion or interference	Folic acid* Iron Vitamin B$_{12}$* Vitamin C Zinc
✓ May be Beneficial: Supportive interaction	Cayenne Licorice
⊘ Avoid: Adverse interaction	Coleus* *Ginkgo biloba* Vitamin E
Side effect reduction/prevention	None known
Reduced drug absorption/bioavailability	None known

Interactions with Dietary Supplements

Folic acid

Increased loss of folic acid in urine has been reported in rheumatoid arthritis patients.[1] Reduced blood levels of the vitamin have also been reported in people with arthritis who take aspirin.[2] Some doctors recommend for people with arthritis who regularly take aspirin to supplement 400 mcg of folic acid per day—an amount frequently found in multivitamins.

Iron

Gastrointestinal (GI) bleeding is a common side effect of taking aspirin. A person with aspirin-induced GI bleeding may not always have symptoms (like stomach pain) or obvious signs of blood in their stool. Such bleeding causes loss of iron from the body. Long-term blood loss due to regular use of aspirin can lead to iron-deficiency anemia. Lost iron can be replaced with iron supplements. Iron supplementation should be used only in cases of iron deficiency verified with laboratory tests.

Vitamin B$_{12}$

In a study of people hospitalized with heart disease, those who had been taking aspirin were nearly twice as likely as nonusers to have a low or marginally low blood level of vitamin B$_{12}$.[3] That finding by itself does not prove that taking aspirin causes vitamin B$_{12}$ deficiency. However, aspirin is known to damage the stomach in some cases, and the stomach plays a key role in vitamin B$_{12}$ absorption (by secreting hydrochloric acid and intrinsic factor).

Vitamin C

Taking aspirin has been associated with increased loss of vitamin C in urine and has been linked to depletion of vitamin C.[4] People who take aspirin regularly should consider supplementing at least a few hundred milligrams of vitamin C per day. Such an amount is often found in a multivitamin.

Vitamin E

Although vitamin E is thought to act like a blood thinner, very little research has supported this idea. In fact, a double-blind trial found that very high amounts of vitamin E do not increase the effects of the powerful blood-thinning drug **warfarin** (page 281).[5] Nonetheless, a double-blind study of smokers found the combination of aspirin plus 50 IU per day of vitamin E led to a statistically significant increase in bleeding gums compared with taking aspirin alone (affecting one person in three versus one in four with just aspirin).[6] The authors concluded that vitamin E might, especially if combined with aspirin, increase the risk of bleedings.

Zinc

Intake of 3 grams of aspirin per day has been shown to decrease blood levels of zinc.[7] Aspirin appeared to increase loss of zinc in the urine in this study, and the effect was noted beginning three days after starting aspirin.

Interactions with Herbs

Cayenne (*Capsicum annuum, Capsicum frutescens*)

Cayenne contains the potent chemical capsaicin, which acts on special nerves found in the stomach lining. In two rat studies, researchers reported that stimulation of these nerves by capsaicin might protect against the damage aspirin can cause to the stomach.[8, 9] In a study of 18 healthy human volunteers, a single dose of 600 mg aspirin taken after ingestion of 20 grams of chili pepper was found to cause less damage to the lining of

Aspirin

the stomach and duodenum (part of the small intestine) than aspirin without chili pepper.[10] However, cayenne may cause stomach irritation in some individuals with stomach inflammation (gastritis) or ulcers and should be used with caution.

Coleus (Coleus forskohlii)
There are theoretical grounds to believe that coleus could increase the effect of anti-platelet medicines such as aspirin, possibly leading to spontaneous bleeding. However, this has never been documented to occur. Controlled human research is needed to determine whether people taking aspirin should avoid coleus.

Ginkgo biloba
There have been two case reports suggesting a possible interaction between ginkgo and an anticoagulant drug or aspirin leading to increased bleeding.[11, 12] In the first, a 78-year-old woman taking **warfarin** (page 281) developed bleeding within the brain following the concomitant use of ginkgo (the amount used is not given in the case report). In the second, a 70-year-old man developed slow bleeding behind the iris of the eye (spontaneous hyphema) following use of ginkgo (80 mg per day) together with aspirin (325 mg per day). While this interaction is unproven, anyone taking anticoagulant medications or aspirin should inform their physician before using ginkgo.

Licorice (DGL) (Glycyrrhiza glabra)
The flavonoids found in the extract of licorice known as DGL (deglycyrrhizinated licorice) are helpful for avoiding the irritating actions aspirin has on the stomach and intestines. One study found that 350 mg of chewable DGL taken together with each dose of aspirin reduced gastrointestinal bleeding caused by the aspirin.[13] DGL has been shown in controlled human research to be as effective as drug therapy (**cimetidine** [page 61]) in healing stomach ulcers.[14] One animal study also showed that DGL and the acid-blocking drug Tagamet (cimetidine) work together more effectively than either alone for preventing negative actions of aspirin.[15]

ATAZANAVIR

Common names: Reyataz

Atazanavir is used in combination with other antiviral drugs to treat HIV infection.

Summary of Interactions for Atazanavir
In some cases, an herb or supplement may appear in more than one category, which may seem contradictory. For clarification, read the full article for details about the summarized interactions.

✓	May be Beneficial: Supportive interaction	Food
⊘	Avoid: Reduced drug absorption/ bioavailability	St. John's wort
	Depletion or interference	None known
	Side effect reduction/prevention	None known
	Adverse interaction	None known

Interactions with Herbs
St. John's wort (Hypericum perforatum)
Taking St. John's wort when taking atazanavir might result in reduced blood levels of the drug, which could lead to reduced effectiveness and eventual resistance. Individuals taking atazanavir should avoid taking St. John's wort at the same time.

Interactions with Foods and Other Compounds
Food
Taking atazanavir with food increases the absorption of the drug, which results in greater effectiveness. Therefore, atazanavir should be taken with a meal.

ATENIXCO

Contains the following ingredients:
Atenolol (page 28)
Chlorthalidone

ATENOLOL

Common names: Antipressan, Apo-Atenolol, Atenix, Gen-Atenolol, Novo-Atenol, Nu-Atenolol, PMS-Atenolol, Rho-Atenolol, Scheinpharm Atenolol, Tenolin, Tenormin, Totamol

Combination drugs: AtenixCo, Beta-Adalat, Co-Tendione, Kalten, Tenben, Tenchlor, Tenif, Tenoret 50, Tenoretic, Totaretic

Atenolol is a beta-blocker drug used to treat some heart conditions, reduce the symptoms of angina pectoris (chest pain), lower blood pressure in people with hypertension, and treat people after heart attacks.

Summary of Interactions for Atenolol

In some cases, an herb or supplement may appear in more than one category, which may seem contradictory. For clarification, read the full article for details about the summarized interactions.

⊘ Avoid: Adverse interaction	High-potassium foods* Pleurisy root* Potassium supplements* Tobacco
Depletion or interference	None known
Side effect reduction/prevention	None known
Supportive interaction	None known
Reduced drug absorption/bioavailability	None known

Interactions with Dietary Supplements

Potassium

Some beta-adrenergic blockers (called "nonselective" beta blockers) decrease the uptake of potassium from the blood into the cells,[1] leading to excess potassium in the blood, a potentially dangerous condition known as hyperkalemia.[2] People taking beta-blockers should therefore avoid taking potassium supplements, or eating large quantities of fruit (e.g., bananas), unless directed to do so by their doctor.

Interactions with Herbs

Pleurisy root

As pleurisy root and other plants in the *Aesclepius* species contain cardiac glycosides, it is best to avoid use of pleurisy root with heart medications such as atenolol.[3]

Interactions with Foods and Other Compounds

Food

Atenolol may be taken with or without food.[4]

Alcohol

Atenolol may cause drowsiness, dizziness, lightheadedness, or blurred vision.[5] Alcohol may intensify these effects and increase the risk of accidental injury. To prevent problems, people taking atenolol should avoid alcohol.

Tobacco

In a double-blind study of ten cigarette smokers with angina treated with atenolol for one week, angina episodes were significantly reduced during the non-smoking phase compared to the smoking phase.[6] People with angina taking atenolol who do not smoke should avoid starting. Those who smoke should consult with their prescribing doctor about quitting.

ATORVASTATIN

Common names: Lipitor

Atorvastatin is a member of the HMG-CoA reductase inhibitor family of drugs that blocks the body's production of cholesterol. Atorvastatin is used to lower elevated cholesterol.

Summary of Interactions for Atorvastatin

In some cases, an herb or supplement may appear in more than one category, which may seem contradictory. For clarification, read the full article for details about the summarized interactions.

✓ May be Beneficial: Depletion or interference	Coenzyme Q_{10}
⊘ Avoid: Adverse interaction	Grapefruit or grapefruit juice Vitamin A*
ⓘ Check: Other	**Magnesium hydroxide** (page 166) Magnesium oxide Magnesium-containing **antacids** (page 18) Niacin
Side effect reduction/prevention	None known
Supportive interaction	None known
Reduced drug absorption/bioavailability	None known

Interactions with Dietary Supplements

Coenzyme Q_{10}

In a group of patients beginning treatment with atorvastatin, the average concentration of coenzyme Q_{10} in blood plasma decreased within 14 days, and had fallen by approximately 50% after 30 days of treatment.[1] Many doctors recommend that people taking HMG-CoA reductase inhibitor drugs such as atorvastatin also supplement with approximately 100 mg CoQ_{10} per day, although lower amounts, such as 10 to 30 mg per day, might conceivably be effective in preventing the decline in CoQ_{10} levels.

Magnesium-containing antacids

A magnesium- and aluminum-containing **antacid** (page 18) was reported to interfere with atorvastatin absorption.[2] People can avoid this interaction by taking atorvastatin two hours before or after any aluminum/magnesium-containing antacids. Some magnesium supplements such as **magnesium hydroxide** (page 166) are also antacids.

Niacin

Niacin is the form of vitamin B_3 used to lower cholesterol. Ingestion of large amounts of niacin along with **lovastatin** (page 163) (a drug closely related to atorvastatin) or with atorvastatin itself may cause muscle disorders (myopathy) that can become serious (rhabdomyolysis).[3, 4] Such problems appear to be uncommon when HMG-CoA reductase inhibitors are combined with niacin.[5, 6] Moreover, concurrent use of niacin with HMG-CoA reductase inhibitors has been reported to enhance the cholesterol-lowering effect of the drugs.[7, 8] Individuals taking atorvastatin should consult their physician before taking niacin.

Vitamin A

A study of 37 people with high cholesterol treated with diet and HMG-CoA reductase inhibitors found blood vitamin A levels increased over two years of therapy.[9] Until more is known, people taking HMG-CoA reductase inhibitors, including atorvastatin, should have blood levels of vitamin A monitored if they intend to supplement vitamin A.

Interactions with Foods and Other Compounds

Food

Atorvastatin is best absorbed when taken without food[10] in the morning.[11] However, it has been reported to be equally well absorbed when taken with or without food.[12]

Grapefruit or grapefruit juice

Grapefruit contains substances that may inhibit the body's ability to break down atorvastatin; consuming grapefruit or grapefruit juice might therefore increase the potential toxicity of the drug. There is one case report of a woman developing severe muscle damage from simvastatin (a drug similar to atorvastatin) after she began eating one grapefruit per day.[13] Although there have been no reports of a grapefruit–atorvastatin interaction, to be on the safe side, people taking atorvastatin should not eat grapefruit or drink grapefruit juice.

ATROPINE

Common names: Minims Atropine Sulphate

Atropine is an alkaloid (a family of chemicals with pharmacologic activity and a common structure) that affects the nervous system. It is found in deadly nightshade (*Atropa belladonna*) and other plants. Some effects of atropine include blurred vision, dilated pupils, constipation, dry mouth, and dry eyes.

Atropine is available as a prescription drug, synthesized in the laboratory. It is used to help restore or control heart function. It is used in combination with other drugs to treat other health problems including diarrhea and excessive salivation (saliva production). Atropine drops (Isopto Atropine and others) are used to dilate pupils for eye exams.

Summary of Interactions for Atropine

In some cases, an herb or supplement may appear in more than one category, which may seem contradictory. For clarification, read the full article for details about the summarized interactions.

⃠ Avoid: Reduced drug absorption/ bioavailability	Tannin-containing herbs* such as green tea, black tea, uva ursi, black walnut, red raspberry, oak, and witch hazel
Depletion or interference	None known
Side effect reduction/prevention	None known
Supportive interaction	None known
Adverse interaction	None known

Interactions with Herbs

Tannin-containing herbs

Tannins are a group of unrelated chemicals that give plants an astringent taste. Herbs containing high amounts of tannins, such as green tea (*Camellia sinensis*), black tea, uva ursi (*Arctostaphylos uva-ursi*), black walnut (*Juglans nigra*), red raspberry (*Rubus idaeus*), oak (*Quercus* spp.), and witch hazel (*Hamamelis virginiana*), may interfere with the absorption of atropine taken by mouth.[1]

AUGMENTIN

Contains the following ingredients:
Amoxicillin (page 13)
Clavulanate

AUREOCORT

Contains the following ingredients:
Chlortetracycline
Triamcinolone

AZATHIOPRINE

Common names: Azamune, Immunoprin, Imuran, Oprisine

Azathioprine is used to prevent organ rejection following kidney transplant and to treat severe cases of rheumatoid arthritis.

Summary of Interactions for Azathioprine

In some cases, an herb or supplement may appear in more than one category, which may seem contradictory. For clarification, read the full article for details about the summarized interactions.

✓ May be Beneficial: Depletion or interference	Folic acid
Side effect reduction/prevention	None known
Supportive interaction	None known
Reduced drug absorption/bioavailability	None known
Adverse interaction	None known

Interaction with Herbs

Folic acid
People receiving dialysis for kidney failure often have low blood levels of folic acid. However, folic acid blood levels should return to normal following kidney transplant. A preliminary study of people taking azathioprine to prevent organ rejection revealed that blood levels of folic acid remained well below those of individuals not taking the drug. The highest blood folic acid level was observed in an individual who had not taken azathioprine for two years.[1] Controlled studies are

needed to determine whether people taking azathioprine should supplement with folic acid.

AZELASTINE

Common names: Astelin, Rhinolast

Azelastine nasal spray is used to treat the symptoms of seasonal allergies of the nose, such as sneezing, itching, and runny nose. Preliminary studies also show that azelastine might prevent mouth ulceration resulting from cancer **chemotherapy** (page 54).

Summary of Interactions for Azelastine

In some cases, an herb or supplement may appear in more than one category, which may seem contradictory. For clarification, read the full article for details about the summarized interactions.

🚫 Avoid: Adverse interaction	Alcohol
Depletion or interference	None known
Side effect reduction/prevention	None known
Supportive interaction	None known
Reduced drug absorption/bioavailability	None known

Interaction with Food and Other Compounds

Alcohol
Drinking alcoholic beverages while using azelastine may increase side effects such as drowsiness, dizziness, and poor coordination.[1] Therefore, people using azelastine nasal spray should avoid drinking alcohol, especially when they must stay alert.

AZITHROMYCIN

Common names: Zithromax

Azithromycin is a macrolide **antibiotic** (page 19) used to treat a variety of bacterial infections.

Summary of Interactions for Azithromycin

In some cases, an herb or supplement may appear in more than one category, which may seem contradictory. For clarification, read the full article for details about the summarized interactions.

Azithromycin

✓ May be Beneficial: Depletion or interference	Vitamin K*
✓ May be Beneficial: Side effect reduction/prevention	Bifidobacterium longum* Lactobacillus acidophilus* Lactobacillus casei* Saccharomyces boulardii* Saccharomyces cerevisiae* Vitamin K*
✓ May be Beneficial: Supportive interaction	Saccharomyces boulardii*
ⓘ Check: Other	Digitalis Magnesium
Reduced drug absorption/bioavailability	None known
Adverse interaction	None known

Interactions with Dietary Supplements

Magnesium

A magnesium- and aluminum-containing **antacid** (page 18) was reported to interfere with azithromycin absorption in a study of ten healthy people.[1] People can avoid this interaction by taking azithromycin two hours before or after any aluminum/magnesium-containing products. It has not yet been shown that magnesium compounds typically found in supplements affect absorption of this drug.

Probiotics

A common side effect of antibiotics is diarrhea, which may be caused by the elimination of beneficial bacteria normally found in the colon. Controlled studies have shown that taking probiotic microorganisms—such as *Lactobacillus casei, Lactobacillus acidophilus, Bifidobacterium longum,* or *Saccharomyces boulardii*—helps prevent antibiotic-induced diarrhea.[2]

The diarrhea experienced by some people who take antibiotics also might be due to an overgrowth of the bacterium *Clostridium difficile,* which causes a disease known as pseudomembranous colitis. Controlled studies have shown that supplementation with harmless yeast—such as *Saccharomyces boulardii*[3] or *Saccharomyces cerevisiae* (baker's or brewer's yeast)[4]—helps prevent recurrence of this infection. In one study, taking 500 mg of *Saccharomyces boulardii* twice daily enhanced the effectiveness of the antibiotic vancomycin in preventing recurrent clostridium infection.[5] Therefore, people taking antibiotics who later develop diarrhea might benefit from supplementing with saccharomyces organisms.

Treatment with antibiotics also commonly leads to an overgrowth of yeast *(Candida albicans)* in the vagina (candida vaginitis) and the intestines (sometimes referred to as "dysbiosis"). Controlled studies have shown that *Lactobacillus acidophilus* might prevent candida vaginitis.[6]

Vitamin K

Several cases of excessive bleeding have been reported in people who take antibiotics.[7, 8, 9, 10] This side effect may be the result of reduced vitamin K activity and/or reduced vitamin K production by bacteria in the colon. One study showed that people who had taken broad-spectrum antibiotics had lower liver concentrations of vitamin K_2 (menaquinone), though vitamin K_1 (phylloquinone) levels remained normal.[11] Several antibiotics appear to exert a strong effect on vitamin K activity, while others may not have any effect. Therefore, one should refer to a specific antibiotic for information on whether it interacts with vitamin K. Doctors of natural medicine sometimes recommend vitamin K supplementation to people taking antibiotics. Additional research is needed to determine whether the amount of vitamin K_1 found in some multivitamins is sufficient to prevent antibiotic-induced bleeding. Moreover, most multivitamins do not contain vitamin K.

Interactions with Herbs

Digitalis (Digitalis lanata, Digitalis purpurea)

Digitalis refers to a family of plants commonly called foxglove that contain digitalis glycosides, chemicals with actions and toxicities similar to the prescription drug **digoxin** (page 90).

Erythromycin (page 106) and **clarithromycin** (page 68) (drugs closely related to azithromycin) can increase the serum level of digitalis glycosides, increasing the therapeutic effects as well as the risk of side effects.[12] While this interaction has not been reported with azithromycin, until more is known, azithromycin and digitalis-containing products should be used only under the direct supervision of a doctor trained in their use.

Interactions with Foods and Other Compounds

Food

Azithromycin suspension should be taken on an empty stomach, one hour before or two hours after food.[13] Azithromycin tablets may be taken with or without food and should be swallowed whole, without cutting, chewing, or crushing.[14]

AZT

Common names: Apo-Zidovudine, Azidothymidine, Novo-AZT, Retrovir, ZDV, Zidovudine

Combination drug: Combivir

AZT inhibits reproduction of retroviruses, including the human immunodeficiency virus (HIV). HIV is considered the cause of acquired immune deficiency syndrome (AIDS). AZT is one of a number of drugs used to treat HIV infection and AIDS.

Summary of Interactions for AZT

In some cases, an herb or supplement may appear in more than one category, which may seem contradictory. For clarification, read the full article for details about the summarized interactions.

✓ May be Beneficial: Depletion or interference	Carnitine* Copper Vitamin B$_{12}$
✓ May be Beneficial: Side effect reduction/prevention	Riboflavin
✓ May be Beneficial: Supportive interaction	Thymopentin Zinc
ⓘ Check: Other	N-acetyl cysteine Vitamin E
Reduced drug absorption/bioavailability	None known
Adverse interaction	None known

Interactions with Dietary Supplements

General nutrition

Preliminary human research suggests AZT therapy may cause a reduction in copper and zinc blood levels. Animal studies suggest that vitamin E may improve the efficacy of AZT.[1] The practical importance of these findings remains unclear.

Carnitine

Preliminary information suggests that muscle damage sometimes caused by AZT is at least partially due to depletion of carnitine in the muscles by the drug.[2] It has been reported that most patients taking AZT have depleted carnitine levels that can be restored with carnitine supplementation (6 grams per day).[3]

N-acetyl cysteine

Animal research suggests that zinc and N-acetyl cysteine supplementation may protect against AZT toxic-

ity.[4] It is not known whether oral supplementation with these nutrients would have similar effects in people taking AZT.

Vitamin B$_{12}$

Vitamin B$_{12}$ deficiency in HIV infected persons may be more common in those taking AZT.[5] HIV infected people with low vitamin B$_{12}$ levels were shown in one study to be more likely to develop blood-related side effects (particularly anemia) from taking AZT.[6]

Riboflavin

Persons with AIDS have developed lactic acidosis and fatty liver while taking AZT and other drugs in its class. AZT can inhibit crucial DNA-related riboflavin activity, which may be normalized by riboflavin supplementation. A 46-year-old woman with AIDS and lactic acidosis received a single dose of 50 mg of riboflavin, after which her laboratory tests returned to normal and her lactic acidosis was completely resolved.[7] More research is needed to confirm the value of riboflavin for preventing and treating this side effect.

Thymopentin

Thymopentin is a small protein that comes from a natural hormone in the body known as thymopoietin. This hormone stimulates production of the white blood cells known as T lymphocytes. Combination of thymopentin with AZT tended to decrease the rate at which HIV-infected persons progressed to AIDS.[8] Thymopentin alone did not seem to have a benefit in this study. Since thymopentin is administered by injections into the skin, people should consult with a doctor as to the availability of this substance.

Zinc

A study found that adding 200 mg zinc per day to AZT treatment decreased the number of *Pneumocystis carinii* pneumonia and *Candida* infections in people with AIDS compared with people treated with AZT alone.[9] The zinc also improved weight and CD4 cell levels. The amount of zinc used in this study was very high and should be combined with 1–2 mg of copper to reduce the risk of immune problems from the zinc long term.

BACLOFEN

Common names: Apo-Baclofen, Baclospas, Balgifen, Gen-Baclofen, Lioresal, Liotec, Novo-Baclofen, Nu-Baclo, PMS-Baclofen

Baclofen is used to treat muscle spasms associated with multiple sclerosis and spinal cord injury, and it may help with face pain due to trigeminal neuralgia. It is in a class of drugs known as centrally acting skeletal muscle relaxants.

Summary of Interactions for Baclofen

In some cases, an herb or supplement may appear in more than one category, which may seem contradictory. For clarification, read the full article for details about the summarized interactions.

Depletion or interference	None known
Side effect reduction/prevention	None known
Supportive interaction	None known
Reduced drug absorption/bioavailability	None known
Adverse interaction	None known

Interactions with Foods and Other Compounds
Food

Baclofen absorption is not affected by food, but the drug should be taken with a meal to minimize stomach upset.[1]

Alcohol

Drinking alcohol may enhance the side effects of baclofen, such as drowsiness, dizziness, weakness, and fatigue.[2] Therefore, people taking baclofen should avoid alcoholic beverages, especially if staying alert is necessary.

BARBITURATES

Common names: Aluratec, Amobarbital, Amylbarbitone, Amytal, Aprobarbital, Brevital, Busodium, Butabarbital, Butisol, Mebaral, Mephobarbital, Metharbital, Methohexital, Nembutal, Pentobarbital, Pentothal, Pentothal, Phenobarbitone, Quinalbarbitone, Secobarbital, Seconal Sodium, Seconal, Sodium Pentothal, Soneryl, Talbutal, Thiamylal, Thiopental, Tuinal

Barbiturates are a family of drugs that depress nerve activity in the brain, which produces changes in mental activity ranging from mild sedation and sleep, to deep coma. They are used to treat anxiety, insomnia, seizure disorders, and migraine headaches. In addition, some barbiturates are used in surgery as general **anesthetics** (page 129).

Interactions involving barbiturates in general are described on this page. For interactions involving a specific barbiturate, refer to the highlighted drugs listed below.

- Amobarbital (Amytal)
- Aprobarbital (Alurate)
- Butabarbital (Butisol)

- **Butalbital** (page 44) (Fiorinal, Fioricet)
- Mephobarbital (Mebaral)
- Methohexital (Brevital)
- Pentobarbital (Nembutal)
- **Phenobarbital** (page 215) (Luminal)
- Secobarbital (Seconal)
- Thiopental (Pentothal)

Summary of Interactions for Barbiturates

In some cases, an herb or supplement may appear in more than one category, which may seem contradictory. For clarification, read the full article for details about the summarized interactions.

⊘ Avoid: Adverse interaction	Alcohol
Depletion or interference	None known
Side effect reduction/prevention	None known
Supportive interaction	None known
Reduced drug absorption/bioavailability	None known

Interactions common to many, if not all, Barbiturates are described in this article. Interactions reported for only one or several drugs in this class may not be listed in this article. Some drugs listed in this article are linked to articles specific to that respective drug; please refer to those individual drug articles. The information in this article may not necessarily apply to drugs in this class for which no separate article exists. If you are taking a Barbiturate for which no separate article exists, talk with your doctor or pharmacist.

Interactions with Foods and Other Compounds
Alcohol

Drinking alcoholic beverages while taking barbiturates increases side effects, such as drowsiness, confusion, and dizziness;[1] if taken in excess, this combination may result in death. Consequently, people taking barbiturates should avoid drinking alcohol.

BENAZEPRIL

Common names: Lotensin

Combination drug: Lotrel

Benazepril is an **angiotensin-converting enzyme (ACE) inhibitor** (page 17) drug used to treat high blood pressure.

Summary of Interactions for Benazepril

In some cases, an herb or supplement may appear in more than one category, which may seem contradictory.

For clarification, read the full article for details about the summarized interactions.

✓ May be Beneficial: Depletion or interference	Zinc*
✓ May be Beneficial: Side effect reduction/prevention	Iron
⊘ Avoid: Adverse interaction	High-potassium foods* Potassium supplements* Salt substitutes*
Supportive interaction	None known
Reduced drug absorption/bioavailability	None known

Interactions with Dietary Supplements

Potassium

An uncommon yet potentially serious side effect of taking ACE inhibitors is increased blood potassium levels.[1, 2, 3] This problem is more likely to occur in people with advanced kidney disease. Taking potassium supplements,[4] potassium-containing salt substitutes (No Salt, Morton Salt Substitute, and others),[5, 6, 7] or large amounts of high-potassium foods at the same time as ACE inhibitors could cause life-threatening problems.[8] Therefore, people should consult their healthcare practitioner before supplementing additional potassium and should have their blood levels of potassium checked periodically while taking ACE inhibitors.

Zinc

In a study of 34 people with hypertension, six months of **captopril** (page 47) or **enalapril** (page 103) (ACE inhibitors related to benazepril) treatment led to decreased zinc levels in certain white blood cells,[9] raising concerns about possible ACE inhibitor–induced zinc depletion.

While zinc depletion has not been reported with benazepril, until more is known, it makes sense for people taking benazepril long term to consider, as a precaution, taking a zinc supplement or a multimineral tablet containing zinc. (Such multiminerals usually contain no more than 99 mg of potassium, probably not enough to trigger the above-mentioned interaction.) Supplements containing zinc should also contain copper, to protect against a zinc-induced copper deficiency.

Iron

In a double-blind study of patients who had developed a cough attributed to an ACE inhibitor, supplementation with iron (in the form of 256 mg of ferrous sulfate per day) for four weeks reduced the severity of the cough by a statistically significant 45%, compared with a non-significant 8% improvement in the placebo group.[10]

Interactions with Foods and Other Compounds

Food

Benazepril may be taken with or without food.[11]

BENZAMYCIN

This drug is a combination of two active ingredients, benzoyl peroxide and **erythromycin** (page 106), which are applied topically to treat mild to moderate acne. Benzoyl peroxide breaks down and removes the outer layer of skin and exerts antibacterial activity. Erythromycin is used as an antibacterial agent.

Summary of Interactions for Benzamycin

In some cases, an herb or supplement may appear in more than one category, which may seem contradictory. For clarification, read the full article for details about the summarized interactions.

✓ May be Beneficial: Side effect reduction/prevention	Vitamin E*
✓ May be Beneficial: Supportive interaction	Zinc
Depletion or interference	None known
Reduced drug absorption/bioavailability	None known
Adverse interaction	None known

Interactions with Dietary Supplements

Vitamin E

Animal studies show that benzoyl peroxide promotes tumor growth, yet the significance of this finding in humans is unknown. A test tube study showed that when exposed to vitamin E, human skin cells were more resistant to damage caused by benzoyl peroxide.[1] Controlled research is needed to determine whether use of benzoyl peroxide products by humans promotes tumor growth and whether vitamin E might prevent this damage.

Zinc

Using a topical zinc solution with topical erythromycin increases the effectiveness of the antibiotic in the treatment of inflammatory acne.[2]

BENZODIAZEPINES

Common names: Alti-Alprazolam, Alti-Clonazepam, Alti-Triazolam, Apo-Alpraz, Apo-Chlordiazepoxide, Apo-Clonazepam, Apo-Diazepam, Apo-Flurazepam, Apo-Lorazepam, Apo-Temazepam, Apo-Triazo, Ativan, Bromazepam, Centrax, Chlordiazepoxide, Clonazepam, Clonpam, Clorazepate, Dalmane, Dialar, Diastat, Diazemuls, Diazepam, Dizac, Doral, Estazolam, Flunitrazepam, Flurazepam, Gen-Alprazolam, Gen-Clonazepam, Gen-Temazepam, Gen-Triazolam, Halazepam, Klonopin, Lexotan, Libritabs, Librium, Loprazolam, Lorazepam, Lormetazepam, Midazolam, Mogadon, Nitrazepam, Novo-Alprazol, Novo-Lorazem, Novo-Poxide, Novo-Temazepam, Nu-Alpraz, Nu-Clonazepam, Nu-Loraz, Nu-Temazepam, Paxipam, PMS-Clonazepam, PMS-Temazepam, Prazepam, ProSom, Quazepam, Restoril, Rho-Clonazepam, Rimapam, Rivotril, Rohypnol, Somnite, Somnol, Stesolid, Temazepam, Tensium, Tropium, Valcalir, Valium, Versed, Vivol

✓ May be Beneficial: Supportive interaction	Vinpocetine
⊘ Avoid: Adverse interaction	Alcohol St. John's wort (alprazolam)
Depletion or interference	None known
Side effect reduction/prevention	None known
Reduced drug absorption/bioavailability	None known

Interactions common to many, if not all, Benzodiazepines are described in this article. Interactions reported for only one or several drugs in this class may not be listed in this article. Some drugs listed in this article are linked to articles specific to that respective drug; please refer to those individual drug articles. The information in this article may not necessarily apply to drugs in this class for which no separate article exists. If you are taking a Benzodiazepine for which no separate article exists, talk with your doctor or pharmacist.

Benzodiazepines are a family of drugs used to treat insomnia, anxiety, panic attacks, muscle spasms, and seizure disorders. One benzodiazepine, midazolam, is used as a general anesthetic.

Interactions involving benzodiazepines in general are described on this page. For interactions involving a specific benzodiazepine, refer to the highlighted drugs listed below.

- **Alprazolam** (page 9) (Xanax)
- Chlordiazepoxide (Librium, Libritabs)
- Clonazepam (Klonopin)
- **Clorazepate Dipotassium** (page 73) (Tranxene)
- Diazepam (Valium)
- Estazolam (ProSom)
- Flunitrazepam (Rohypnol)
- Flurazepam (Dalmane)
- Lorazepam (Ativan)
- Midazolam (Versed)
- **Oxazepam** (page 204) (Serax)
- Quazepam (Doral)
- Temazepam (Restoril)
- **Triazolam** (page 269) (Halcion)

Summary of Interactions for Benzodiazepines

In some cases, an herb or supplement may appear in more than one category, which may seem contradictory. For clarification, read the full article for details about the summarized interactions.

Interactions with Dietary Supplements
Vinpocetine

In a preliminary trial, an extract of periwinkle called vinpocetine was shown to produce minor improvements in short-term memory among people taking flunitrazepam, a benzodiazepine.[1] Further study is needed to determine if vinpocetine would be a helpful adjunct to use of benzodiazepines.

Interactions with Herbs
Kava (Piper methysticum)

Kava is an herb used to treat anxiety disorder. One individual who took a benzodiazepine (**alprazolam** [page 9]) and kava together, along with two other medications (**cimetidine** [page 61] and **terazosin** [page 253]) was hospitalized in a lethargic and disoriented condition.[2] Further research is needed to determine whether the combination of kava and benzodiazepines produces an adverse interaction. However, individuals should not take benzodiazepines and kava together unless supervised by a doctor.

St. John's wort (Hypericum perforatum)

In a study of healthy volunteers, administration of St. John's wort along with alprazolam decreased blood levels of alprazolam, compared with the levels when alprazolam was taken by itself.[3] Individuals taking alprazolam should not take St. John's wort without supervision by a doctor.

Interactions with Foods and Other Compounds
Alcohol

Drinking alcoholic beverages while taking benzodiazepines may increase side effects, such as drowsiness, confusion, and dizziness;[4] if taken in excess, this combination may result in death. Consequently, people taking benzodiazepines should avoid drinking alcohol.

BENZONATATE

Common names: Tessalon Perles

Benzonatate is a non-narcotic drug used to treat cough, including chronic cough in cancer patients who have not responded to narcotic drugs.

Summary of Interactions for Benzonatate

In some cases, an herb or supplement may appear in more than one category, which may seem contradictory. For clarification, read the full article for details about the summarized interactions.

Depletion or interference	None known
Side effect reduction/prevention	None known
Supportive interaction	None known
Reduced drug absorption/bioavailability	None known
Adverse interaction	None known

BENZTROPINE

Common names: Apo-Benztropine, Cogentin

Benztropine is used in the treatment of Parkinson's disease and to treat adverse reactions to anti-psychotic drugs.

Summary of Interactions

In some cases, an herb or supplement may appear in more than one category, which may seem contradictory. For clarification, read the full article for details about the summarized interactions.

✓ May be Beneficial: Supportive interaction	L-tryptophan* Niacin*
Depletion or interference	None known
Side effect reduction/prevention	None known
Reduced drug absorption/bioavailability	None known
Adverse interaction	None known

Interactions with Dietary Supplements

L-tryptophan and niacin

Akathisia is an adverse reaction to anti-psychotic drugs, where a person has an uncontrollable desire to be in constant motion. One preliminary report suggested that 4,000 mg of L-tryptophan and 25 mg niacin per day taken with benztropine enhances the treatment of akathisia.[1] Controlled studies are necessary to determine whether L-tryptophan and niacin supplements might benefit most people taking benztropine who experience adverse reactions to anti-psychotic drugs.

BETA-ADALAT

Contains the following ingredients:
Atenolol (page 28)
Nifedipine (page 189)

BETA-ADRENERGIC BLOCKERS

Common names: Betagan, Brevibloc, Carteolol, Cartrol, Celectol, Celiprolol, Esmolol, Levatol, Levobunolol, Metipranolol, Nebilet, Nebivolol, Ocupress, OptiPranolol, Oxprenolol, Penbutolol, Pindolol, Slow-Trasicor, Trasicor, Visken

Beta-adrenergic blockers or "beta blockers" are a family of drugs used to treat high blood pressure, angina, heart arrhythmia, tremors, alcohol withdrawal, glaucoma, and other conditions. They are also used to prevent migraine headaches, stage fright, and second heart attacks.

Interactions that are common to all beta-adrenergic blockers are described below. For interactions involving a specific beta-adrenergic blocker, refer to the highlighted drugs listed below.

Oral forms
- **Acebutolol** (page 3) (Sectral)
- **Atenolol** (page 28) (Tenormin)
- **Betaxolol** (page 38) (Kerlone)
- **Bisoprolol** (page 41) (Zebeta)
- Carteolol (Cartrol)
- Esmolol (Brevibloc)
- **Labetalol** (page 151) (Normodyne, Trandate)
- **Metoprolol** (page 176) (Lopressor)
- **Nadolol** (page 185) (Corgard)
- Penbutolol (Levatol)
- Pindolol (Visken)
- **Propranolol** (page 224) (Inderal)

- **Sotalol** (page 242) (Betapace)
- **Timolol** (page 263) (Blocadren)

Ophthalmic forms
- Betaxolol (Betoptic)
- Carteolol (Ocupress)
- Levobunolol (Betagan)
- Metipranolol (OptiPranolol)
- Timolol (Timoptic)

Summary of Interactions for Beta-Adrenergic Blockers

In some cases, an herb or supplement may appear in more than one category, which may seem contradictory. For clarification, read the full article for details about the summarized interactions.

⊘ Avoid: Adverse interaction	High-potassium foods Pleurisy root Potassium supplements
Depletion or interference	None known
Side effect reduction/prevention	None known
Supportive interaction	None known
Reduced drug absorption/bioavailability	None known

Interactions common to many, if not all, Beta-Adrenergic Blockers are described in this article. Interactions reported for only one or several drugs in this class may not be listed in this article. Some drugs listed in this article are linked to articles specific to that respective drug; please refer to those individual drug articles. The information in this article may not necessarily apply to drugs in this class for which no separate article exists. If you are taking a Beta-Adrenergic Blocker for which no separate article exists, talk with your doctor or pharmacist.

Interactions with Dietary Supplements
Potassium

Some beta-adrenergic blockers (called "nonselective" beta blockers) decrease the uptake of potassium from the blood into the cells,[1] leading to excess potassium in the blood, a potentially dangerous condition known as hyperkalemia.[2] People taking beta-blockers should therefore avoid taking potassium supplements, or eating large quantities of fruit (e.g., bananas), unless directed to do so by their doctor.

Interactions with Herbs
Pleurisy root

As pleurisy root and other plants in the *Aesclepius* genus contain cardiac glycosides, it is best to avoid use of pleurisy root with heart medications such as beta-blockers.[3]

BETAXOLOL

Common names: Betopic, Kerlone

Betaxolol is used orally to treat high blood pressure and in the eye to treat glaucoma. It belongs to a family of drugs known as **beta-adrenergic blockers** (page 37).

Summary of Interactions for Betaxolol

In some cases, an herb or supplement may appear in more than one category, which may seem contradictory. For clarification, read the full article for details about the summarized interactions.

⊘ Avoid: Adverse interaction	High-potassium foods* Pleurisy root* Potassium supplements*
Depletion or interference	None known
Side effect reduction/prevention	None known
Supportive interaction	None known
Reduced drug absorption/bioavailability	None known

Interactions with Dietary Supplements
Potassium

Some beta-adrenergic blockers (called "nonselective" beta blockers) decrease the uptake of potassium from the blood into the cells,[1] leading to excess potassium in the blood, a potentially dangerous condition known as hyperkalemia.[2] People taking beta-blockers should therefore avoid taking potassium supplements, or eating large quantities of fruit (e.g., bananas), unless directed to do so by their doctor.

Interactions with Herbs
Pleurisy root

As pleurisy root and other plants in the *Aesclepius* genus contain cardiac glycosides, it is best to avoid use of pleurisy root with heart medications such as beta-blockers.[3]

BETNOVATE-C

Contains the following ingredients:
Betamethasone
Clioquinol

BETNOVATE-N

Contains the following ingredients:
Betamethasone
Neomycin (page 187)

BILE ACID SEQUESTRANTS

Common names: Alti-Cholestyramine, Anion-Exchange Resins, Cholestyramine, Colestyramine, Novo-Cholamine, PMS-Cholestyramine, Prevalite, Questran

Cholestyramine (Questran) and **colestipol** (page 76) (Colestid) are bile acid sequestrants—a class of drugs that binds bile acids, prevents their reabsorption from the digestive system, and reduces cholesterol levels. Cholestyramine and colestipol are two of many drugs used to lower cholesterol levels in people with high cholesterol.

Bile acids are produced in the liver from cholesterol and secreted into the small intestine to help with the absorption of dietary fat and cholesterol. Bile acid sequestrants bind bile acids in the small intestine and carry them out of the body. This causes the body to use more cholesterol to make more bile acids, which are secreted into the small intestine, bound to bile acid sequestrants, and carried out of the body. The end result is lower cholesterol levels. Bile acid sequestrants also prevent absorption of some dietary cholesterol.

The information in this article pertains to bile acid sequestrants in general. The interactions reported here may not apply to all the Also Indexed As terms. Talk to your doctor or pharmacist if you are taking any of these drugs.

Summary of Interactions for Bile Acid Sequestrants

In some cases, an herb or supplement may appear in more than one category, which may seem contradictory. For clarification, read the full article for details about the summarized interactions.

✓ May be Beneficial: Depletion or interference	Beta-carotene and other carotenoids Calcium* Folic acid Vitamin A Vitamin D Vitamin E Vitamin K Zinc*

Side effect reduction/prevention	None known
Supportive interaction	None known
Reduced drug absorption/bioavailability	None known
Adverse interaction	None known

Interactions with Dietary Supplements

Vitamins and Minerals

Bile acid sequestrants may prevent absorption of folic acid and the fat-soluble vitamins A, D, E, and K.[1, 2] Other medications and vitamin supplements should be taken one hour before or four to six hours after bile acid sequestrants for optimal absorption.[3] Animal studies suggest calcium and zinc may also be depleted by taking cholestyramine.[4]

Carotenoids

Use of colestipol for six months has been shown to significantly lower blood levels of carotenoids including beta-carotene.[5]

Interactions with Foods and Other Compounds

Food

Bile acid sequestrants should be taken with plenty of water before meals.[6]

BIRLEY

Contains the following ingredients:
Magnesium
Sodium bicarbonate (page 240)

BISACODYL

Common names: Apo-Bisacodyl, Bisacolax, Carters Little Pills, Correctol, Dulcolax, Feen-A-Mint, PMS-Bisacodyl, Soflax EX

Bisacodyl, a stimulant-type laxative used to treat constipation, is available as a nonprescription product. All laxatives, including bisacodyl, should be used for a maximum of one week to prevent laxative dependence and loss of normal bowel function.

Summary of Interactions for Bisacodyl

In some cases, an herb or supplement may appear in more than one category, which may seem contradictory. For clarification, read the full article for details about the summarized interactions.

✓ May be Beneficial: Depletion or interference	Potassium
Side effect reduction/prevention	None known
Supportive interaction	None known
Reduced drug absorption/bioavailability	None known
Adverse interaction	None known

Interactions with Dietary Supplements
Potassium and other nutrients
Prolonged and frequent use of stimulant laxatives, including bisacodyl, may cause excessive and unwanted loss of water, potassium, and other nutrients from the body.[1, 2] Bisacodyl should be used for a maximum of one week, or as directed on the package label. Excessive use of any laxative can cause depletion of many nutrients. In order to protect against multiple nutrient deficiencies, it is important to not overuse laxatives.[3] People with constipation should consult with their doctor or pharmacist before using bisacodyl.

Interactions with Foods and Other Compounds
Food
Bisacodyl tablets are enteric coated to pass through the stomach and dissolve in the small intestine. Milk, dairy products, vegetables, almonds, chestnuts, and other foods can cause the enteric coating to dissolve in the stomach, leading to irritation and cramping.[4] People should take bisacodyl one hour before or two hours after meals to avoid this problem.

BISMAG

Contains the following ingredients:
　　Magnesium
　　Sodium bicarbonate (page 240)

BISMA-REX

Contains the following ingredients:
　　Bismuth (page 40)
　　Calcium
　　Magnesium
　　Peppermint oil

BISMUTH SUBSALICYLATE

Common names: Bismatrol, Bismed Liquid, Bismylate, BSS, Pepto-Bismol

Combination drugs: Bisma-Rex, Helidac, Moorland, Roter

Bismuth subsalicylate is a nonprescription drug used to relieve indigestion without constipation, nausea, and abdominal cramps. It is also used to control diarrhea and traveler's diarrhea. Bismuth subsalicylate is used together with prescription **antibiotics** (page 19) and stomach acid-blocking drugs to treat gastric and duodenal ulcers associated with *Helicobacter pylori* infection.

Summary of Interactions for Bismuth Subsalicylate
In some cases, an herb or supplement may appear in more than one category, which may seem contradictory. For clarification, read the full article for details about the summarized interactions.

🚫 Avoid: Adverse interaction	Salicylate-containing herbs* such as meadowsweet, poplar, willow, and wintergreen Sarsaparilla
Depletion or interference	None known
Side effect reduction/prevention	None known
Supportive interaction	None known
Reduced drug absorption/bioavailability	None known

Interactions with Herbs
Sarsaparilla (Smilax spp.)
Sarsaparilla may increase the absorption of digitalis and bismuth, increasing the chance of toxicity.[1]

Salicylate-containing herbs
Bismuth subsalicylate contains salicylates. Various herbs including meadowsweet (*Filipendula ulmaria*), poplar (*Populus tremuloides*), willow (*Salix alba*), and wintergreen (*Gaultheria procumbens*) contain salicylates as well. Though similar to **aspirin** (page 26), plant salicylates have been shown to have different actions in test tube studies.[2] Furthermore, salicylates are poorly absorbed and likely do not build up to levels sufficient to cause negative interactions that aspirin

might.[3] No reports have been published of negative interactions between salicylate-containing plants and aspirin or aspirin-containing drugs.[4] Therefore concerns about combining salicylate-containing herbs remain theoretical, and the risk of causing problems appears to be low.

BISODOL EXTRA STRONG MINT TABLETS

Contains the following ingredients:
    Calcium
    Magnesium
    Sodium bicarbonate (page 240)

BISODOL HEARTBURN RELIEF TABLETS

Contains the following ingredients:
    Alginic acid
    Aluminium
    Magnesium
    Sodium bicarbonate (page 240)

BISODOL INDIGESTION RELIEF POWDER

Contains the following ingredients:
    Magnesium
    Sodium bicarbonate (page 240)

BISODOL INDIGESTION RELIEF TABLETS

Contains the following ingredients:
    Calcium
    Magnesium
    Sodium bicarbonate (page 240)

BISODOL WIND RELIEF TABLETS

Contains the following ingredients:
    Calcium
    Dimethicone
    Magnesium
    Sodium bicarbonate (page 240)

BISOPROLOL

Common names: Cardicor, Emcor, Monocor, Zebeta

Combination drugs: Monozide, Ziac

Bisoprolol is a beta-blocker drug used to lower blood pressure in people with hypertension.

Summary of Interactions for Bisoprolol

In some cases, an herb or supplement may appear in more than one category, which may seem contradictory. For clarification, read the full article for details about the summarized interactions.

⊘ Avoid: Adverse interaction	High-potassium foods* Pleurisy root Potassium supplements*
Depletion or interference	None known
Side effect reduction/prevention	None known
Supportive interaction	None known
Reduced drug absorption/bioavailability	None known

Interactions with Dietary Supplements
Potassium
Some beta-adrenergic blockers (called "nonselective" beta blockers) decrease the uptake of potassium from the blood into the cells,[1] leading to excess potassium in the blood, a potentially dangerous condition known as hyperkalemia.[2] People taking beta-blockers should therefore avoid taking potassium supplements, or eating large quantities of fruit (e.g., bananas), unless directed to do so by their doctor.

Bisoprolol

Interactions with Herbs
Pleurisy root
As pleurisy root and other plants in the *Aesclepius* species contain cardiac glycosides, it is best to avoid use of pleurisy root with heart medications such as bisoprolol.[3]

Interactions with Foods and Other Compounds
Food
Bisoprolol may be taken with or without food.[4]

Alcohol
Bisoprolol may cause drowsiness, dizziness, lightheadedness, or blurred vision.[5] Alcohol may intensify these effects and increase the risk of accidental injury. To prevent problems, people taking bisoprolol should avoid alcohol.

BISPHOSPHONATES

Common names: Aredia Dry Powder, Bonefos, Clodronate, Didronel, Etidronate, Loron, Pamidronate, Skelid, Tiludronate, Tiludronic Acid

Bisphosphonates are a family of drugs used to treat osteoporosis and Paget's disease of bone, a chronic disorder that typically results in enlarged and deformed bones.

For interactions involving specific bisphosphonates, refer to the highlighted drugs listed below.
- **Alendronate** (page 7) (Fosamax)
- Etidronate (Didronel)
- Pamidronate (Aredia)
- **Risedronate** (page 232) (Actonel)
- Tiludronate (Skelid)

> For interactions involving a specific Bisphosphonate, see the individual drug article. For interactions involving a Bisphosphonate for which no separate article exists, talk to your doctor or pharmacist.

BOOTS DOUBLE ACTION INDIGESTION MIXTURE

Contains the following ingredients:
    Aluminium
    Dimethicone
    Magnesium

BOOTS DOUBLE ACTION INDIGESTION TABLETS

Contains the following ingredients:
    Aluminium
    Dimethicone
    Magnesium

BOOTS INDIGESTION TABLETS

Contains the following ingredients:
    Calcium
    Magnesium
    Sodium bicarbonate (page 240)

BRIMONIDINE

Common names: Alphagan

Brimonidine is a drug applied topically to the eyes to treat glaucoma.

Summary of Interactions for Brimonidine
In some cases, an herb or supplement may appear in more than one category, which may seem contradictory. For clarification, read the full article for details about the summarized interactions.

⊘ Avoid: Reduced drug absorption/ bioavailability	Yohimbe*
Depletion or interference	None known
Side effect reduction/prevention	None known
Supportive interaction	None known
Adverse interaction	None known

Interactions with Herbs
Yohimbe
The active ingredients in yohimbe can block the actions of brimonidine in certain human tissues,[1] thus reducing the drug's beneficial effects. Adequate human studies involving the eye are lacking, and until more information is available, yohimbe should be avoided in people using brimonidine.

Interactions with Foods and Other Compounds
Alcohol
Although human studies are lacking, preliminary studies suggest alcohol may enhance the effects of brimonidine.[2] Until more is known, individuals using brimonidine should avoid alcoholic beverages.

BROMPHENIRAMINE

Common names: Dimetane, Dimetapp Allergy, Dimotane, Nasahist B, ND-Stat, Oraminic II, Parabromodylamine maleate

Combination drugs: DayQuil Allergy Relief, Dimetapp

Brompheniramine is an antihistamine used to relieve allergic rhinitis (seasonal allergy) symptoms including sneezing, runny nose, itching, and watery eyes. It is also used to treat immediate allergic reactions. Brompheniramine is available in nonprescription products alone and in combination with other nonprescription drugs to treat symptoms of allergy, colds, and upper respiratory infections.

Summary of Interactions for Brompheniramine
In some cases, an herb or supplement may appear in more than one category, which may seem contradictory. For clarification, read the full article for details about the summarized interactions.

⊘ Avoid: Adverse interaction	Henbane*
Depletion or interference	None known
Side effect reduction/prevention	None known
Supportive interaction	None known
Reduced drug absorption/bioavailability	None known

Interactions with Herbs
Henbane (Hyoscyamus niger)
Antihistamines, including brompheniramine, can cause "anticholinergic" side effects such as dryness of mouth and heart palpitations. Henbane also has anticholinergic activity and side effects. Therefore, use with brompheniramine could increase the risk of anticholinergic side effects,[1] though apparently no interactions have yet been reported with brompheniramine and henbane. Henbane should not be taken except by prescription from a physician trained in its use, as it is extremely toxic.

Interactions with Foods and Other Compounds
Alcohol
Brompheniramine causes drowsiness.[2] Alcohol may intensify this effect and increase the risk of accidental injury.[3] To prevent problems, people taking brompheniramine or brompheniramine-containing products should avoid alcohol.

BUPROPION

Common names: Wellbutrin SR, Wellbutrin, Zyban

Bupropion is used to treat people with depression and to aid in smoking cessation treatment.

Summary of Interactions for Bupropion
In some cases, an herb or supplement may appear in more than one category, which may seem contradictory. For clarification, read the full article for details about the summarized interactions.

✓ May be Beneficial: Supportive interaction	Yohimbe*
⊘ Avoid: Adverse interaction	Alcohol
Depletion or interference	None known
Side effect reduction/prevention	None known
Reduced drug absorption/bioavailability	None known

Interactions with Herbs
Yohimbe
A 50-year-old woman who was unresponsive to traditional antidepressant therapy was reported to have a marked and persistent improvement in mood when yohimbine was added to her bupropion therapy.[1] Further research is necessary to determine the significance of this finding.

Interactions with Foods and Other Compounds
Alcohol
Unlike most other antidepressant drugs, there is no evidence that alcohol causes significant changes in blood levels of bupropion.[2] However, people taking bupropion who are also attempting to discontinue chronic alcohol consumption have been reported to sometimes experience convulsions.[3]

BUSPIRONE

Common names: Apo-Buspirone, BuSpar, Buspirex, Bustab, Gen-Buspirone, Novo-Buspirone, Nu-Buspirone, PMS-Buspirone

Buspirone is used to treat anxiety disorders and less commonly to treat symptoms of premenstrual syndrome.

Summary of Interactions for Buspirone

In some cases, an herb or supplement may appear in more than one category, which may seem contradictory. For clarification, read the full article for details about the summarized interactions.

⊘ Avoid: Adverse interaction	Kava
Depletion or interference	None known
Side effect reduction/prevention	None known
Supportive interaction	None known
Reduced drug absorption/bioavailability	None known

Interactions with Herbs

Kava (Piper methysticum)
Kava is an herb used to treat anxiety disorder. Although no direct interactions have been reported, buspirone should not be used together with kava unless with medical supervision.

Interactions with Foods and Other Compounds

Food
Food reduces metabolism of buspirone, increasing serum buspirone levels.[1] Buspirone should be taken at the same time each day, always with food or always without food.

Alcohol
Buspirone may cause drowsiness and dizziness.[2] Alcohol may compound these effects and increase the risk of accidental injury. To prevent problems, people taking buspirone should avoid alcohol.

BUTALBITAL

Combination drugs: Fioricet, Fiorinal, Phrenilin

Butalbital is in a class of drugs known as barbiturates and is used to treat tension headaches. There are currently no reported nutrient or herb interactions involving butalbital. See **barbiturates** (page 34) for interactions common to this class of drugs, though they have not yet been investigated for butalbital.

Summary of Interactions for Butalbital

In some cases, an herb or supplement may appear in more than one category, which may seem contradictory. For clarification, read the full article for details about the summarized interactions.

⊘ Avoid: Adverse interaction	Alcohol
Depletion or interference	None known
Side effect reduction/prevention	None known
Supportive interaction	None known
Reduced drug absorption/bioavailability	None known

Interactions with Foods and Other Compounds

Alcohol
Drinking alcoholic beverages while taking barbiturates increases side effects, such as drowsiness, confusion, and dizziness;[1, 2] if taken in excess, this combination may result in death. Consequently, people taking barbiturates should avoid drinking alcohol.

CAFFEINE

Common names: Cafcit, Caffedrine, Enerjets, NoDoz, Quick Pep, Snap Back, Stay Alert, Vivarin

Combination drugs: Anacin, Darvon Compound, Fioricet, Fiorinal

Caffeine is a central nervous system stimulant drug used as an aid to stay awake, for mental alertness due to fatigue, and as an adjunct with other drugs for pain relief. Caffeine is available alone as a nonprescription drug, in combination with other nonprescription drugs, and in prescription drug combinations for relief of pain and headache.

Summary of Interactions for Caffeine

In some cases, an herb or supplement may appear in more than one category, which may seem contradictory. For clarification, read the full article for details about the summarized interactions.

✓ May be Beneficial: Depletion or interference	Calcium
⊘ Avoid: Adverse interaction	Ephedra Tobacco
ⓘ Check: Other	Guaraná
Side effect reduction/prevention	None known
Supportive interaction	None known
Reduced drug absorption/bioavailability	None known

Interactions with Dietary Supplements

Calcium

In 205 healthy postmenopausal women, caffeine consumption (three cups of coffee per day) was associated with bone loss in women with calcium intake of less than 800 mg per day.[1] In a group of 980 postmenopausal women, lifetime caffeine intake equal to two cups of coffee per day was associated with decreased bone density in those who did not drink at least one glass of milk daily during most of their life.[2] However, in 138 healthy postmenopausal women, long-term dietary caffeine (coffee) intake was not associated with bone density.[3] Until more is known, postmenopausal women should limit caffeine consumption and consume a total of approximately 1,500 mg of calcium per day (from diet and supplements).

Interactions with Herbs

Guaraná (Paullinia cupana)

Guaraná is a plant with a high caffeine content. Combining caffeine drug products and guaraná increases caffeine-induced side effects.

Ephedra

Until 2004, many herbal weight loss and quick energy products combined caffeine or caffeine-containing herbs with ephedra. This combination may lead to dangerously increased heart rate and blood pressure and should be avoided by people with heart conditions, hypertension, diabetes, or thyroid disease.[4]

Interactions with Foods and Other Compounds

Food

Caffeine is found in coffee, tea, soft drinks, and chocolate. To reduce side effects, people taking caffeine-containing drug products should limit their intake of caffeine-containing foods/beverages.

Tobacco

Smoking can increase caffeine metabolism,[5] decreasing effectiveness. Smokers who use caffeine-containing drug products may require higher amounts of caffeine to achieve effectiveness.

CALCITONIN

Common names: Calcimar, Miacalcin Nasal

Calcitonin is a hormone found naturally in the body. As a drug inhaled through the nose, it is used primarily to treat certain types of osteoporosis as well as to provide symptomatic relief from pain due to acute fractures or compression of the bones in the spine.

Summary of Interactions for Calcitonin

In some cases, an herb or supplement may appear in more than one category, which may seem contradictory. For clarification, read the full article for details about the summarized interactions.

✓ May be Beneficial: Supportive interaction	Calcium
Depletion or interference	None known
Side effect reduction/prevention	None known
Reduced drug absorption/bioavailability	None known
Adverse interaction	None known

Interactions with Dietary Supplements

Calcium

Supplementation with 1,500 mg per day of calcium enhances the effects of nasal calcitonin on bone mass of the lumbar spine.[1] Women who take a calcitonin nasal product for osteoporosis should also take calcium.

CALCIUM ACETATE

Common names: Phosex, PhosLo

Calcium acetate is used to prevent high phosphorus blood levels in people with kidney failure.

Summary of Interactions for Calcium Acetate

In some cases, an herb or supplement may appear in more than one category, which may seem contradictory. For clarification, read the full article for details about the summarized interactions.

✓ May be Beneficial: Depletion or interference	Zinc
✓ May be Beneficial: Supportive interaction	Food
⊘ Avoid: Adverse interaction	**Antacids** (page 18) (calcium-containing) Calcium
Side effect reduction/prevention	None known
Reduced drug absorption/bioavailability	None known

Calcium Acetate

Interactions with Dietary Supplements
Calcium

People with kidney failure may develop high blood levels of calcium while taking calcium acetate. Since calcium acetate is a source of supplemental calcium, people taking the drug should avoid taking additional calcium supplements.[1] People experiencing adverse effects of high blood calcium—such as loss of appetite, mental depression, poor memory, and muscle weakness—should notify their healthcare practitioner.

Zinc

People with renal failure or on hemodialysis often have low blood levels of zinc, which may produce symptoms such as abnormal taste or smell, reduced sexual functions, and poor immunity. One controlled study showed that taking zinc at the same time as calcium acetate reduces absorption of zinc.[2] Therefore, people should avoid taking calcium acetate and zinc supplements together. Another controlled study revealed that neither short-term nor long-term treatment with calcium acetate results in reduced blood zinc levels.[3] Thus, while calcium acetate reduces the amount of zinc absorbed from supplements, long-term treatment with the drug does not appear to affect overall zinc status. However, people with renal failure who experience symptoms of zinc deficiency might benefit from supplementing with zinc, regardless of whether or not they take calcium acetate.

Interaction with Foods and Other Compounds
Food

Taking calcium acetate with food reduces absorption of phosphorus, which is the goal of therapy.[4] Therefore, calcium acetate should be taken with a meal.

Antacids *(page 18) (Calcium-containing)*

Calcium-containing antacids, when taken together with calcium acetate, may result in abnormally high blood levels of calcium.[5] Consequently, people taking calcium acetate should avoid taking calcium-containing antacids.

CALCIUM RICH ROLAIDS

Contains the following ingredients:
  Calcium carbonate
  Magnesium hydroxide (page 166)

CALCIUM-CHANNEL BLOCKERS

Common names: Bepadin, Bepridil, Cardene SR, Cardene, DynaCirc, Isradipine, Lacidipine, Lercanidipine, Motens, Nicardipine, Nimodipine, Nimotop, Nisoldipine, Prescal, Sular, Syscor MR, Vascor, Zanidip

Calcium-channel blockers are a family of drugs used to treat angina, high blood pressure, heart arrhythmia, heart failure, and Raynaud's disease, as well as to prevent migraine headaches.

For interactions involving specific calcium-channel blocking drugs, refer to the highlighted medications listed below.
- **Amlodipine** (page 13) (Norvasc)
- Bepridil (Bepadin, Vascor)
- **Diltiazem** (page 92) (Cardizem, Dilacor XR, Tiazac)
- **Felodipine** (page 113) (Plendil)
- Isradipine (DynaCirc)
- Nicardipine (Cardene)
- **Nifedipine** (page 189) (Adalat, Procardia)
- Nimodipine (Nimotop)
- Nisoldipine (Sular)
- **Verapamil** (page 280) (Calan, Covera H-S, Isoptin, Verelan)

Summary of Interactions for Calcium-Channel Blockers

In some cases, an herb or supplement may appear in more than one category, which may seem contradictory. For clarification, read the full article for details about the summarized interactions.

⊘ Avoid: Adverse interaction	Pleurisy root
Depletion or interference	None known
Side effect reduction/prevention	None known
Supportive interaction	None known
Reduced drug absorption/bioavailability	None known

Interactions common to many, if not all, Calcium-Channel Blockers are described in this article. Interactions reported for only one or several drugs in this class may not be listed in this article. Some drugs listed in this article are linked to articles specific to that respective drug; please refer to those individual drug articles. The information in this article may not necessarily apply to drugs in this class for which no separate article exists. If you are taking a Calcium-Channel Blocker for which no separate article exists, talk with your doctor or pharmacist.

Interactions with Herbs
Pleurisy root

As pleurisy root and other plants in the *Aesclepius* genus contain cardiac glycosides, it is best to avoid use of pleurisy root with heart medications such as calcium channel blockers.[1]

CALMURID HC

Contains the following ingredients:
Hydrocortisone
Lactic acid (page 152)
Urea

CANDESARTAN

Common names: Amias, Atacand

Candesartan is used to treat high blood pressure, and is in a class of drugs known as angiotensin II receptor antagonists. At the time of this writing, no evidence of nutrient or herb interactions involving candesartan was found in the medical literature.

Summary of Interactions for Candesartan

In some cases, an herb or supplement may appear in more than one category, which may seem contradictory. For clarification, read the full article for details about the summarized interactions.

Depletion or interference	None known
Side effect reduction/prevention	None known
Supportive interaction	None known
Reduced drug absorption/bioavailability	None known
Adverse interaction	None known

CANESTEN HC

Contains the following ingredients:
Clotrimazole (page 73)
Hydrocortisone

CAPTO-CO

Contains the following ingredients:
Captopril (page 47)
Hydrochlorothiazide

CAPTOPRIL

Common names: Acepril, Alti-Capropril, Apo-Capto, Capoten, Ecopace, Gen-Captopril, Hyteneze, Kaplon, Novo-Captoril, Nu-Capto, Tensopril

Combination drugs: Acezide, Capto-Co, Captozide, Co-Zidocapt

Captopril is an **angiotensin-converting enzyme (ACE) inhibitor** (page 17)—a family of drugs used to treat high blood pressure and some types of heart failure. Captopril is also used to slow the progression of kidney disease in people with diabetes.

Summary of Interactions for Captopril

In some cases, an herb or supplement may appear in more than one category, which may seem contradictory. For clarification, read the full article for details about the summarized interactions.

✓ May be Beneficial: Depletion or interference	Zinc
✓ May be Beneficial: Side effect reduction/prevention	Iron
⊘ Avoid: Adverse interaction	High-potassium foods* Potassium supplements* Salt substitutes*
Supportive interaction	None known
Reduced drug absorption/bioavailability	None known

Interactions with Dietary Supplements
Potassium

An uncommon yet potentially serious side effect of taking ACE inhibitors is increased blood potassium levels.[1, 2, 3] This problem is more likely to occur in people with advanced kidney disease. Taking potassium supplements,[4] potassium-containing salt substitutes (No Salt, Morton Salt Substitute, and others),[5, 6, 7] or large amounts of high-potassium foods at the same time as ACE inhibitors could cause life-threatening problems.[8] Therefore, individuals should consult their healthcare practitioner before supplementing additional potassium and should have their blood levels of potassium checked periodically while taking ACE inhibitors.

Zinc

Preliminary research has found significant loss of zinc in urine triggered by taking captopril.[9] In this trial, depletion of zinc reduced red blood cell levels of zinc. Although details remain unclear, it now appears that chronic use of captopril may lead to a zinc deficiency.[10]

It makes sense for people taking captopril long term to consider taking a zinc supplement or a multimineral tablet containing zinc as a precaution. (Such multiminerals usually contain no more than 99 mg of potassium, probably not enough to trigger the above-mentioned interaction.) Supplements containing zinc should also contain copper, to protect against a zinc-induced copper deficiency.

Iron

In a double-blind study of patients who had developed a cough attributed to an ACE inhibitor, supplementation with iron (in the form of 256 mg of ferrous sulfate per day) for four weeks reduced the severity of the cough by a statistically significant 45%, compared with a nonsignificant 8% improvement in the placebo group.[11]

CAPTOZIDE

Contains the following ingredients:
Captopril (page 47)
Hydrochlorothiazide

CARACE PLUS

Contains the following ingredients:
Hydrochlorothiazide
Lisinopril (page 156)

CARBELLON

Contains the following ingredients:
Charcoal
Magnesium
Peppermint oil

CARBIDOPA

Common names: Lodosyn

See also: **Carbidopa/Levodopa** (page 49)

Carbidopa is used together with the drug **levodopa** (page 154) to reduce symptoms of Parkinson's disease.

Summary of Interactions for Carbidopa

In some cases, an herb or supplement may appear in more than one category, which may seem contradictory. For clarification, read the full article for details about the summarized interactions.

✓	May be Beneficial: Depletion or interference	Niacin*
✓	May be Beneficial: Supportive interaction	Vitamin C*
⊘	Avoid: Reduced drug absorption/ bioavailability	Iron
ⓘ	Check: Other	5-HTP, Vitamin B$_6$ (see text)
	Side effect reduction/prevention	None known
	Adverse interaction	None known

Interactions with Dietary Supplements

Iron

Iron supplements taken with carbidopa may interfere with the action of the drug.[1]

5-Hydroxytryptophan (5-HTP)

5-HTP and carbidopa have been reported to improve intention myoclonus (a neuromuscular disorder) in some human cases but not others.[2, 3, 4] Several cases of scleroderma-like illness have been reported in patients using carbidopa and 5-HTP for intention myoclonus.[5, 6, 7]

Niacin

A study in animals has found that carbidopa inhibits an enzyme involved in the synthesis of niacin in the body.[8] In addition, there is evidence that niacin synthesis is decreased in people taking carbidopa and other drugs in its class,[9] raising the concern that people taking these drugs could be at risk of niacin deficiency, even if not frankly deficient. Further studies will be required determine if niacin supplementation is appropriate in people taking carbidopa.

Vitamin B$_6$

Test tube,[10] animal,[11] and preliminary human studies[12] suggest that carbidopa may cause depletion of vitamin B$_6$. However, the use of carbidopa with **levodopa** (page 154) reduces the vitamin B$_6$-depleting effects of levodopa.[13] More research is needed to determine whether vitamin B$_6$ supplementation is advisable when taking carbidopa.

Vitamin C

A combination of **carbidopa/levodopa** (page 49) and vitamin C may be useful for people with Parkinson's disease whose motor complications are not effectively managed with conventional drug treatment. This combination was administered to people with Parkinson's disease for 16.8 months in an unblinded, uncontrolled study.[14] The researchers reported that participants who completed the study experienced substantial increases in the number of hours with good functional capacity and were able to reduce their intake of other anti-Parkinsonian drugs. However, 62% of the participants withdrew from the study, citing difficulty in performing voluntary movements as the main reason. Until more research is performed, this drug-nutrient combination must be viewed as preliminary.

CARBIDOPA/LEVODOPA

Common names: Apo-Levocarb, Atamet, Co-Careldopa, Endo Levodopa/Carbidopa, Half Sinemet, Nu-Levocarb, Sinemet

Levodopa (page 154) is required by the brain to produce dopamine, an important neurotransmitter. People with Parkinson's disease have depleted levels of dopamine, leading to debilitating symptoms. Levodopa is given to increase production of dopamine, which in turn reduces the symptoms of Parkinson's disease. When taken by mouth, most levodopa is broken down by the body before it reaches the brain. Sinemet combines levodopa with **carbidopa** (page 48), a drug that prevents the breakdown, allowing levodopa to reach the brain to increase dopamine levels.

Summary of Interactions for Carbidopa/Levodopa

In some cases, an herb or supplement may appear in more than one category, which may seem contradictory. For clarification, read the full article for details about the summarized interactions.

✓	May be Beneficial: Depletion or interference	Niacin*
✓	May be Beneficial: Supportive interaction	Vitamin C*
⊘	Avoid: Reduced drug absorption/ bioavailability	Iron
ⓘ	Check: Other	5-HTP Vitamin B₆
	Side effect reduction/prevention	None known
	Adverse interaction	None known

Interactions with Dietary Supplements

Vitamin B₆

Vitamin B₆ supplementation above 5–10 mg per day reduces the effectiveness of levodopa.[1] However, combining levodopa with carbidopa prevents this adverse effect, so vitamin B₆ supplements may safely be taken with Sinemet (carbidopa/levodopa).

Iron

Iron supplements taken with carbidopa interfere with the action of the drug.[2] People taking carbidopa should not supplement iron without consulting the prescribing physician.

5-Hydroxytryptophan (5-HTP)

Several cases of scleroderma-like illness have been reported in patients using carbidopa and 5-HTP.[3, 4, 5] People taking carbidopa should not supplement 5-HTP without consulting the prescribing physician.

Niacin

A study in animals has found that carbidopa inhibits an enzyme involved in the synthesis of niacin in the body.[6] In addition, there is evidence that niacin synthesis is decreased in people taking carbidopa and other drugs in its class.[7] Further studies are needed to determine whether niacin supplementation is appropriate in people taking carbidopa.

Vitamin C

Combining levodopa-carbidopa and vitamin C may be useful for people with Parkinson's disease whose motor complications are not effectively managed with conventional drug treatment. This combination was administered to people with Parkinson's disease in a preliminary study.[8] The researchers reported several improvements in participants who completed the study; however, 62% of the participants withdrew from the study, most citing difficulty in performing normal movements. Until more research is performed, this drug-nutrient combination must be viewed as experimental.

Interactions with Foods and Other Compounds

Food

Food, especially foods high in protein, can alter levodopa absorption.[9, 10] However, Sinemet is often taken with food to avoid stomach upset. Sinemet and Sinemet CR should be taken at the same time, always with or always without food, every day.

CARDEC DM

Cardec DM is a combination drug containing carbinoxamine (an antihistamine similar to **diphenhydramine** [page 93]) plus pseudoephedrine and **dextromethorphan** (page 87). It is used to treat symptoms associated with the common cold and hay fever.

Summary of Interactions for Cardec DM

In some cases, an herb or supplement may appear in more than one category, which may seem contradictory. For clarification, read the full article for details about the summarized interactions.

⊘ Avoid: Reduced drug absorption/ bioavailability	Tannin-containing herbs* such as green tea, black tea, uva ursi, black walnut, red raspberry, oak, and witch hazel
⊘ Avoid: Adverse interaction	**Caffeine** (page 44) Ephedra
ⓘ Check: Other	Vitamin C
Depletion or interference	None known
Side effect reduction/prevention	None known
Supportive interaction	None known

Interactions with Herbs

Ephedra

Ephedra is the plant from which ephedrine was originally isolated. Until 2004, ephedra—also called ma huang—was used in many herbal products including supplements promoted for weight loss. To prevent potentially serious interactions, people taking Cardec DM should avoid using ephedra-containing drug products and should read product labels carefully for ma huang or ephedra content. Native North American ephedra, sometimes called Mormon tea, contains no ephedrine.

Tannin-containing herbs

Tannins are a group of unrelated chemicals that give plants an astringent taste. Herbs containing high amounts of tannins may interfere with the absorption of ephedrine or pseudoephedrine taken by mouth.[1] Herbs containing high levels of tannins include green tea, black tea, uva ursi (*Arctostaphylos uva-ursi*), black walnut (*Juglans nigra*), red raspberry (*Rubus idaeus*), oak (*Quercus* spp.), and witch hazel (*Hamamelis virginiana*).

Interactions with Foods and Other Compounds

Alcohol

Drinking alcohol while taking carbinoxamine can result in enhanced side effects such as drowsiness and dizziness.[2] Consequently, people who are taking Cardec DM should avoid drinking alcoholic beverages, especially when staying alert is necessary.

Food

Foods that acidify the urine may increase the elimination of ephedrine from the body, potentially reducing the action of the drug.[3] Urine-acidifying foods include eggs, peanuts, meat, chicken, vitamin C (greater than 5 grams per day), wheat-containing foods, and others.

Foods that alkalinize the urine may slow the elimination of ephedrine from the body, potentially increasing the actions and side effects of the drug.[4] Urine-alkalinizing foods include dairy products, nuts, vegetables (except corn and lentils), most fruits, and others.

Caffeine (page 44)

Caffeine, which is found in coffee, tea, chocolate, guaraná (*Paullinia cupana*), and some nonprescription and supplement products, can amplify the side effects of ephedrine and pseudoephedrine. People should avoid combination products containing ephedrine/ pseudoephedrine/ephedra and caffeine.

CARISOPRODOL

Common names: Carisoma, Isomeprobamate, Rela, Soma

Combination drugs: Soma Compound, Soma Compound with Codeine

Carisoprodol is a drug used as an adjunct to rest and physical therapy for relief of muscle pain. Carisoprodol is available by prescription alone and in combinations with other drugs.

Summary of Interactions for Carisoprodol

In some cases, an herb or supplement may appear in more than one category, which may seem contradictory. For clarification, read the full article for details about the summarized interactions.

Depletion or interference	None known
Side effect reduction/prevention	None known
Supportive interaction	None known
Reduced drug absorption/bioavailability	None known
Adverse interaction	None known

Interactions with Foods and Other Compounds

Food
Carisoprodol may be taken with food to prevent stomach upset.[1]

Alcohol
Carisoprodol may cause dizziness or drowsiness.[2] Alcohol may intensify these effects and increase the risk of accidental injury. To prevent problems, people taking carisoprodol or carisoprodol-containing products should avoid alcohol.

CARVEDILOL

Common names: Creg, Eucardic

Carvedilol is used to treat mild to moderate heart failure and high blood pressure.

Summary of Interactions for Carvedilol

In some cases, an herb or supplement may appear in more than one category, which may seem contradictory. For clarification, read the full article for details about the summarized interactions.

✓ May be Beneficial: Side effect reduction/prevention	Food
✓ May be Beneficial: Supportive interaction	Low-salt diet
Depletion or interference	None known
Reduced drug absorption/bioavailability	None known
Adverse interaction	None known

Interaction with Foods and Other Compounds

Food
Taking carvedilol with food slows the speed, but not the overall extent of absorption of the drug. Though taking carvedilol with food does not reduce the effectiveness of the drug, it might reduce the incidence of a common side effect known as orthostatic hypotension.[1] Therefore, people should take carvedilol with a meal.

Salt restriction
In one controlled clinical trial, lowering dietary salt intake increased the fall in blood pressure obtained with carvedilol.[2] Therefore, people taking carvedilol to treat high blood pressure should consider eating a diet low in salt to improve the outcome of drug therapy.

CELECOXIB

Common names: Celebrex

Celecoxib is used to treat rheumatoid arthritis and osteoarthritis; it is in a class of medications known as selective COX-2 inhibitor **nonsteroidal anti-inflammatory drugs** (page 193) (NSAIDs).

Summary of Interactions for Celecoxib

In some cases, an herb or supplement may appear in more than one category, which may seem contradictory. For clarification, read the full article for details about the summarized interactions.

✓ May be Beneficial: Depletion or interference	Potassium Sodium
⊘ Avoid: Adverse interaction	Willow*
ⓘ Check: Other	**Lithium** (page 157)
Side effect reduction/prevention	None known
Supportive interaction	None known
Reduced drug absorption/bioavailability	None known

Interactions with Dietary Supplements

Sodium and potassium
Controlled studies indicate that individuals on low-salt diets who take celecoxib retain sodium and potassium, which might result in higher than normal blood levels of these minerals.[1] More research is needed to determine whether potassium supplements might produce unwanted side effects in people taking celecoxib. Until more information is available, people taking celecoxib should have their sodium and potassium blood levels monitored by their healthcare practitioner.

Lithium (page 157)
Lithium is a mineral that may be present in some supplements and is also used in large amounts to treat mood disorders such as manic-depression. Taking celecoxib together with the mineral can result in significant

increases in lithium blood levels,[2] which might cause unwanted side effects. Consequently, people taking celecoxib and lithium-containing supplements should consult their healthcare practitioner about having their lithium blood levels checked regularly.

Interactions with Herbs

Willow (Salix alba)

Willow bark contains salicin, which is related to **aspirin** (page 26). Both salicin and aspirin produce anti-inflammatory effects after they have been converted to salicylic acid in the body. Taking aspirin and celecoxib together increases the likelihood of developing stomach and intestinal ulcers.[3] Though no studies have investigated a similar interaction between willow bark and celecoxib, people taking the drug should avoid the herb until more information is available.

CEPHALOSPORINS

Common names: Ancef, Anspor, Apo-Cefaclor, Apo-Cephalex, Azactam, Aztreonam, Baxan, Ceclor, Cedax, Cefaclor, Cefadroxil, Cefamandole, Cefazolin, Cefdinir, Cefepime, Cefixime, Cefizox, Cefobid, Cefonicid, Cefoperazone, Ceforanide, Cefotan, Cefotaxime, Cefotetan, Cefoxitin, Cefpodoxime, Cefprozil, Ceftazidime, Ceftibuten, Ceftin, Ceftizoxime, Ceftriaxone, Cefuroxime, Cefzil, Cephadrine, Cephadyl, Cephalexin, Cephalothin, Cephapirin, Ceporex, Ceptaz, Claforan, Distaclor, Duricef, Fortaz, Keflet, Keflex, Keflin, Keftab, Keftid, Kefurox, Kefzol, Kiflone, Mandol, Maxipime, Mefoxin, Meropenem, Merrem I.V., Monocid, Novo-Lexin, Nu-Cefaclor, Nu-Cephalex, Omnicef, Orelox, PMS-Cefaclor, PMS-Cephalexin, Precef, Rocephin, Scheinpharm Cefaclor, Suprax, Tazicef, Tazidime, Tenkorex, Ultracef, Vantin, Velosef, Zinacef, Zinnat

Cephalosporins and related drugs are a family of antibiotics used to treat a wide range of bacterial infections occurring in the body. Each drug within the family kills specific bacteria; therefore, healthcare practitioners prescribe cephalosporins based on the individual's current needs. Interactions that are common to antibacterial drugs may be found in the article on **antibiotics** (page 19).

There are interactions that are common to **antibacterial drugs** (page 19) and interactions involving a specific cephalosporin or related medication. For the latter interactions, refer to the highlighted drug listed below.

- Aztreonam (Azactam for injection)
- Cefaclor (Ceclor)
- Cefadroxil (Duricef)
- Cefamandole (Mandol)
- Cefazolin (Ancef, Kefzol)
- Cefdinir (Omnicef)
- Cefepime (Maxipime)
- Cefixime (Suprax)
- Cefoperazone (Cefobid)
- Cefotaxime (Claforan)
- Cefotetan (Cefotan)
- Cefoxitin (Mefoxin)
- Cefpodoxime (Vantin)
- Cefprozil (Cefzil)
- Ceftazidime (Ceptaz, Fortaz, Tazicef, Tazidime)
- Ceftibuten (Cedax)
- Ceftizoxime (Cefizox)
- Ceftriaxone (Rocephin)
- Cefuroxime (Ceftin, Kefurox, Zinacef)
- Cephalexin (Keflex, Keftab)
- Cephapirin (Cefadyl)
- Cephradine (Anspor, Velocef)
- Imipenem and Cilastatin (Primaxin I.V.)
- **Loracarbef** (page 161) (Lorabid)
- Meropenem (Merrem I.V.)

Summary of Interactions for Cephalosporins

In some cases, an herb or supplement may appear in more than one category, which may seem contradictory. For clarification, read the full article for details about the summarized interactions.

✓ May be Beneficial: Depletion or interference	Vitamin K*
✓ May be Beneficial: Side effect reduction/prevention	*Bifidobacterium longum* *Lactobacillus acidophilus* *Lactobacillus casei* *Saccharomyces boulardii* *Saccharomyces cerevisiae* Vitamin K
✓ May be Beneficial: Supportive interaction	*Saccharomyces boulardii*
Reduced drug absorption/bioavailability	None known
Adverse interaction	None known

Interactions common to many, if not all, Cephalosporins are described in this article. Interactions reported for only one or several drugs in this class may not be listed in this article. Some drugs listed in this article are linked to articles specific to that respective drug; please refer to those individual drug articles. The information in this article may not necessarily apply to drugs in this class for which no separate article exists. If you are taking a Cephalosporin for which no separate article exists, talk with your doctor or pharmacist.

Interactions with Dietary Supplements

Probiotics

A common side effect of antibiotics is diarrhea, which may be caused by the elimination of beneficial bacteria normally found in the colon. Controlled studies have shown that taking probiotic microorganisms—such as *Lactobacillus casei, Lactobacillus acidophilus, Bifidobacterium longum,* or *Saccharomyces boulardii*—helps prevent antibiotic-induced diarrhea.[1]

The diarrhea experienced by some people who take antibiotics also might be due to an overgrowth of the bacterium *Clostridium difficile,* which causes a disease known as pseudomembranous colitis. Controlled studies have shown that supplementation with harmless yeast—such as *Saccharomyces boulardii*[2] or *Saccharomyces cerevisiae* (baker's or brewer's yeast)[3]—helps prevent recurrence of this infection. In one study, taking 500 mg of *Saccharomyces boulardii* twice daily enhanced the effectiveness of the antibiotic vancomycin in preventing recurrent clostridium infection.[4] Therefore, people taking antibiotics who later develop diarrhea might benefit from supplementing with saccharomyces organisms.

Treatment with antibiotics also commonly leads to an overgrowth of yeast *(Candida albicans)* in the vagina (candida vaginitis) and the intestines (sometimes referred to as "dysbiosis"). Controlled studies have shown that *Lactobacillus acidophilus* might prevent candida vaginitis.[5]

Vitamin K

Several cases of excessive bleeding have been reported in people who take antibiotics.[6, 7, 8, 9] This side effect may be the result of reduced vitamin K activity and/or reduced vitamin K production by bacteria in the colon. One study showed that people who had taken broad-spectrum antibiotics had lower liver concentrations of vitamin K_2 (menaquinone), though vitamin K_1 (phylloquinone) levels remained normal.[10] Several antibiotics appear to exert a strong effect on vitamin K activity, while others may not have any effect. Therefore, one should refer to a specific antibiotic for information on whether it interacts with vitamin K. Doctors of natural medicine sometimes recommend vitamin K supplementation to people taking antibiotics. Additional research is needed to determine whether the amount of vitamin K_1 found in some multivitamins is sufficient to prevent antibiotic-induced bleeding. Moreover, most multivitamins do not contain vitamin K.

CERIVASTATIN

Common names: Baycol

Warning: On August 8, 2001, Bayer Pharmaceutical Division voluntarily withdrew Baycol (cerivastatin) from the U.S. market because of reports of sometimes fatal rhabdomyolysis, a severe muscle adverse reaction from this cholesterol-lowering (lipid-lowering) product. Bayer is taking similar action in all other countries except Japan.

Cerivastatin is used to lower elevated blood cholesterol and triglyceride levels when low-fat diets and lifestyle changes are ineffective. It is in a family of drugs known as HMG-CoA reductase inhibitors.

Summary of Interactions for Cerivastatin

In some cases, an herb or supplement may appear in more than one category, which may seem contradictory. For clarification, read the full article for details about the summarized interactions.

ⓘ Check: Other	Niacin
Depletion or interference	None known
Side effect reduction/prevention	None known
Supportive interaction	None known
Reduced drug absorption/bioavailability	None known
Adverse interaction	None known

Interactions with Dietary Supplements

Niacin

Some sources have reported that taking niacin together with HMG-CoA reductase inhibitors may result in serious muscle damage.[1] However, niacin has also been used in combination with statin drugs without ill effects, and has been found to enhance the cholesterol-lowering effect of these drugs.[2, 3] Persons taking cerivastatin or any other HMG-CoA reductase inhibitor should consult with their doctor before taking niacin.

CETIRIZINE

Common names: Apo-Cetirizine, Reactine, Zyrtec

Cetirizine is a selective antihistamine used to relieve allergic rhinitis (seasonal allergy) symptoms including sneezing, runny nose, itching, and watery eyes. It is also used to treat people with idiopathic urticaria.

Summary of Interactions for Cetirizine
In some cases, an herb or supplement may appear in more than one category, which may seem contradictory. For clarification, read the full article for details about the summarized interactions.

Depletion or interference	None known
Side effect reduction/prevention	None known
Supportive interaction	None known
Reduced drug absorption/bioavailability	None known
Adverse interaction	None known

Interactions with Foods and Other Compounds
Food
Cetirizine may be taken with or without food.[1]

Alcohol
Selective antihistamines, including cetirizine, may cause drowsiness or dizziness, although it is less likely than with nonselective antihistamines.[2] Alcohol can intensify drowsiness and dizziness, increasing the risk of accidental injury. People taking cetirizine should use alcohol only with caution.

CHEMOTHERAPY

Chemotherapy typically involves the use of several antineoplastic (anticancer) drugs to treat cancer, though some people are treated with single medications. While the drugs in this family are toxic to cancer cells, many are also toxic to healthy cells, which gives rise to numerous side effects. A few drugs used in chemotherapy enhance immune function, while some alter hormonal activity. One anticancer drug, **methotrexate** (page 169), is also used to treat severe cases of rheumatoid arthritis. For interactions involving specific anticancer drugs, refer to the highlighted medications listed below.

Alkylating agents
- Busulfan (Myleran)
- Carboplatin (Paraplatin for Injection)
- Carmustine (BiCNU for Injection)
- Chlorambucil (Leukeran)
- **Cisplatin** (page 64) (Platinol, Platinol-AQ Injection)
- **Cyclophosphamide** (page 79) (Cytoxan, Neosar)
- Ifosfamide (Ifex for Injection)

- Lomustine (CeeNu)
- Mechlorethamine (Mustargen for Injection)
- Melphalan (Alkeran)
- Pipobroman (Vercyte)
- Polifeprosan 20 with Carmustine (Gliadel Wafer)
- Streptozocin (Zanosar for Injection)
- Thiotepa (Thioplex for Injection)
- Uracil Mustard

Antineoplastic antibiotics
- Bleomycin (Blenoxane)
- Dactinomycin (Cosmegen for Injection)
- Daunorubicin (Cerubidine for Injection, DaunoXome Injection)
- Doxorubicin (Adriamycin Injection, Rubex for Injection, Doxil Injection)
- Idarubicin (Idamycin)
- Mitomycin (Mutamycin for Injection)
- Mitoxantrone (Novantrone Injection)
- Pentostatin (Nipent)
- Plicamycin (Mithracin)

Antimetabolites
- Capecitabine (Xeloda)
- Cladribine (Leustatin Injection)
- Cytarabine (Cytosar-U for Injection, Tarabine PFS Injection, DepoCyt Injection)
- Floxuridine (FUDR for Injection)
- Fludarabine (Fludara for Injection)
- **Fluorouracil** (page 116) (Adrucil for Injection, Efudex, Fluoroplex)
- Mercaptopurine (Purinethol)
- **Methotrexate** (page 169) (Folex for Injection, Rheumatrex)
- Thioguanine (Tabloid)

Hormonal agonists/antagonists
- **Anastrozole** (page 16) (Arimidex)
- Bicalutamide (Casodex)
- Diethylstilbestrol (Stilphostrol)
- Estramustine (Emcyt)
- Flutamide (Eulexin)
- Goserelin (Zoladex)
- Leuprolide (Lupron Injection)
- Megestrol (Megace)
- Nilutamide (Nilandron)
- **Tamoxifen** (page 251) (Nolvadex)
- Testolactone (Teslac)
- Toremifene (Fareston)

Mitotic inhibitors
- Etoposide (VePesid)
- Teniposde (Vumon Injection)

- Vinblastine (Alkaban-AQ Injection, Velban for Injection, Velsar for Injection)
- Vincristine (Oncovin Injection, Vincasar PFS Injection)

Immunomodulators
- Aldesleukin (Proleukin for Injection)
- Levamisole (Ergamisol)

Miscellaneous Antineoplastics
- Altretamine (Hexalen)
- Asparaginase (Elspar)
- **Docetaxel** (page 95) (Taxotere for Injection)
- Hydroxyurea (Hydrea)
- **Interferon** (page 144) alpha (Roferon-A Injection, Intron A for Injection, Alferon N Injection)
- Irinotecan
- Mitotane (Lysodren)
- **Paclitaxel** (page 205) (Paxene, Taxol)
- Procarbazine (Matulane)

Summary of Interactions for Chemotherapy

In some cases, an herb or supplement may appear in more than one category, which may seem contradictory. For clarification, read the full article for details about the summarized interactions.

✓ May be Beneficial: Depletion or interference	Multiple nutrients (malabsorption) Taurine
✓ May be Beneficial: Side effect reduction/prevention	Beta-carotene (mouth sores)* Chamomile (mouth sores) Eleuthero (see text) Ginger (nausea) Glutamine (mouth sores) L-Carnitine* Melatonin (see text) N-acetyl cysteine (NAC) Spleen peptide extract (see text) Thymus peptides (see text) Vitamin E, topical (mouth sores) Zinc (taste alterations)

✓ May be Beneficial: Supportive interaction	Antioxidants* Melatonin Milk thistle PSK
⊘ Avoid: Reduced drug absorption/bioavailability	St. John's wort
⊘ Avoid: Adverse interaction	See **Methotrexate** (page 169) (Folic acid)
ⓘ Check: Other	Echinacea Multivitamin-mineral Vitamin A Vitamin C

Interactions common to many, if not all, Chemotherapy drugs are described in this article. Interactions reported for only one or several drugs in this class may not be listed in this article. Some drugs listed in this article are linked to articles specific to that respective drug; please refer to those individual drug articles. The information in this article may not necessarily apply to drugs in this class for which no separate article exists. If you are taking a Chemotherapy drug for which no separate article exists, talk with your doctor or pharmacist.

Interactions with Dietary Supplements

Antioxidants

Chemotherapy can injure cancer cells by creating oxidative damage. As a result, some oncologists recommend that patients avoid supplementing antioxidants if they are undergoing chemotherapy. Limited test tube research occasionally does support the idea that an antioxidant can interfere with oxidative damage to cancer cells.[1] However, most scientific research does not support this supposition.

A modified form of vitamin A has been reported to work synergistically with chemotherapy in test tube research.[2] Vitamin C appears to increase the effectiveness of chemotherapy in animals[3] and with human breast cancer cells in test tube research.[4] In a double-blind study, Japanese researchers found that the combination of vitamin E, vitamin C, and N-acetyl cysteine (NAC)—all antioxidants—protected against chemotherapy-induced heart damage without interfering with the action of the chemotherapy.[5]

A comprehensive review of antioxidants and chemotherapy leaves open the question of whether supplemental antioxidants definitely help people with chemotherapy side effects, but it clearly shows that antioxidants need not be avoided for fear that the actions of chemotherapy are interfered with.[6] Although research remains incomplete, the idea that people taking chemotherapy should avoid antioxidants is not supported by scientific research.

A new formulation of selenium (Seleno-Kappacarrageenan) was found to reduce kidney damage and white blood cell–lowering effects of **cisplatin** (page 64) in one human study. However, the level used in this study (4,000 mcg per day) is potentially toxic and should only be used under the supervision of a doctor.[7]

Glutathione, the main antioxidant found within cells, is frequently depleted in individuals on chemotherapy and/or radiation. Preliminary studies have found that intravenously injected glutathione may decrease some of the adverse effects of chemotherapy and radiation, such as diarrhea.[8]

Glutamine

Though cancer cells use glutamine as a fuel source, studies in humans have not found that glutamine stimulates growth of cancers in people taking chemotherapy.[9, 10] In fact, animal studies show that glutamine may actually decrease tumor growth while increasing susceptibility of cancer cells to radiation and chemotherapy,[11, 12] though such effects have not yet been studied in humans.

Glutamine has successfully reduced chemotherapy-induced mouth sores. In one trial, people were given 4 grams of glutamine in an oral rinse, which was swished around the mouth and then swallowed twice per day.[13] Thirteen of fourteen people in the study had fewer days with mouth sores as a result. These excellent results have been duplicated in some,[14] but not all,[15] double-blind research. In another study, patients receiving high-dose **paclitaxel** (page 205) and melphalan had significantly fewer episodes of oral ulcers and bleeding when they took 6 grams of glutamine four times daily along with the chemotherapy.[16]

One double-blind trial suggested that 6 grams of glutamine taken three times per day can decrease diarrhea caused by chemotherapy.[17] However, other studies using higher amounts or intravenous glutamine have not reported this effect.[18, 19]

Intravenous use of glutamine in people undergoing bone marrow transplants, a procedure sometimes used to allow very high amounts of chemotherapy to be used, has led to reduced hospital stays, leading to a savings of over $21,000 for each patient given glutamine.[20]

Magnesium and potassium

Some chemotherapy drugs (e.g., cisplatin) may cause excessive loss of magnesium and potassium in the urine.[21] Three case reports and one review article suggest that both potassium and magnesium supplementation may be necessary to increase low potassium levels.[22, 23] In one case report, a 32-year-old man with testicular cancer developed severe magnesium deficiency after receiving cisplatin therapy for nine weeks.[24] The magnesium deficiency resulted in seizures that were corrected by a combination of injected and oral magnesium therapy. Magnesium deficiency, as seen in this case, is a potentially dangerous medical condition that should only be treated by a doctor.

Melatonin

High amounts of melatonin have been combined with a variety of chemotherapy drugs to reduce their side effects or improve drug efficacy. One study gave melatonin at night in combination with the drug triptorelin to men with metastatic prostate cancer.[25] All of these men had previously become unresponsive to triptorelin. The combination decreased PSA levels—a marker of prostate cancer progression—in eight of fourteen patients, decreased some side effects of triptorelin, and helped nine of fourteen to live longer than one year. The outcome of this preliminary study suggests that melatonin may improve the efficacy of triptorelin even after the drug has apparently lost effectiveness.

N-acetyl cysteine (NAC)

NAC, an amino acid–like supplement that possesses antioxidant activity, has been used in four human studies to decrease the kidney and bladder toxicity of the chemotherapy drug ifosfamide.[26, 27, 28, 29] These studies used 1–2 grams NAC four times per day. There was no sign that NAC interfered with the efficacy of ifosfamide in any of these studies. Intakes of NAC over 4 grams per day may cause nausea and vomiting.

The newer anti-nausea drugs prescribed for people taking chemotherapy lead to greatly reduced nausea and vomiting for most people. Nonetheless, these drugs often do not totally eliminate all nausea. Natural substances used to reduce nausea should not be used instead of prescription anti-nausea drugs. Rather, under the guidance of a doctor, they should be added to those drugs if needed. At least one trial suggests that NAC, at 1,800 mg per day, may reduce nausea and vomiting caused by chemotherapy.[30]

Spleen extract

Patients with inoperable head and neck cancer were treated with a spleen peptide preparation (Polyerga) in a double-blind trial during chemotherapy with cisplatin and 5-FU.[31] The spleen preparation had a significant stabilizing effect on certain white blood cells. People taking it also experienced stabilized body weight and a reduction in the fatigue and inertia that usually accompany this combination of chemotherapy agents.

Beta-carotene and vitamin E

Chemotherapy frequently causes mouth sores. In one trial, people were given approximately 400,000 IU of beta-carotene per day for three weeks and then 125,000 IU per day for an additional four weeks.[32] Those taking beta-carotene still suffered mouth sores, but the mouth sores developed later and tended to be less severe than mouth sores that formed in people receiving the same chemotherapy without beta-carotene.

In a study of chemotherapy-induced mouth sores, six of nine patients who applied vitamin E directly to their mouth sores had complete resolution of the sores compared with one of nine patients who applied placebo.[33] Others have confirmed the potential for vitamin E to help people with chemotherapy-induced mouth sores.[34] Applying vitamin E only once per day was helpful to only some groups of patients in another trial,[35] and not all studies have found vitamin E to be effective.[36] Until more is known, if vitamin E is used in an attempt to reduce chemotherapy-induced mouth sores, it should be applied topically twice per day and should probably be in the tocopherol (versus tocopheryl) form.

Vitamin A

A controlled French trial reported that when postmenopausal late-stage breast cancer patients were given very large amounts of vitamin A (350,000–500,000 IU per day) along with chemotherapy, remission rates were significantly better than when the chemotherapy was not accompanied by vitamin A.[37] Similar results were not found in premenopausal women. The large amounts of vitamin A used in the study are toxic and require clinical supervision.

Zinc

Irradiation treatment, especially of head and neck cancers, frequently results in changes to normal taste sensation.[38, 39] Zinc supplementation may be protective against taste alterations caused or exacerbated by irradiation. A double-blind trial found that 45 mg of zinc sulfate three times daily reduced the alteration of taste sensation during radiation treatment and led to significantly greater recovery of taste sensation after treatment was concluded.[40]

Multivitamin-mineral

Many chemotherapy drugs can cause diarrhea, lack of appetite, vomiting, and damage to the gastrointestinal tract. Recent anti-nausea prescription medications are often effective. Nonetheless, nutritional deficiencies still occur.[41] It makes sense for people undergoing chemotherapy to take a high-potency multivitamin-mineral to protect against deficiencies.

Taurine

Taurine has been shown to be depleted in people taking chemotherapy.[42] It remains unclear how important this effect is or if people taking chemotherapy should take taurine supplements.

L-carnitine

In a preliminary study, supplementation with 2 grams of L-carnitine twice a day for seven days relieved chemotherapy-induced fatigue in 90% of people who had been treated with the chemotherapy drugs cisplatin or ifosfamide.[43] However, because there was no placebo group in the study, one cannot rule out the possibility that the fatigue resolved spontaneously.

Thymus peptides

Peptides or short proteins derived from the thymus gland, an important immune organ, have been used in conjunction with chemotherapy drugs for people with cancer. One study using thymosin fraction V in combination with chemotherapy, compared with chemotherapy alone, found significantly longer survival times in the thymosin fraction V group.[44] A related substance, thymostimulin, decreased some side effects of chemotherapy and increased survival time compared with chemotherapy alone.[45] A third product, thymic extract TP1, was shown to improve immune function in people treated with chemotherapy compared with effects of chemotherapy alone.[46] Thymic peptides need to be administered by injection. People interested in their combined use with chemotherapy should consult a doctor.

Interactions with Herbs

Echinacea (Echinacea purpurea, Echinacea angustifolia)

Echinacea is a popular immune-boosting herb that has been investigated for use with chemotherapy. One study investigated the actions of **cyclophosphamide** (page 79), echinacea, and thymus gland extracts to treat advanced cancer patients. Although small and uncontrolled, this trial suggested that the combination modestly extended the life span of some patients with inoperable cancers.[47] Signs of restoration of immune function were seen in these patients.

Eleuthero (Eleutherococcus senticosus)

Russian research has looked at using eleuthero with chemotherapy. One study of patients with melanoma found that chemotherapy was less toxic when eleuthero was given simultaneously. Similarly, women with inoperable breast cancer given eleuthero were reported to tolerate more chemotherapy.[48] Eleuthero treatment was also associated with improved immune function in women with breast cancer treated with chemotherapy and radiation.[49]

Milk thistle (Silybum marianum)

Milk thistle's major flavonoids, known collectively as silymarin, have shown synergistic actions with the chemotherapy drugs **cisplatin** (page 64) and **doxorubicin** (page 100) (Adriamycin) in test tubes.[50] Silymarin also offsets the kidney toxicity of cisplatin in animals.[51] Silymarin has not yet been studied in humans treated with cisplatin. There is some evidence that silymarin may not interfere with some chemotherapy in humans with cancer.[52]

Ginger (Zingiber officinale)

Ginger can be helpful in alleviating nausea and vomiting caused by chemotherapy.[53, 54] Ginger, as tablets, capsules, or liquid herbal extracts, can be taken in 500 mg amounts every two or three hours, for a total of 1 gram per day.

German chamomile (Matricaria recutita)

A liquid preparation of German chamomile has been shown to reduce the incidence of mouth sores in people receiving radiation and systemic chemotherapy treatment in an uncontrolled study. When 15 drops of chamomile liquid was taken in 100 ml of warm water at least three times daily, the radiation amount required to produce mouth sores doubled, and their overall incidence and severity decreased.[55]

PSK (Coriolus versicolor)

The mushroom *Coriolus versicolor* contains an immune-stimulating substance called polysaccharide krestin, or PSK. PSK has been shown in several studies to help cancer patients undergoing chemotherapy. One study involved women with estrogen receptor-negative breast cancer. PSK combined with chemotherapy significantly prolonged survival time compared with chemotherapy alone.[56] Another study followed women with breast cancer who were given chemotherapy with or without PSK. The PSK-plus-chemotherapy group had a 25% better chance of survival after ten years compared with those taking chemotherapy without PSK.[57] Another study investigated people who had surgically removed colon cancer. They were given chemotherapy with or without PSK. Those given PSK

had a longer disease-free period and longer survival time.[58] Three grams of PSK were taken orally each day in these studies.

Although PSK is rarely available in the United States, hot-water extract products made from *Coriolus versicolor* mushrooms are available. These products may have activity related to that of PSK, but their use with chemotherapy has not been studied.

Administration of St. John's wort has been shown to reduce blood levels of the active form of the anticancer drug irinotecan.[59] Consequently, individuals taking irinotecan should not take St. John's wort.

Interactions with Foods and Other Compounds
Fruit drinks

Often, people who undergo chemotherapy develop aversions to certain foods, sometimes making it permanently difficult to eat those foods. Exposing people to what researchers have called a "scapegoat stimulus" just before the administration of chemotherapy can direct the food aversion to the "scapegoat" food instead of more important parts of the diet. In one trial, fruit drinks administered just before chemotherapy were most effective in protecting against aversions to other foods.[60]

Ingestion of grapefruit juice along with etoposide has been found to reduce blood levels of the drug.[61] Studies with certain other medications suggest that grapefruit juice may affect drug availability, even if it is consumed at a different time of the day. Therefore, individuals taking etoposide should probably avoid grapefruit and grapefruit juice.

CHLORHEXIDINE

Common names: Chlorhexidine mouthwash, Chlorohex, Corsodyl, Eludril, Oro-Clense, Peridex, Periochip, Periogard Oral Rinse

Combination drug: Nystaform-HC

Chlorhexidine is used to prevent and treat the redness, swelling, and bleeding gums associated with gingivitis. It is classified as an antimicrobial drug.

Summary of Interactions for Chlorhexidine

In some cases, an herb or supplement may appear in more than one category, which may seem contradictory. For clarification, read the full article for details about the summarized interactions.

✓ May be Beneficial: Depletion or interference	Vitamin K*
✓ May be Beneficial: Side effect reduction/prevention	Bifidobacterium longum* Lactobacillus acidophilus* Lactobacillus casei* Saccharomyces boulardii* Saccharomyces cerevisiae* Vitamin K*
✓ May be Beneficial: Supportive interaction	Saccharomyces boulardii*
⃠ Avoid: Adverse interaction	Iron
ⓘ Check: Other	Zinc
Reduced drug absorption/bioavailability	None known

Interactions with Dietary Supplements

Iron
Tooth staining is a common side effect of using chlorhexidine. One controlled study showed that people who took iron immediately after using chlorhexidine developed severe staining within two weeks.[1] Therefore, individuals using chlorhexidine might prevent this side effect by taking iron supplements an hour before or two hours after using the drug.

Probiotics
A common side effect of antibiotics is diarrhea, which may be caused by the elimination of beneficial bacteria normally found in the colon. Controlled studies have shown that taking probiotic microorganisms—such as Lactobacillus casei, Lactobacillus acidophilus, Bifidobacterium longum, or Saccharomyces boulardii—helps prevent antibiotic-induced diarrhea.[2]

The diarrhea experienced by some people who take antibiotics also might be due to an overgrowth of the bacterium Clostridium difficile, which causes a disease known as pseudomembranous colitis. Controlled studies have shown that supplementation with harmless yeast—such as Saccharomyces boulardii[3] or Saccharomyces cerevisiae (baker's or brewer's yeast)[4]—helps prevent recurrence of this infection. In one study, taking 500 mg of Saccharomyces boulardii twice daily enhanced the effectiveness of the antibiotic vancomycin in preventing recurrent clostridium infection.[5] Therefore, people taking antibiotics who later develop diarrhea might benefit from supplementing with saccharomyces organisms.

Treatment with antibiotics also commonly leads to an overgrowth of yeast (Candida albicans) in the vagina (candida vaginitis) and the intestines (sometimes referred to as "dysbiosis"). Controlled studies have shown that Lactobacillus acidophilus might prevent candida vaginitis.[6]

Vitamin K
Several cases of excessive bleeding have been reported in people who take antibiotics.[7, 8, 9, 10] This side effect may be the result of reduced vitamin K activity and/or reduced vitamin K production by bacteria in the colon. One study showed that people who had taken broad-spectrum antibiotics had lower liver concentrations of vitamin K_2 (menaquinone), though vitamin K_1 (phylloquinone) levels remained normal.[11] Several antibiotics appear to exert a strong effect on vitamin K activity, while others may not have any effect. Therefore, one should refer to a specific antibiotic for information on whether it interacts with vitamin K. Doctors of natural medicine sometimes recommend vitamin K supplementation to people taking antibiotics. Additional research is needed to determine whether the amount of vitamin K_1 found in some multivitamins is sufficient to prevent antibiotic-induced bleeding. Moreover, most multivitamins do not contain vitamin K.

Zinc
Using a zinc solution at the same time as chlorhexidine may increase the anti-plaque activity of the drug[12] and may reduce the possibility of staining.[13] Whether taking a zinc supplement at the same time as chlorhexidine produces the same beneficial effects is unknown.

Interaction with Foods and Other Compounds

Coffee and tea
Controlled studies show that drinking coffee and tea enhances the tooth-staining effect of chlorhexidine.[14] People using chlorhexidine may prevent tooth staining if they consume coffee and tea an hour before or after using the drug, or if they avoid these beverages altogether.

CHLORPHENIRAMINE

Common names: Aller-Chlor, Boots Allergy Relief Antihistamine Tablets, Calimal, Chlor-Trimeton Allergy, Chlor-Tripolon, Chlorphenamine, Piriton, Teldrin

Combination drugs: Alka-Seltzer Plus, Chlor-Trimeton 12 Hour, Contac 12 Hour, Theraflu, Triaminic-12, Tussionex, Tylenol Cold, Tylenol Multi-Symptom Hot Medication

Chlorpheniramine is an antihistamine used to relieve allergic rhinitis (seasonal allergy) symptoms including sneezing, runny nose, itching, and watery eyes. It is also used to treat immediate allergic reactions. Chlorpheniramine is available in nonprescription products alone and in combination with other nonprescription drugs, to treat symptoms of allergy, colds, and upper respiratory infections.

Summary of Interactions for Chlorpheniramine

In some cases, an herb or supplement may appear in more than one category, which may seem contradictory. For clarification, read the full article for details about the summarized interactions.

⊘ Avoid: Adverse interaction	Henbane*
Depletion or interference	None known
Side effect reduction/prevention	None known
Supportive interaction	None known
Reduced drug absorption/bioavailability	None known

Interactions with Herbs

Henbane (Hyoscyamus niger)
Antihistamines, including chlorpheniramine, can cause "anticholinergic" side effects such as dryness of mouth and heart palpitations. Henbane also has anticholinergic activity and side effects. Therefore, use of henbane with chlorpheniramine could increase the risk of anticholinergic side effects,[1] though apparently no interactions have yet been reported. Henbane should not be taken except by prescription from a physician trained in its use, as it is extremely toxic.

Interactions with Foods and Other Compounds

Alcohol
Chlorpheniramine causes drowsiness.[2] Alcohol may intensify this effect and increase the risk of accidental injury.[3] To prevent problems, people taking chlorpheniramine or chlorpheniramine-containing products should avoid alcohol.

CHLOR-TRIMETON 12 HOUR

Contains the following ingredients:
Chlorpheniramine (page 59)
Pseudoephedrine

CHLORZOXAZONE

Common names: Paraflex, Parafon Forte DSC, Strifon

Chlorzoxazone is used to treat acute painful muscle conditions. It is a type of drug called a centrally acting skeletal muscle relaxant.

Summary of Interactions for Chlorzoxazone

In some cases, an herb or supplement may appear in more than one category, which may seem contradictory. For clarification, read the full article for details about the summarized interactions.

⊘ Avoid: Reduced drug absorption/ bioavailability	Broccoli Brussels sprouts Chinese cabbage Garlic Tea Watercress
⊘ Avoid: Adverse interaction	Alcohol **Caffeine** (page 44)*
Depletion or interference	None known
Side effect reduction/prevention	None known
Supportive interaction	None known

Interactions with Foods and Other Compounds

Food
Test tube studies show that watercress, garlic, tea, and cruciferous vegetables, such as Brussels sprouts, broccoli, and Chinese cabbage, block the breakdown of chlorzoxazone into inactive compounds.[1, 2] Controlled human research is needed to determine whether these interactions are important in people taking chlorzoxazone.

Alcohol
Drinking alcoholic beverages while taking chlorzoxazone may enhance side effects of the drug, such as drowsiness, dizziness, and light-headedness.[3] In addition, test tube studies show that alcohol might increase the elimination of chlorzoxazone from the body.[4] Consequently, people who are taking chlorzoxazone should avoid drinking alcohol.

Smoking
Studies show that cigarette smoking increases the elimination of chlorzoxazone from the body.[5] Problems could occur if people either start or stop smoking while taking chlorzoxazone: individuals who stop smoking

may experience increased side effects, while those who start smoking may notice that the drug is less effective.

Caffeine *(page 44)*

Controlled studies show that chlorzoxazone reduces the elimination of caffeine from the body,[6] which could cause side effects of caffeine, such as restlessness and insomnia. If side effects occur, some individuals may need to avoid caffeinated beverages, such as coffee and tea, while taking chlorzoxazone.

CHOLESTEROL-LOWERING DRUGS

Cholesterol-lowering drugs are used to treat individuals who have higher-than-normal levels of cholesterol in their blood. Drugs in this family are prescribed to reduce the risk for cardiovascular disease or death associated with atherosclerosis, when diet restriction, lifestyle changes, and weight reduction are insufficient.

For interactions involving specific cholesterol-lowering drugs, refer to the highlighted medications listed below.

Bile Acid Sequestrants *(page 39)*
- Cholestyramine (Questran)
- Colesevelam (Welchol)
- **Colestipol** (page 76) (Colestid)

HMG CoA Reductase Inhibitors
- **Atorvastatin** (page 29) (Lipitor)
- **Cerivastatin** (page 53) (Baycol)
- **Fluvastatin** (page 122) (Lescol)
- **Lovastatin** (page 163) (Mevacor)
- **Pravastatin** (page 220) (Pravachol)
- **Simvastatin** (page 239) (Zocor)

Miscellaneous Cholesterol-Lowering Agents
- **Clofibrate** (page 71) (Atromid-S)
- **Gemfibrozil** (page 127) (Lopid)
- **Fenofibrate** (page 114) (Tricor)
- Nicotinic acid

For interactions involving a specific Cholesterol-Lowering Drug, see the individual drug article. For interactions involving a Cholesterol-Lowering Drug for which no separate article exists, talk to your doctor or pharmacist.

CIMETIDINE

Common names: Acitak, Apo-Cimetidine, Dyspamet, Galenamet, Gen-Cimetidine, Novo-Cimetine, Nu-Cimet, Peptimax, Peptol, Phimetine, PMS-Cimetidine, Tagamet, Tagamet HB, Ultec, Zita

Cimetidine is a member of the H-2 blocker (histamine blocker) family of drugs that prevents the release of acid into the stomach. Cimetidine is used to treat stomach and duodenal ulcers, reflux of stomach acid into the esophagus, and Zollinger-Ellison syndrome. Cimetidine is available as a prescription drug and as a nonprescription over-the-counter product for relief of heartburn.

Summary of Interactions for Cimetidine

In some cases, an herb or supplement may appear in more than one category, which may seem contradictory. For clarification, read the full article for details about the summarized interactions.

✓ May be Beneficial: Depletion or interference	Iron Vitamin B$_{12}$ Vitamin D	
⊘ Avoid: Reduced drug absorption/bioavailability	Magnesium	
⊘ Avoid: Adverse interaction	**Caffeine** (page 44)*	
Side effect reduction/prevention	None known	
Supportive interaction	None known	

Interactions with Dietary Supplements

Iron

Stomach acid may facilitate iron absorption. H-2 blocker drugs reduce stomach acid and are associated with decreased dietary iron absorption.[1] People with ulcers may also be iron deficient due to blood loss and benefit from iron supplementation. Iron levels in the blood can be checked with lab tests.

Magnesium

In healthy volunteers, a **magnesium hydroxide** (page 166)/**aluminum hydroxide** (page 10) antacid, taken with cimetidine, decreased cimetidine absorption by 20 to 25%.[2] People can avoid this interaction by taking cimetidine two hours before or after any aluminum/magnesium-containing antacids, including magnesium hydroxide found in some vitamin/mineral supplements. However, the available studies do not clearly indicate if magnesium hydroxide was the problem and may not need to be avoided.

Vitamin B₁₂

Hydrochloric acid is needed to release vitamin B_{12} from food so it can be absorbed by the body. Cimetidine, which reduces stomach acid, may decrease the amount of vitamin B_{12} available for the body to absorb.[3] The vitamin B_{12} found in supplements is available to the body without the need for stomach acid. Lab tests can determine vitamin B_{12} levels in people.

Vitamin D

Cimetidine may reduce vitamin D activation by the liver.[4] Lab tests can measure activated vitamin D levels in the blood. Forms of vitamin D that do not require liver activation are available, but only by prescription.

Interactions with Foods and Other Compounds
Food

Cimetidine may be taken with or without food.

Caffeine (page 44)

Caffeine is found in coffee, tea, soft drinks, chocolate, guaraná (Paullinia cupana), nonprescription over-the-counter drug products, and supplement products containing caffeine or guaraná. Cimetidine may decrease the clearance of caffeine from the body, causing increased caffeine blood levels and unwanted actions.[5] People taking cimetidine may choose to limit their caffeine intake to avoid problems. They should read food, beverage, drug, and supplement labels carefully for caffeine content.

CIPROFLOXACIN

Common names: Ciloxan, Ciproxin, Cipro

Ciprofloxacin is member of the fluoroquinolone family of **antibiotics** (page 19). It is used to treat bacterial infections. Ciprofloxacin penetrates many hard-to-reach tissues in the body and kills a wide variety of bacteria.

Summary of Interactions for Ciprofloxacin

In some cases, an herb or supplement may appear in more than one category, which may seem contradictory. For clarification, read the full article for details about the summarized interactions.

✓	May be Beneficial: Depletion or interference	Vitamin K*
✓	May be Beneficial: Side effect reduction/prevention	Bifidobacterium longum* Lactobacillus acidophilus* Lactobacillus casei* Saccharomyces boulardii* Saccharomyces cerevisiae* Vitamin K*
✓	May be Beneficial: Supportive interaction	Saccharomyces boulardii*
🚫	Avoid: Reduced drug absorption/ bioavailability	Calcium, Copper, Iron, Magnesium, Manganese, Zinc (if taken at the same time) Dandelion* Fennel Yogurt
🚫	Avoid: Adverse interaction	**Caffeine** (page 44)

Interactions with Dietary Supplements
Minerals

Minerals such as aluminum, calcium, copper, iron, magnesium, manganese, and zinc can bind to ciprofloxacin, greatly reducing the absorption of the drug.[1, 2, 3, 4] Because of the mineral content, people are advised to take ciprofloxacin two hours after consuming dairy products (milk, cheese, yogurt, ice cream, and others), **antacids** (page 18) (Maalox, Mylanta, Tums, Rolaids, and others), and mineral-containing supplements.[5]

Probiotics

A common side effect of antibiotics is diarrhea, which may be caused by the elimination of beneficial bacteria normally found in the colon. Controlled studies have shown that taking probiotic microorganisms—such as Lactobacillus casei, Lactobacillus acidophilus, Bifidobacterium longum, or Saccharomyces boulardii—helps prevent antibiotic-induced diarrhea.[6]

The diarrhea experienced by some people who take antibiotics also might be due to an overgrowth of the bacterium Clostridium difficile, which causes a disease known as pseudomembranous colitis. Controlled studies have shown that supplementation with harmless yeast—such as *Saccharomyces boulardii*[7] or *Saccharomyces cerevisiae* (baker's or brewer's yeast)[8]—helps prevent recurrence of this infection. In one study, taking 500 mg of *Saccharomyces boulardii* twice daily enhanced the effectiveness of the antibiotic vancomycin in preventing recurrent clostridium infection.[9] Therefore, people taking antibiotics who later develop diarrhea might benefit from supplementing with saccharomyces organisms.

Treatment with antibiotics also commonly leads to an overgrowth of yeast *(Candida albicans)* in the vagina (candida vaginitis) and the intestines (sometimes referred to as "dysbiosis"). Controlled studies have shown that *Lactobacillus acidophilus* might prevent candida vaginitis.[10]

Vitamin K

Several cases of excessive bleeding have been reported in people who take antibiotics.[11, 12, 13, 14] This side effect may be the result of reduced vitamin K activity and/or reduced vitamin K production by bacteria in the colon. One study showed that people who had taken broad-spectrum antibiotics had lower liver concentrations of vitamin K_2 (menaquinone), though vitamin K_1 (phylloquinone) levels remained normal.[15] Several antibiotics appear to exert a strong effect on vitamin K activity, while others may not have any effect. Therefore, one should refer to a specific antibiotic for information on whether it interacts with vitamin K. Doctors of natural medicine sometimes recommend vitamin K supplementation to people taking antibiotics. Additional research is needed to determine whether the amount of vitamin K_1 found in some multivitamins is sufficient to prevent antibiotic-induced bleeding. Moreover, most multivitamins do not contain vitamin K.

Interactions with Herbs

Dandelion (Taraxacum officinale)

In an animal study, administration of an extract of the whole plant dandelion (actually *Taraxacum mongolicum*, a close relative of the more common western dandelion, *Taraxacum officinale*) concomitantly with ciprofloxacin decreased absorption of the drug.[16] The authors found this was due to the high mineral content of the dandelion herb. Until further information is available, ciprofloxacin should not be taken within two hours of any dandelion supplement including teas.

Fennel (Foeniculum vulgare)

Preliminary research in animals has shown that fennel may reduce the absorption of ciprofloxacin.[17] This interaction may be due to the rich mineral content of the herb; it has not yet been reported in humans. People taking ciprofloxacin should avoid supplementing with fennel-containing products until more is known.

Interactions with Foods and Other Compounds

Food

Food in general[18] and yogurt in particular has been found to reduce absorption of ciprofloxacin. Ciprofloxacin should be taken two hours before eating.[19]

Calcium supplements are known to interfere with the absorption of ciprofloxacin. The same interference has been shown to occur when calcium-fortified orange juice is taken at the same time as ciprofloxacin.[20]

Caffeine (page 44)

Caffeine is found in coffee, tea, soft drinks, chocolate, guaraná *(Paullinia cupana),* nonprescription drug products, and supplement products containing caffeine. Ciprofloxacin may decrease the elimination of caffeine from the body, causing increased caffeine blood levels and unwanted actions.[21] People taking ciprofloxacin may choose to limit their caffeine intake to avoid problems. They should read food, beverage, drug, and supplement labels carefully for caffeine content.

CISAPRIDE

Common names: Prepulsid, Propulsid

Cisapride is a gastrointestinal stimulant drug used to treat people with nighttime heartburn due to reflux of stomach acid into the esophagus. It is also used to increase movement of gastrointestinal contents in conditions of lack of spontaneous gastrointestinal movement.

Summary of Interactions for Cisapride

In some cases, an herb or supplement may appear in more than one category, which may seem contradictory. For clarification, read the full article for details about the summarized interactions.

⊘ Avoid: Reduced drug absorption/ bioavailability	Tobacco
⊘ Avoid: Adverse interaction	Grapefruit juice Red wine
Depletion or interference	None known
Side effect reduction/prevention	None known
Supportive interaction	None known

Cisapride

Interactions with Foods and Other Compounds

Alcohol

Alcohol consumption is associated with nighttime heartburn and may interfere with cisapride therapy.[1] Alcohol causes sleepiness, and cisapride may intensify this effect,[2] increasing the risk of accidental injury. Ingestion of red wine along with cisapride may also increase blood levels of the drug in some individuals, potentially increasing its side effects.[3] People taking cisapride should avoid alcohol.

Tobacco

Smoking is associated with nighttime heartburn and may interfere with cisapride therapy.[4] Smokers taking cisapride may benefit from reducing or quitting smoking.

Grapefruit juice

In a study of healthy males, ingestion of 250 ml (about one cup) of grapefruit juice along with cisapride increased the peak blood level of the drug by an average of 68%.[5] It is not known whether consuming grapefruit juice at a separate time of the day would affect blood levels of cisapride. As this interaction could potentially increase the side effects of cisapride, individuals taking cisapride should avoid grapefruit and its juice.

CISPLATIN

Common names: Platinol

Cisplatin is a **chemotherapy** (page 54) drug used to treat some forms of cancer.

> **Note:** Many of the interactions described below, in the text and in the Summary of Interactions, have been reported only for specific chemotherapeutic drugs, and may not apply to other chemotherapeutic drugs. There are many unknowns concerning interactions of nutrients, herbs, and chemotherapy drugs. People receiving chemotherapy who wish to supplement with vitamins, minerals, herbs, or other natural substances should always consult a physician.

Summary of Interactions for Cisplatin

In some cases, an herb or supplement may appear in more than one category, which may seem contradictory. For clarification, read the full article for details about the summarized interactions.

✓ May be Beneficial: Depletion or interference	Calcium* Magnesium Multiple nutrients (malabsorption)* Phosphate* Potassium Sodium* Taurine*
✓ May be Beneficial: Side effect reduction/prevention	Beta-carotene* (mouth sores) Chamomile* (mouth sores) Eleuthero* (see text) Ginger* (nausea) Glutamine* (mouth sores) Glutathione (i.v. only) Melatonin (see text) N-acetyl cysteine (NAC)* Selenium Spleen peptide extract* (see text) Thymus peptides* (see text) Vitamin E (oral) Vitamin E* topical, (mouth sores) Zinc* (taste alterations)
✓ May be Beneficial: Supportive interaction	Antioxidants* Melatonin Milk thistle* PSK*
ⓘ Check: Other	Echinacea* Glutathione (i.v. only) Multivitamin-mineral* Vitamin A* Vitamin C*
Reduced drug absorption/bioavailability	None known
Adverse interaction	None known

Interactions with Dietary Supplements

Antioxidants

Chemotherapy can injure cancer cells by creating oxidative damage. As a result, some oncologists recommend that patients avoid supplementing antioxidants if they are undergoing chemotherapy. Limited test tube research occasionally does support the idea that an antioxidant can interfere with oxidative damage to cancer cells.[1] However, most scientific research does not support this supposition.

A modified form of vitamin A has been reported to work synergistically with chemotherapy in test tube research.[2] Vitamin C appears to increase the effectiveness of chemotherapy in animals[3] and with human breast cancer cells in test tube research.[4] In a double-blind study, Japanese researchers found that the combination of vitamin E, vitamin C, and N-acetyl cysteine (NAC)—all antioxidants—protected against chemotherapy-induced heart damage without interfering with the action of the chemotherapy.[5]

A comprehensive review of antioxidants and chemotherapy leaves open the question of whether supplemental antioxidants definitely help people with chemotherapy side effects, but it clearly shows that antioxidants need not be avoided for fear that the actions of chemotherapy are interfered with.[6] Although research remains incomplete, the idea that people taking chemotherapy should avoid antioxidants is not supported by scientific research.

Beta-carotene and vitamin E
Chemotherapy frequently causes mouth sores. In one trial, people were given approximately 400,000 IU of beta-carotene per day for three weeks and then 125,000 IU per day for an additional four weeks.[7] Those taking beta-carotene still suffered mouth sores, but the mouth sores developed later and tended to be less severe than mouth sores that formed in people receiving the same chemotherapy without beta-carotene.

In a study of chemotherapy-induced mouth sores, six of nine patients who applied vitamin E directly to their mouth sores had complete resolution of the sores compared with one of nine patients who applied placebo.[8] Others have confirmed the potential for vitamin E to help people with chemotherapy-induced mouth sores.[9] Applying vitamin E only once per day was helpful to only some groups of patients in another trial,[10] and not all studies have found vitamin E to be effective.[11] Until more is known, if vitamin E is used in an attempt to reduce chemotherapy-induced mouth sores, it should be applied topically twice per day and should probably be in the tocopherol (versus tocopheryl) form.

In a preliminary study, the addition of oral vitamin E (300 IU per day) to cisplatin chemotherapy signifi-cantly reduced the incidence of drug-induced damage to the nervous system (neurotoxicity).[12]

Calcium and phosphate
Cisplatin may cause kidney damage, resulting in depletion of calcium and phosphate.[13]

Glutamine
Though cancer cells use glutamine as a fuel source, studies in humans have not found that glutamine stimulates growth of cancers in people taking chemotherapy.[14, 15] In fact, animal studies show that glutamine may actually decrease tumor growth while increasing susceptibility of cancer cells to radiation and chemotherapy,[16, 17] though such effects have not yet been studied in humans.

Glutamine has successfully reduced chemotherapy-induced mouth sores. In one trial, people were given 4 grams of glutamine in an oral rinse, which was swished around the mouth and then swallowed twice per day.[18] Thirteen of fourteen people in the study had fewer days with mouth sores as a result. These excellent results have been duplicated in some,[19] but not all,[20] double-blind research. In another study, patients receiving high-dose **paclitaxel** (page 205) and melphalan had significantly fewer episodes of oral ulcers and bleeding when they took 6 grams of glutamine four times daily along with the chemotherapy.[21]

One double-blind trial suggested that 6 grams of glutamine taken three times per day can decrease diarrhea caused by chemotherapy.[22] However, other studies using higher amounts or intravenous glutamine have not reported this effect.[23, 24]

Intravenous use of glutamine in people undergoing bone marrow transplants, a procedure sometimes used to allow very high amounts of chemotherapy to be used, has led to reduced hospital stays, leading to a savings of over $21,000 for each patient given glutamine.[25]

Glutathione
High-dose cisplatin therapy is associated with kidney toxicity and damage, which may be reduced by glutathione administration.[26, 27, 28, 29] Nerve damage is another frequent complication of high amounts of cisplatin. Preliminary evidence has shown that glutathione injections may protect nerve tissue during cisplatin therapy without reducing cisplatin's anti-tumor activity.[30, 31, 32] There is no evidence that glutathione taken by mouth has the same benefits.

Magnesium and potassium
Cisplatin may cause excessive loss of magnesium and potassium in the urine.[33, 34] Preliminary reports suggest

that both potassium and magnesium supplementation may be necessary to increase low potassium levels.[35, 36] Severe magnesium deficiency caused by cisplatin therapy has been reported to result in seizures.[37] Severe magnesium deficiency is a potentially dangerous medical condition that should only be treated by a doctor. People receiving cisplatin chemotherapy should ask their prescribing doctor to closely monitor magnesium and potassium status.

Melatonin

Melatonin supplementation (20 mg per day) has decreased toxicity and improved effectiveness of **chemotherapy** (page 54) with cisplatin plus etoposide and cisplatin plus 5-FU.[38]

Multivitamin-mineral

Many chemotherapy drugs can cause diarrhea, lack of appetite, vomiting, and damage to the gastrointestinal tract. Recent anti-nausea prescription medications are often effective. Nonetheless, nutritional deficiencies still occur.[39] It makes sense for people undergoing chemotherapy to take a high-potency multivitamin-mineral to protect against deficiencies.

N-acetyl cysteine (NAC)

NAC, an amino acid–like supplement that possesses antioxidant activity, has been used in four human studies to decrease the kidney and bladder toxicity of the chemotherapy drug ifosfamide.[40, 41, 42, 43] These studies used 1–2 grams NAC four times per day. There was no sign that NAC interfered with the efficacy of ifosfamide in any of these studies. Intakes of NAC over 4 grams per day may cause nausea and vomiting.

The newer anti-nausea drugs prescribed for people taking chemotherapy lead to greatly reduced nausea and vomiting for most people. Nonetheless, these drugs often do not totally eliminate all nausea. Natural substances used to reduce nausea should not be used instead of prescription anti-nausea drugs. Rather, under the guidance of a doctor, they should be added to those drugs if needed. At least one trial suggests that NAC at 1,800 mg per day may reduce nausea and vomiting caused by chemotherapy.[44]

Selenium

In one human study, administration of 4,000 mcg per day of a selenium product, Seleno-Kappacarrageenan, reduced the kidney damage and white blood cell–lowering effects of cisplatin.[45] The amount of selenium used in this study is potentially toxic and should only be used under the supervision of a doctor. In another study, patients being treated with cisplatin and cyclophosphamide for ovarian cancer were given a multivitamin preparation, with or without 200 mcg of selenium per day. Compared with the group not receiving selenium, those receiving selenium had a smaller reduction in white blood cell count and fewer chemotherapy side effects such as nausea, hair loss, weakness, and loss of appetite.[46]

Spleen extract

Patients with inoperable head and neck cancer were treated with a spleen peptide preparation (Polyerga) in a double-blind trial during chemotherapy with cisplatin and 5-FU.[47] The spleen preparation had a significant stabilizing effect on certain white blood cells. People taking it also experienced stabilized body weight and a reduction in the fatigue and inertia that usually accompany this combination of chemotherapy agents.

Sodium

Cisplatin may cause depletion of sodium due to kidney damage which sometimes occurs in people treated with cisplatin.[48]

Taurine

Taurine has been shown to be depleted in people taking chemotherapy.[49] It remains unclear how important this effect is or if people taking chemotherapy should take taurine supplements.

Thymus peptides

Peptides or short proteins derived from the thymus gland, an important immune organ, have been used in conjunction with chemotherapy drugs for people with cancer. One study using thymosin fraction V in combination with chemotherapy, compared with chemotherapy alone, found significantly longer survival times in the thymosin fraction V group.[50] A related substance, thymostimulin, decreased some side effects of chemotherapy and increased survival time compared with chemotherapy alone.[51] A third product, thymic extract TP1, was shown to improve immune function in people treated with chemotherapy compared with effects of chemotherapy alone.[52] Thymic peptides need to be administered by injection. People interested in their combined use with chemotherapy should consult a doctor.

Vitamin A

A controlled French trial reported that when postmenopausal late-stage breast cancer patients were given very large amounts of vitamin A (350,000–500,000 IU per day) along with chemotherapy, remission rates were significantly better than when the chemotherapy was not accompanied by vitamin A.[53] Similar results were not found in premenopausal women. The large amounts of vitamin A used in the study are toxic and require clinical supervision.

Zinc

Irradiation treatment, especially of head and neck cancers, frequently results in changes to normal taste sensation.[54, 55] Zinc supplementation may be protective against taste alterations caused or exacerbated by irradiation. A double-blind trial found that 45 mg of zinc sulfate three times daily reduced the alteration of taste sensation during radiation treatment and led to significantly greater recovery of taste sensation after treatment was concluded.[56]

Interactions with Herbs

Echinacea (Echinacea purpurea, Echinacea angustifolia)

Echinacea is a popular immune-boosting herb that has been investigated for use with chemotherapy. One study investigated the actions of **cyclophosphamide** (page 79), echinacea, and thymus gland extracts to treat advanced cancer patients. Although small and uncontrolled, this trial suggested that the combination modestly extended the life span of some patients with inoperable cancers.[57] Signs of restoration of immune function were seen in these patients.

Eleuthero (Eleutherococcus senticosus)

Russian research has looked at using eleuthero with chemotherapy. One study of patients with melanoma found that chemotherapy was less toxic when eleuthero was given simultaneously. Similarly, women with inoperable breast cancer given eleuthero were reported to tolerate more chemotherapy.[58] Eleuthero treatment was also associated with improved immune function in women with breast cancer treated with chemotherapy and radiation.[59]

Milk thistle (Silybum marianum)

Milk thistle's major flavonoids, known collectively as silymarin, have shown synergistic actions with the chemotherapy drugs cisplatin and **doxorubicin** (page 100) (Adriamycin) in test tubes.[60] Silymarin also offsets the kidney toxicity of cisplatin in animals.[61] Silymarin has not yet been studied in humans treated with cisplatin. There is some evidence that silymarin may not interfere with some chemotherapy in humans with cancer.[62]

Ginger (Zingiber officinale)

Ginger can be helpful in alleviating nausea and vomiting caused by chemotherapy.[63, 64] Ginger, as tablets, capsules, or liquid herbal extracts, can be taken in 500 mg amounts every two or three hours, for a total of 1 gram per day.

German chamomile (Matricaria recutita)

A liquid preparation of German chamomile has been shown to reduce the incidence of mouth sores in people receiving radiation and systemic chemotherapy treatment in an uncontrolled study. [65]

PSK (Coriolus versicolor)

The mushroom *Coriolus versicolor* contains an immune-stimulating substance called polysaccharide krestin, or PSK. PSK has been shown in several studies to help cancer patients undergoing chemotherapy. One study involved women with estrogen receptor-negative breast cancer. PSK combined with chemotherapy significantly prolonged survival time compared with chemotherapy alone.[66] Another study followed women with breast cancer who were given chemotherapy with or without PSK. The PSK-plus-chemotherapy group had a 25% better chance of survival after ten years compared with those taking chemotherapy without PSK.[67] Another study investigated people who had surgically removed colon cancer. They were given chemotherapy with or without PSK. Those given PSK had a longer disease-free period and longer survival time.[68] Three grams of PSK were taken orally each day in these studies.

Although PSK is rarely available in the United States, hot-water extract products made from *Coriolus versicolor* mushrooms are available. These products may have activity related to that of PSK, but their use with chemotherapy has not been studied.

Interactions with Foods and Other Compounds

Fruit drinks

Often, people who undergo chemotherapy develop aversions to certain foods, sometimes making it permanently difficult to eat those foods. Exposing people to what researchers have called a "scapegoat stimulus" just before the administration of chemotherapy can direct the food aversion to the "scapegoat" food instead of more important parts of the diet. In one trial, fruit drinks administered just before chemotherapy were most effective in protecting against aversions to other foods.[69]

CITALOPRAM

Common names: Celexa, Cipramil

Citalopram is used to treat mental depression and is in a class of drugs known as selective serotonin reuptake inhibitor (SSRI) antidepressants.

Summary of Interactions for Citalopram

In some cases, an herb or supplement may appear in more than one category, which may seem contradictory. For clarification, read the full article for details about the summarized interactions.

✓ May be Beneficial: Side effect reduction/prevention	*Ginkgo biloba*
ⓘ Check: Other	**Lithium** (page 157)
Depletion or interference	None known
Supportive interaction	None known
Reduced drug absorption/bioavailability	None known
Adverse interaction	None known

Interactions with Dietary Supplements
Lithium (page 157)

Lithium is a mineral that may be present in some supplements and is also used in large amounts to treat mood disorders such as manic-depression. Taking lithium at the same time as citalopram can either increase the effectiveness of citalopram or increase the likelihood of developing side effects.[1] Therefore, people taking citalopram together with lithium-containing supplements should contact their healthcare practitioner if they experience side effects, such as nausea, dry mouth, or sleep disturbances.

Interactions with Herbs
Ginkgo biloba

Ginkgo biloba extract (GBE) may reduce the side effects experienced by some persons taking SSRIs such as **fluoxetine** (page 120) or **sertraline** (page 237). An open-label study with elderly, depressed persons found that 200–240 mg of GBE daily was effective in alleviating sexual side effects in both men and women taking SSRIs.[2] One case study reported that 180–240 mg of GBE daily reduced genital anesthesia and sexual side effects secondary to fluoxetine use in a 37-year-old woman.[3]

CLARITHROMYCIN

Common names: Biaxin, Klaricid XL, Klaricid

Clarithromycin is a macrolide **antibiotic** (page 19) used to treat a variety of bacterial infections.

Summary of Interactions for Clarithromycin

In some cases, an herb or supplement may appear in more than one category, which may seem contradictory. For clarification, read the full article for details about the summarized interactions.

✓ May be Beneficial: Depletion or interference	Vitamin K*
✓ May be Beneficial: Side effect reduction/prevention	*Bifidobacterium longum** *Lactobacillus acidophilus** *Lactobacillus casei** *Saccharomyces boulardii** *Saccharomyces cerevisiae** Vitamin K*
✓ May be Beneficial: Supportive interaction	*Saccharomyces boulardii**
ⓘ Check: Other	Digitalis
Reduced drug absorption/bioavailability	None known
Adverse interaction	None known

Interactions with Dietary Supplements
Probiotics

A common side effect of antibiotics is diarrhea, which may be caused by the elimination of beneficial bacteria normally found in the colon. Controlled studies have shown that taking probiotic microorganisms—such as *Lactobacillus casei, Lactobacillus acidophilus, Bifidobacterium longum,* or *Saccharomyces boulardii*—helps prevent antibiotic-induced diarrhea.[1]

The diarrhea experienced by some people who take antibiotics also might be due to an overgrowth of the bacterium *Clostridium difficile,* which causes a disease known as pseudomembranous colitis. Controlled studies have shown that supplementation with harmless yeast—such as *Saccharomyces boulardii*[2] or *Saccharomyces cerevisiae* (baker's or brewer's yeast)[3]—helps prevent recurrence of this infection. In one study, taking 500 mg of *Saccharomyces boulardii* twice daily enhanced the effectiveness of the antibiotic vancomycin in preventing recurrent clostridium infection.[4] Therefore, people taking antibiotics who later develop diarrhea might benefit from supplementing with saccharomyces organisms.

Treatment with antibiotics also commonly leads to an overgrowth of yeast *(Candida albicans)* in the vagina (candida vaginitis) and the intestines (sometimes referred to as "dysbiosis"). Controlled studies have shown that *Lactobacillus acidophilus* might prevent candida vaginitis.[5]

Vitamin K
Several cases of excessive bleeding have been reported in people who take antibiotics.[6, 7, 8, 9] This side effect may be the result of reduced vitamin K activity and/or reduced vitamin K production by bacteria in the colon. One study showed that people who had taken broad-spectrum antibiotics had lower liver concentrations of vitamin K_2 (menaquinone), though vitamin K_1 (phylloquinone) levels remained normal.[10] Several antibiotics appear to exert a strong effect on vitamin K activity, while others may not have any effect. Therefore, one should refer to a specific antibiotic for information on whether it interacts with vitamin K. Doctors of natural medicine sometimes recommend vitamin K supplementation to people taking antibiotics. Additional research is needed to determine whether the amount of vitamin K_1 found in some multivitamins is sufficient to prevent antibiotic-induced bleeding. Moreover, most multivitamins do not contain vitamin K.

Interactions with Herbs
Digitalis (Digitalis lanata, Digitalis purpurea)
Digitalis refers to a family of plants commonly called foxglove that contain digitalis glycosides, chemicals with actions and toxicities similar to the prescription drug **digoxin** (page 90).

Clarithromycin can increase the serum level of digitalis glycosides, increasing the therapeutic effects as well as the risk of side effects.[11] Clarithromycin and digitalis-containing products should be used only under the direct supervision of a doctor.

Interactions with Foods and Other Compounds
Food
Clarithromycin may be taken with or without food and may be taken with milk.[12] Clarithromycin tablets should be swallowed whole, without cutting, chewing, or crushing.[13]

CLARITIN-D

Contains the following ingredients:
> **Loratadine** (page 162)
> Pseudoephedrine

CLEMASTINE

Common names: Aller-eze, Antihist-1, Tavegil, Tavist, Tavist Allergy

Combination drug: Tavist-D

Clemastine is an antihistamine used to relieve allergic rhinitis (seasonal allergy) symptoms including sneezing, runny nose, itching, and watery eyes. It is also used to treat itching and swelling associated with uncomplicated allergic skin reactions. Clemastine is available in nonprescription products alone and in a combination formula to treat symptoms of allergy, colds, and upper respiratory infections.

Summary of Interactions for Clemastine
In some cases, an herb or supplement may appear in more than one category, which may seem contradictory. For clarification, read the full article for details about the summarized interactions.

⊘ Avoid: Adverse interaction	Henbane*
Depletion or interference	None known
Side effect reduction/prevention	None known
Supportive interaction	None known
Reduced drug absorption/bioavailability	None known

Interactions with Herbs
Henbane (Hyoscyamus niger)
Antihistamines, including clemastine, can cause "anticholinergic" side effects such as dryness of mouth and heart palpitations. Henbane also has anticholinergic activity and side effects. Therefore, use with clemastine could increase the risk of anticholinergic side effects,[1] though apparently no interactions have yet been reported with clemastine and henbane. Henbane should not be taken except by prescription from a physician trained in its use, as it is extremely toxic.

Interactions with Foods and Other Compounds
Alcohol
Clemastine causes drowsiness.[2] Alcohol may intensify this effect and increase the risk of accidental injury.[3] To

prevent problems, people taking clemastine or clemastine-containing products should avoid alcohol.

CLIMAGEST

Contains the following ingredients:
Estradiol (page 108)
Norethisterone

CLIMESSE

Contains the following ingredients:
Estradiol (page 108)
Norethisterone

CLINDAMYCIN ORAL

Common names: Cleocin, Dalacin C

Oral clindamycin is used for serious bacterial infections of the lungs, skin, abdomen, and female genital tract. It is a kind of **antibiotic** (page 19) called a lincosamide.

Summary of Interactions for Clindamycin Oral

In some cases, an herb or supplement may appear in more than one category, which may seem contradictory. For clarification, read the full article for details about the summarized interactions.

✓	May be Beneficial: Depletion or interference	Vitamin K*
✓	May be Beneficial: Side effect reduction/prevention	Bifidobacterium longum* Lactobacillus acidophilus* Lactobacillus casei* Probiotics* Saccharomyces boulardii* Saccharomyces cerevisiae* Vitamin K*
✓	May be Beneficial: Supportive interaction	Saccharomyces boulardii*
	Reduced drug absorption/bioavailability	None known
	Adverse interaction	None known

Interactions with Dietary Supplements

Probiotics

A common side effect of antibiotics is diarrhea, which may be caused by the elimination of beneficial bacteria normally found in the colon. Controlled studies have shown that taking probiotic microorganisms—such as *Lactobacillus casei, Lactobacillus acidophilus, Bifidobacterium longum,* or *Saccharomyces boulardii*—helps prevent antibiotic-induced diarrhea.[1]

The diarrhea experienced by some people who take antibiotics also might be due to an overgrowth of the bacterium *Clostridium difficile*, which causes a disease known as pseudomembranous colitis. Controlled studies have shown that supplementation with harmless yeast—such as *Saccharomyces boulardii*[2] or *Saccharomyces cerevisiae* (baker's or brewer's yeast)[3]—helps prevent recurrence of this infection. In one study, taking 500 mg of *Saccharomyces boulardii* twice daily enhanced the effectiveness of the antibiotic vancomycin in preventing recurrent clostridium infection.[4] Therefore, people taking antibiotics who later develop diarrhea might benefit from supplementing with saccharomyces organisms.

Treatment with antibiotics also commonly leads to an overgrowth of yeast *(Candida albicans)* in the vagina (candida vaginitis) and the intestines (sometimes referred to as "dysbiosis"). Controlled studies have shown that *Lactobacillus acidophilus* might prevent candida vaginitis.[5]

Vitamin K

Several cases of excessive bleeding have been reported in people who take antibiotics.[6, 7, 8, 9] This side effect may be the result of reduced vitamin K activity and/or reduced vitamin K production by bacteria in the colon. One study showed that people who had taken broad-spectrum antibiotics had lower liver concentrations of vitamin K_2 (menaquinone), though vitamin K_1 (phylloquinone) levels remained normal.[10] Several antibiotics appear to exert a strong effect on vitamin K activity, while others may not have any effect. Therefore, one should refer to a specific antibiotic for information on whether it interacts with vitamin K. Doctors of natural medicine sometimes recommend vitamin K supplementation to people taking antibiotics. Additional research is needed to determine whether the amount of vitamin K_1 found in some multivitamins is sufficient to prevent antibiotic-induced bleeding. Moreover, most multivitamins do not contain vitamin K.

CLINDAMYCIN TOPICAL

Common names: Cleocin T, Clindaderm, Dalacin T Topical, Dalacin Vaginal Cream

Clindamycin is an antibiotic applied to the skin to treat acne. While only a small percentage of topical clindamycin is absorbed through skin, side effects such as diarrhea, bloody diarrhea, colitis, and pseudomembranous colitis have been reported. Individuals who experience any of these symptoms should contact their healthcare practitioner.

Summary of Interactions Clindamycin Topical

In some cases, an herb or supplement may appear in more than one category, which may seem contradictory. For clarification, read the full article for details about the summarized interactions.

✓ May be Beneficial: Depletion or interference	Vitamin K*
✓ May be Beneficial: Side effect reduction/prevention	Bifidobacterium longum* Lactobacillus acidophilus* Lactobacillus casei* Probiotics* Saccharomyces boulardii* Saccharomyces cerevisiae* Vitamin K*
✓ May be Beneficial: Supportive interaction	Saccharomyces boulardii* Zinc
Reduced drug absorption/bioavailability	None known
Adverse interaction	None known

Interactions with Dietary Supplements
Probiotics

A common side effect of antibiotics is diarrhea, which may be caused by the elimination of beneficial bacteria normally found in the colon. Controlled studies have shown that taking probiotic microorganisms—such as *Lactobacillus casei, Lactobacillus acidophilus, Bifidobacterium longum,* or *Saccharomyces boulardii*—helps prevent antibiotic-induced diarrhea.[1]

The diarrhea experienced by some people who take antibiotics also might be due to an overgrowth of the bacterium *Clostridium difficile*, which causes a disease known as pseudomembranous colitis. Controlled studies have shown that supplementation with harmless yeast—such as *Saccharomyces boulardii*[2] or *Saccharomyces cerevisiae* (baker's or brewer's yeast)[3]—helps prevent recurrence of this infection. In one study, taking 500 mg of *Saccharomyces boulardii* twice daily enhanced the effectiveness of the antibiotic vancomycin in preventing recurrent clostridium infection.[4] Therefore, people taking antibiotics who later develop diarrhea might benefit from supplementing with saccharomyces organisms.

Treatment with antibiotics also commonly leads to an overgrowth of yeast *(Candida albicans)* in the vagina (candida vaginitis) and the intestines (sometimes referred to as "dysbiosis"). Controlled studies have shown that *Lactobacillus acidophilus* might prevent candida vaginitis.[5]

Vitamin K

Several cases of excessive bleeding have been reported in people who take antibiotics.[6, 7, 8, 9] This side effect may be the result of reduced vitamin K activity and/or reduced vitamin K production by bacteria in the colon. One study showed that people who had taken broad-spectrum antibiotics had lower liver concentrations of vitamin K_2 (menaquinone), though vitamin K_1 (phylloquinone) levels remained normal.[10] Several antibiotics appear to exert a strong effect on vitamin K activity, while others may not have any effect. Therefore, one should refer to a specific antibiotic for information on whether it interacts with vitamin K. Doctors of natural medicine sometimes recommend vitamin K supplementation to people taking antibiotics. Additional research is needed to determine whether the amount of vitamin K_1 found in some multivitamins is sufficient to prevent antibiotic-induced bleeding. Moreover, most multivitamins do not contain vitamin K.

Zinc

The effectiveness of topically applied clindamycin for inflammatory acne is enhanced when zinc is added to the topical formula, according to a recent review.[11]

CLOFIBRATE

Common names: Atromid-S

Clofibrate is a drug used to lower cholesterol in people with high blood cholesterol. It is rarely used, due to the possibility of liver damage and the availability of safer, more effective drugs.

Summary of Interactions for Clofibrate

In some cases, an herb or supplement may appear in more than one category, which may seem contradictory. For clarification, read the full article for details about the summarized interactions.

✓ May be Beneficial: Depletion or interference	Vitamin B$_{12}$*
✓ May be Beneficial: Side effect reduction/prevention	Milk thistle*
Supportive interaction	None known
Reduced drug absorption/bioavailability	None known
Adverse interaction	None known

Interactions with Dietary Supplements
Vitamin B$_{12}$
Clofibrate has been reported to reduce absorption of vitamin B$_{12}$.[1]

Interactions with Herbs
Milk thistle (Silybum marianum)
Although there have been no clinical studies, use of milk thistle with clofibrate may theoretically lower the risk of liver side effects associated with the drug. People may take a standardized milk thistle extract supplying 70–80% silymarin at an amount of 200 mg three times per day.

CLONIDINE

Common names: Apo-Clonidine, Catapres, Dixarit, Duraclon, Novo-Clonidine, Nu-Clonidine

Combination drug: Combipres

Clonidine is a drug that blocks signals in the brain controlling heart rate and blood pressure. It is used to lower blood pressure in people with hypertension. It is available alone in oral tablets, skin patches (Catapres-TTS), and in a form for intravenous (iv) injection; and in an oral combination product. Clonidine is used with narcotics to treat severe pain and as an adjunct to alcohol withdrawal, narcotic detoxification, and quitting smoking.

Summary of Interactions for Clonidine

In some cases, an herb or supplement may appear in more than one category, which may seem contradictory. For clarification, read the full article for details about the summarized interactions.

✓ May be Beneficial: Supportive interaction	DHEA*
Depletion or interference	None known
Side effect reduction/prevention	None known
Reduced drug absorption/bioavailability	None known
Adverse interaction	None known

Interactions with Dietary Supplements
Dehydroepiandrosterone (DHEA)
DHEA supplementation (50 mg per day) has been shown to restore the response of beta-endorphin (a brain chemical involved in pain and pleasure sensations) to clonidine.[1]

Interactions with Foods and Other Compounds
Alcohol
Alcohol is a central nervous system depressant and can cause drowsiness and dizziness. Clonidine may intensify these effects, increasing the risk of accidental injury.[2] To avoid problems, people taking clonidine should avoid alcohol.

CLOPIDOGREL

Common names: Plavix

Clopidogrel is used to prevent a second heart attack or stroke in people with atherosclerosis, and is known as an anti-platelet drug. At the time of this writing, no evidence of nutrient or herb interactions involving clopidogrel was found in the medical literature.

Summary of Interactions for Clopidogrel

In some cases, an herb or supplement may appear in more than one category, which may seem contradictory. For clarification, read the full article for details about the summarized interactions.

Depletion or interference	None known
Side effect reduction/prevention	None known
Supportive interaction	None known
Reduced drug absorption/bioavailability	None known
Adverse interaction	None known

CLORAZEPATE DIPOTASSIUM

Common names: Apo-Clorazepate, Gen-Xene, Novo-Clopate, Tranxene

Clorazepate is used to treat the symptoms of anxiety, including restlessness, insomnia, and worry; it is also used for convulsions and symptoms associated with acute alcohol withdrawal. It is in a class of drugs known as **benzodiazepines** (page 36).

Summary of Interactions for Clorazepate Dipotassium

In some cases, an herb or supplement may appear in more than one category, which may seem contradictory. For clarification, read the full article for details about the summarized interactions.

✓ May be Beneficial: Supportive interaction	Vinpocetine*
⊘ Avoid: Reduced drug absorption/ bioavailability	Tobacco
⊘ Avoid: Adverse interaction	Alcohol
ⓘ Check: Other	L-tryptophan*
Depletion or interference	None known
Side effect reduction/prevention	None known

Interactions with Dietary Supplements

L-tryptophan
Test tube studies show that L-tryptophan and clorazepate dipotassium interact in the blood in such a way that the actions of the drug may be enhanced when high amounts of L-tryptophan are ingested.[1] Controlled research is needed to determine the significance of this interaction and to investigate possible interactions between clorazepate and 5-hydroxytryptophan, a supplement related to L-tryptophan.

Vinpocetine
In a preliminary trial, an extract of periwinkle called vinpocetine was shown to produce minor improvements in short-term memory among people taking flunitrazepam, a benzodiazepine.[2] Further study is needed to determine if vinpocetine would be a helpful adjunct to use of benzodiazepines, or clorazepate specifically.

Interactions with Foods and Other Compounds

Alcohol
Drinking alcohol while taking clorazepate may enhance drowsiness and slow reaction time,[3] and, according to animal studies, prolong sleep time.[4] Consequently, people taking clorazepate dipotassium should avoid alcoholic beverages.

Smoking
Cigarette smoking decreases the amount of time clorazepate is in the body, lowers blood levels of the drug, and reduces the beneficial effects;[5] therefore, people should avoid smoking while taking the drug. People who quit smoking while taking clorazepate might experience unwanted side effects due to increased blood levels of the drug; gradual reduction in nicotine is preferred.

CLOTRIMAZOLE/ BETAMETHASONE

Common names: Lotrisone

Combination drugs: Canesten HC, Lotriderm

The drug is a combination product containing clotrimazole, an antifungal component, and betamethasone, a **corticosteroid** (page 77) that reduces inflammation. It is a topical agent most often applied to the skin for the treatment of ringworm, jock itch, and athlete's foot accompanied by inflammation. In addition, the combination may be administered as a secondary treatment for yeast infections of the skin caused by *Candida albicans*.

There are currently no reported nutrient or herb interactions involving clotrimazole. However, small amounts of topically applied corticosteroids may enter the blood and interact with other substances. Refer to the article on oral **corticosteroid** (page 77) for potential interactions.

Summary of Interactions for Clotrimazole Bethamethasone

In some cases, an herb or supplement may appear in more than one category, which may seem contradictory. For clarification, read the full article for details about the summarized interactions.

Depletion or interference	None known
Side effect reduction/prevention	None known
Supportive interaction	None known
Reduced drug absorption/bioavailability	None known
Adverse interaction	None known

CLOZAPINE

Common names: Clozaril

Clozapine is an atypical neuroleptic used to control symptoms of schizophrenia when other treatments are ineffective.

Summary of Interactions for Clozapine

In some cases, an herb or supplement may appear in more than one category, which may seem contradictory. For clarification, read the full article for details about the summarized interactions.

✓ May be Beneficial: Depletion or interference	L-tryptophan Selenium
✓ May be Beneficial: Side effect reduction/prevention	N-acetyl cysteine* Vitamin C
⃠ Avoid: Reduced drug absorption/ bioavailability	Glycine
Supportive interaction	None known
Adverse interaction	None known

Interactions with Dietary Supplements
Glycine

The use of glycine may interfere with the efficacy of clozapine as an antipsychotic drug. In a double-blind trial, people with chronic, treatment-resistant schizophrenia were given clozapine (400–1,200 mg per day) and either glycine (30 g per day) or placebo for 12 weeks.[1] The combination of clozapine and glycine was not effective at decreasing symptoms. In contrast, participants who took clozapine *without* glycine had a 35% reduction in some symptoms. Therefore, the combination should be avoided until more is known.

N-acetyl cysteine and vitamin C

Clozapine can inhibit the formation of immune cells that protect the body from invading organisms. Test tube studies show that N-acetyl-cysteine and vitamin C

block the formation of immune cell–damaging compounds produced when clozapine is broken down.[2] Controlled studies are necessary to determine whether supplementing N-acetyl-cysteine and vitamin C might prevent harmful side effects in people taking clozapine.

Selenium

One controlled study showed that taking clozapine can decrease blood levels of selenium, a mineral with antioxidant activity.[3] While more research is needed to determine whether people taking clozapine might require selenium supplementation, until more information is available, some health practitioners recommend supplementation.

L-tryptophan

Some people who take clozapine become mentally depressed after taking the drug for a few weeks. Studies have shown that clozapine can reduce blood levels of the amino acid L-tryptophan, which is often deficient in people with depression.[4] More controlled research is needed to determine whether the interaction is significant and whether individuals taking clozapine might benefit from supplemental L-tryptophan or 5-hydroxytryptophan (5-HTP).

Interactions with Foods and Other Compounds
Alcohol

Drinking alcoholic beverages together with clozapine can cause side effects, such as drowsiness and dizziness.[5] Consequently, people taking clozapine should avoid alcohol, especially when it is necessary to stay alert.

Caffeine (page 44)

Caffeine is a compound found in coffee, colas, and tea, as well as in some over-the-counter products. One 31-year-old woman taking clozapine who consumed nearly 1,000 mg of caffeine daily experienced side effects from the drug.[6] A subsequent study involving individuals with schizophrenia who were stabilized on clozapine, showed that caffeine avoidance resulted in significantly lower blood levels of the drug.[7] Controlled research is needed to determine whether problems might occur when individuals taking clozapine change the amount of caffeine they consume each day. Until more information is available, individuals taking clozapine should talk with their healthcare practitioner before making changes in their caffeine intake.

Smoking

Controlled studies show that smoking cigarettes can significantly reduce blood levels of clozapine,[8] which can become a problem if an individual either starts or stops smoking while taking the drug. Those who start smoking may experience more symptoms of schizophrenia, while those who quit smoking might experience unwanted side effects of the drug. Consequently, people taking clozapine should talk with their healthcare practitioner before making changes in their smoking habit.

COALGESIC

Contains the following ingredients:
Acetaminophen (page 3)
Dextropropoxyphene

COAPROVEL

Contains the following ingredients:
Hydrochlorothiazide
Irbesartan (page 146)

CO-BETALOC

Contains the following ingredients:
Hydrochlorothiazide
Metoprolol (page 176)

CO-BETALOC SA

Contains the following ingredients:
Hydrochlorothiazide
Metoprolol (page 176)

CODEINE

Common names: Codeine Contin, Galcodine Pediatric, Galcodine

Combination drugs: Empirin with Codeine, Fiorinal, Phenergan VC with Codeine, Phenergan with Codeine, Robitussin AC, Soma Compound with Codeine, Tylenol with Codeine

Codeine is a narcotic analgesic (pain reliever) derived from opium. It is used alone and in combination products to treat mild to moderate pain and as a cough suppressant.

Summary of Interactions for Codeine

In some cases, an herb or supplement may appear in more than one category, which may seem contradictory. For clarification, read the full article for details about the summarized interactions.

⊘ Avoid: Reduced drug absorption/ bioavailability	Tannin-containing herbs* such as green tea, black tea, uva ursi, black walnut, red raspberry, oak, and witch hazel
Depletion or interference	None known
Side effect reduction/prevention	None known
Supportive interaction	None known
Adverse interaction	None known

Interactions with Herbs
Tannin-containing herbs
Tannins are a group of unrelated chemicals that give plants an astringent taste. Herbs with large amounts of tannins may interfere with the absorption of codeine and should not be taken together with codeine or codeine-containing products.[1] Herbs containing high levels of tannins include green tea (*Camellia sinensis*), black tea, uva ursi (*Arctostaphylos uva-ursi),* black walnut (*Juglans nigra),* red raspberry (*Rubus idaeus),* oak (*Quercus* spp.), and witch hazel (*Hamamelis virginiana).*

Interactions with Foods and Other Compounds
Food
Codeine commonly causes gastrointestinal (GI) upset. Codeine and codeine-containing products may be taken with food to reduce or prevent GI upset.[2] A common side effect of narcotic analgesics, including codeine, is constipation. Increasing dietary fiber (fruits, vegetables, beans, whole-grain foods, and others) and water intake can ease constipation.

Alcohol
Alcohol causes a loss of coordination, impaired judgment, decreased alertness, drowsiness, and other actions. Narcotic analgesics, including codeine, cause similar loss of control. Combining codeine and alcohol increases the risk of accidental injury. People taking codeine-containing products should avoid alcohol.

Codeine

COLCHICINE

Colchicine reduces the inflammatory (swelling) response and pain in people with gout (high uric acid blood levels leading to painful accumulation of uric acid crystals in and around joints).

Summary of Interactions for Colchicine

In some cases, an herb or supplement may appear in more than one category, which may seem contradictory. For clarification, read the full article for details about the summarized interactions.

✓ May be Beneficial: Depletion or interference	Beta-carotene* Potassium* Vitamin B$_{12}$*
ⓘ Check: Other	Sodium
Side effect reduction/prevention	None known
Supportive interaction	None known
Reduced drug absorption/bioavailability	None known
Adverse interaction	None known

Interactions with Dietary Supplements
Vitamin B$_{12}$
Colchicine may interfere with vitamin B$_{12}$ in the body. Research is inconsistent. Both colchicine and vitamin B$_{12}$ deficiency are reported to cause neuropathies (disorders of the nervous system), but it remains unclear whether neuropathies caused by colchicine could be due to vitamin B$_{12}$ depletion.[1, 2]

Nutrient malabsorption
Colchicine has been associated with impaired absorption of beta-carotene, fat, lactose (milk sugar), potassium, and sodium.[3]

COLESTIPOL

Common names: Colestid

Colestipol is a **bile acid sequestrant** (page 39) (prevents absorption of bile acids in the digestive system). Bile acids may facilitate the absorption of cholesterol. Colestipol is one of many **cholesterol-lowering drugs** (page 61) used in people with high blood cholesterol.

Summary of Interactions for Colestipol

In some cases, an herb or supplement may appear in more than one category, which may seem contradictory. For clarification, read the full article for details about the summarized interactions.

✓ May be Beneficial: Depletion or interference	Beta-carotene Calcium* Carotenoids* Folic acid Vitamin A Vitamin D Vitamin E Vitamin K Zinc*
Side effect reduction/prevention	None known
Supportive interaction	None known
Reduced drug absorption/bioavailability	None known
Adverse interaction	None known

Interactions with Dietary Supplements
Vitamins
Bile acid sequestrants, including colestipol, may prevent absorption of folic acid and the fat-soluble vitamins A, D, E, K.[1, 2] People taking colestipol should consult with their doctor about vitamin malabsorption and supplementation. People should take other drugs and vitamin supplements one hour before or four to six hours after colestipol to improve absorption.[3]

Animal studies suggest calcium and zinc may be depleted by taking cholestyramine, another bile acid sequestrant.[4] Whether these same interactions would occur with colestipol is not known.

Carotenoids
Use of colestipol for six months has been shown to significantly lower blood levels of carotenoids including beta-carotene.[5]

Interactions with Foods and Other Compounds
Water
Bile acid sequestrants should be taken with plenty of water before meals.[6]

CO-MAGALDROX

Contains the following ingredients:
Aluminium hydroxide (page 10)
Magnesium hydroxide (page 166)

COMBIPRES

Contains the following ingredients:
Chlorthalidone
Clonidine (page 72)

COMBIVENT

Contains the following ingredients:
Albuterol (page 6)
Ipratropium Bromide (page 146)

COMBIVIR

Contains the following ingredients:
AZT (page 33)
Lamivudine (page 153)

CONTAC 12 HOUR

Contains the following ingredients:
Chlorpheniramine (page 59)
Phenylpropanolamine (page 218)

CO-PROXAMOL

Contains the following ingredients:
Acetaminophen (page 3)
Dextropropoxyphene

CORGARETIC

Contains the following ingredients:
Bendroflumethiazide
Nadolol (page 185)

CORTICOSTEROIDS

Common names: A-Hydrocort, A-Methapred, Aeroseb-Dex, Alti-Beclomethasone, Amcinonide, Aristocort, Aristospan, Beclodisk, Benisone, Beta-Val, Betamethasone, Betatrex, Bronalide, Celestone, Clobetasol Propionate, Clocortolone Pivalate, Cloderm, Cordran, Corlan, Cortisone, Cortisyl, Cortone, Cyclocort, Decaspray, Delta-cortril Enteric, Depo-Medrol, Desonide, Desowen, Dexsol, Diflorasone Diacetate, Diprolene, Econopred, Elocom, Entocort, Exasone, Filair, Flixonase, Florinef, Florone, Fludrocortisone Acetate, Fluocinolone Acetonide, Fluonid, Fluor-Op, Fluorometholone, Flurandrenolide, FML, Gen-Beclo Aq, Gen-Budesonide Aq, Haldrone, Halog, Hexadrol, HMS Liquifilm, Hydeltrasol, Hydrocortone, Kenacort, Kenalog, Lidex, Luxiq, Maxidex, Maxiflor, Maxivate, Medrone, Medrysone, Nasacort, Nasalide, Nasobec, Orasone, Pediapred, Precortisyl, Prednesol, Prednisolone, Prednisone, Rhinalar, Rhinocort, Rivanase Aq, Solu-Cortef, Solu-Medrol, Synalar, Syntaris, Topicort, Tridesilon, Turbinaire, Uticort, Valisone, Vancenase AQ, Vancenase, Vanceril, Westcort, Zonivent

Combination drugs: Adcortyl with Graneodin, Aureocort, Lotrisone, Tobradex, Tri-Adcortyl

Corticosteroids are a family of drugs that include cortisol (hydrocortisone)—an adrenal hormone found naturally in the body—as well as synthetic drugs. Though natural and synthetic corticosteroids are both potent anti-inflammatory compounds, the synthetics exert a stronger effect. Oral forms of corticosteroids are used to treat numerous autoimmune and inflammatory conditions, including asthma, bursitis, Crohn's disease, skin disorders, tendinitis, ulcerative colitis, and others. They are also used to treat severe allergic reactions and to prevent rejection after organ transplant.

Corticosteroids are available for inhalation by mouth to treat asthma and other conditions of restricted breathing, as well as by nose to treat symptoms of nasal allergies. Topical forms are available to treat skin conditions, such as eczema, psoriasis, insect bites, and hives. Some topical products contain combinations of corticosteroids and **antibiotics** (page 19), and are used to treat ear, eye, and skin infections. For interactions involving oral, inhaled, or topical forms of corticosteroids, refer to the categories listed below.

Oral Corticosteroids (page 200)
• Cortisone
• Hydrocortisone (Cortef)
• Prednisone (Deltasone, Meticorten, Orasone)
• Prednisolone (Delta-Cortef, Pediapred, Prelone)
• Triamcinolone (Aristocort, Kenacort)
• Methylprednisolone (Medrol)
• Dexamethasone (Decadron, Dexone, Hexadrol)
• Betamethasone (Celestone)

Inhaled Corticosteroids (page 143)
• Beclomethasone (Beclovent, Beconase, Vanceril, Vancenase)
• Budesonide (Pulmicort, Rhinocort)

- Mometasone (Nasonex)
- Triamcinolone (Azmacort, Nasacort)
- Flunisolide (AeroBid, Nasalide, Nasarel)
- Fluticasone (Flovent, Flonase)

Topical Corticosteroids (page 265)

- Alclometasone (Aclovate)
- Amcinonide (Cyclocort)
- Augmented betamethasone (Diprolene)
- Betamethasone (Uticort, Diprosone, Maxivate, Teladar, Valisone)
- Clobetasol (Cormax, Embeline E, Temovate)
- Clocortolone (Cloderm)
- Desonide (DesOwen, Tridesilon)
- Desoximetasone (Topicort)
- Dexamethasone (Decadron, Decaspray)
- Diflorasone (Florone, Maxiflor, Psorcon)
- Flucinolone (Synalar, Fluonid)
- Fluocinonide (Lidex, Fluonex)
- Flurandrenolide (Cordran)
- Fluticasone (Cutivate)
- Halcinonide (Halog)
- Halobetasol (Ultravate)
- Hydrocortisone (Anusol-HC, Hytone, Cort-Dome, Cortenema, Cortifoam, Cortaind, Lanacort, Locoid, Westcort)
- Methylprednisolone (Medrol)
- Mometasone (Elocon)
- Prednicarbate (Dermatop)
- Triamcinolone (Aristocort, Kenalog, Flutex)

> For interactions involving a specific Corticosteroid, see the individual drug article. For interactions involving a Corticosteroid for which no separate article exists, talk to your doctor or pharmacist.

COSOPT

Contains the following ingredients:
Dorzolamide (page 99)
Timolol (page 263)

CO-TENDIONE

Contains the following ingredients:
Atenolol (page 28)
Chlorthalidone

COZAAR-COMP

Contains the following ingredients:
Hydrochlorothiazide
Losartan (page 162)

CO-ZIDOCAPT

Contains the following ingredients:
Captopril (page 47)
Hydrochlorothiazide

CROMOLYN SODIUM

Common names: Apo-Cromolyn Sterules Nebulizer Solution, Apo-Cromolyn Nasal Spray, Boots Hayfever Relief Eye Drops, Clariteyes Eye Drops, Crolom, Cromogen Easi-Breathe Aerosol Spray, Cromogen Steri-Neb Nebulizer Solution, Cromoglycate, Cromolyn Nasal Solution, Cromolyn Opthalmic Solution, Fisonair Inhaler, Gastrocrom, Gen-Cromoglycate Sterinebs Nebulizer Solution, Gen-Cromoglycate Nasal Soution, Hay-Crom Eye Drops, Intal, Nasalcrom, Novo-Cromolyn, Nu-Cromolyn, Opticrom, Opticrom Eye Drops, Optrex Eye Drops, PMS-Sodium Cromoglycate, Rynacrom Nasal Spray, Sodium Cromoglicate, Syncroner Inhaler, Vividrin Nasal Spray, Viz-On Eye Drops

Cromolyn is used to prevent chronic asthma and can be helpful for people who experience acute asthma attacks brought on by exercise, allergies, and environmental pollution.

Summary of Interactions for Cromolyn Sodium

In some cases, an herb or supplement may appear in more than one category, which may seem contradictory. For clarification, read the full article for details about the summarized interactions.

Depletion or interference	None known
Side effect reduction/prevention	None known
Supportive interaction	None known
Reduced drug absorption/bioavailability	None known
Adverse interaction	None known

CYCLOBENZAPRINE

Common names: Alti-Cyclobenzaprine, Apo-Cyclobenzaprine, Flexeril, Flexitec, Gen-Cycloprine, Novo-Cycloprine, Nu-Cyclobenzaprine

Cyclobenzaprine is a drug used as an adjunct to rest and physical therapy for relief of spasm.

Summary of Interactions for Cyclobenzaprine

In some cases, an herb or supplement may appear in more than one category, which may seem contradictory. For clarification, read the full article for details about the summarized interactions.

Depletion or interference	None known
Side effect reduction/prevention	None known
Supportive interaction	None known
Reduced drug absorption/bioavailability	None known
Adverse interaction	None known

Interactions with Foods and Other Compounds
Alcohol

Cyclobenzaprine may cause dizziness, drowsiness, or blurred vision.[1] Alcohol may intensify these effects and increase the risk of accidental injury. To prevent problems, people taking cyclobenzaprine should avoid alcohol.

CYCLOPHOSPHAMIDE

Common names: Cytoxan, Endoxana, Neosar, Procytox

Cyclophosphamide is a **chemotherapy** (page 54) drug used primarily to treat various forms of cancer. It is also used less commonly to treat some noncancer diseases.

> **Note:** Many of the interactions described below, in the text and in the Summary of Interactions, have been reported only for specific chemotherapeutic drugs, and may not apply to other chemotherapeutic drugs. There are many unknowns concerning interactions of nutrients, herbs, and chemotherapy drugs. People receiving chemotherapy who wish to supplement with vitamins, minerals, herbs, or other natural substances should always consult a physician.

Summary of Interactions for Cyclophosphamide

In some cases, an herb or supplement may appear in more than one category, which may seem contradictory. For clarification, read the full article for details about the summarized interactions.

✓ May be Beneficial: Side effect reduction/prevention	Antioxidants* (Vitamin A, Vitamin C, Vitamin E) Beta-carotene* (mouth sores) Chamomile* (mouth sores) Eleuthero* (see text) Ginger* (nausea) Glutamine* (mouth sores) Glutathione* (i.v. only) Melatonin* (see text) N-acetyl cysteine* (NAC) Selenium Spleen peptide extract (see text) Thymus peptides* (see text) Vitamin E*, topical (mouth sores) Zinc (taste alterations)
ⓘ Check: Other	Echinacea* Multivitamin-mineral* Vitamin A* Vitamin C*
Depletion or interference	None known
Supportive interaction	None known
Reduced drug absorption/bioavailability	None known
Adverse interaction	None known

Interactions with Dietary Supplements
Antioxidants

Cyclophosphamide requires activation by the liver through a process called oxidation. In theory, antioxidant nutrients (vitamin A, vitamin E, beta-carotene and others) might interfere with the activation of cyclophosphamide. There is no published research linking antioxidant vitamins to reduced cyclophosphamide effectiveness in cancer treatment. In a study of mice with vitamin A deficiency, vitamin A supplementation enhanced the anticancer action of cyclophosphamide.[1] Another animal research report indicated that vitamin C may increase the effectiveness of cyclophosphamide without producing new side effects.[2] Preliminary human research found that adding antioxidants (beta-carotene, vitamin A, and vitamin E) to cyclophosphamide therapy increased the survival of people with small-cell lung cancer treated with cyclophosphamide.[3] It is too early to know if adding antioxidants to cyclophosphamide for cancer treatment is better than cyclophosphamide alone. Vitamin A can be toxic in high amounts.

Intravenous injections of the antioxidant, glutathione, may protect the bladder from damage caused by cyclophosphamide. Preliminary evidence suggests, but cannot confirm, a protective action of glutathione in the bladders of people on cyclophosphamide therapy.[4] There is no evidence that glutathione taken by mouth has the same benefits.

Glutamine

Though cancer cells use glutamine as a fuel source, studies in humans have not found that glutamine stimulates growth of cancers in people taking chemotherapy.[5, 6] In fact, animal studies show that glutamine may actually decrease tumor growth while increasing susceptibility of cancer cells to radiation and chemotherapy,[7, 8] though such effects have not yet been studied in humans.

Glutamine has successfully reduced chemotherapy-induced mouth sores. In one trial, people were given 4 grams of glutamine in an oral rinse, which was swished around the mouth and then swallowed twice per day.[9] Thirteen of fourteen people in the study had fewer days with mouth sores as a result. These excellent results have been duplicated in some,[10] but not all[11] double-blind research. In another study, patients receiving high-dose **paclitaxel** (page 205) and melphalan had significantly fewer episodes of oral ulcers and bleeding when they took 6 grams of glutamine four times daily along with the chemotherapy.[12]

One double-blind trial suggested that 6 grams of glutamine taken three times per day can decrease diarrhea caused by chemotherapy.[13] However, other studies using higher amounts or intravenous glutamine have not reported this effect.[14, 15]

Intravenous use of glutamine in people undergoing bone marrow transplants, a procedure sometimes used to allow very high amounts of chemotherapy to be used, has led to reduced hospital stays, leading to a savings of over $21,000 for each patient given glutamine.[16]

Melatonin

High amounts of melatonin have been combined with a variety of chemotherapy drugs to reduce their side effects or improve drug efficacy. One study gave melatonin at night in combination with the drug triptorelin to men with metastatic prostate cancer.[17] All of these men had previously become unresponsive to triptorelin. The combination decreased PSA levels—a marker of prostate cancer progression—in eight of fourteen patients, decreased some side effects of triptorelin, and helped nine of fourteen to live longer than one year. The outcome of this preliminary study suggests that melatonin may improve the efficacy of triptorelin even after the drug has apparently lost effectiveness.

N-acetyl cysteine (NAC)

NAC, an amino acid–like supplement that possesses antioxidant activity, has been used in four human studies to decrease the kidney and bladder toxicity of the chemotherapy drug ifosfamide.[18, 19, 20, 21] These studies used 1–2 grams NAC four times per day. There was no sign that NAC interfered with the efficacy of ifosfamide in any of these studies. Intakes of NAC over 4 grams per day may cause nausea and vomiting.

The newer anti-nausea drugs prescribed for people taking chemotherapy lead to greatly reduced nausea and vomiting for most people. Nonetheless, these drugs often do not totally eliminate all nausea. Natural substances used to reduce nausea should not be used instead of prescription anti-nausea drugs. Rather, under the guidance of a doctor, they should be added to those drugs if needed. At least one trial suggests that NAC, at 1,800 mg per day may reduce nausea and vomiting caused by chemotherapy.[22]

Selenium

Patients being treated with cyclophosphamide and cisplatin for ovarian cancer were given a multivitamin preparation, with or without 200 mcg of selenium per day. Compared with the group not receiving selenium, those receiving selenium had a smaller reduction in white blood cell count and fewer chemotherapy side effects such as nausea, hair loss, weakness, and loss of appetite.[23]

Spleen extract

Patients with inoperable head and neck cancer were treated with a spleen peptide preparation (Polyerga) in a double-blind trial during chemotherapy with cisplatin and 5-FU.[24] The spleen preparation had a significant stabilizing effect on certain white blood cells. People taking it also experienced stabilized body weight and a reduction in the fatigue and inertia that usually accompany this combination of chemotherapy agents.

Beta-carotene and vitamin E

Chemotherapy frequently causes mouth sores. In one trial, people were given approximately 400,000 IU of beta-carotene per day for three weeks and then 125,000 IU per day for an additional four weeks.[25] Those taking beta-carotene still suffered mouth sores, but the mouth sores developed later and tended to be less severe than mouth sores that formed in people receiving the same chemotherapy without beta-carotene.

In a study of chemotherapy-induced mouth sores, six of nine patients who applied vitamin E directly to their mouth sores had complete resolution of the sores compared with one of nine patients who applied placebo.[26] Others have confirmed the potential for vitamin E to help people with chemotherapy-induced mouth sores.[27] Applying vitamin E only once per day was helpful to only some groups of patients in another trial,[28] and not all studies have found vitamin E to be effective.[29] Until more is known, if vitamin E is used in an attempt to reduce chemotherapy-induced mouth sores, it should be applied topically twice per day and should probably be in the tocopherol (versus tocopheryl) form.

Vitamin A

A controlled French trial reported that when post-menopausal late-stage breast cancer patients were given very large amounts of vitamin A (350,000–500,000 IU per day) along with chemotherapy, remission rates were significantly better than when the chemotherapy was not accompanied by vitamin A.[30] Similar results were not found in premenopausal women. The large amounts of vitamin A used in the study are toxic and require clinical supervision.

Zinc

Irradiation treatment, especially of head and neck cancers, frequently results in changes to normal taste sensation.[31, 32] Zinc supplementation may be protective against taste alterations caused or exacerbated by irradiation. A double-blind trial found that 45 mg of zinc sulfate three times daily reduced the alteration of taste sensation during radiation treatment and led to significantly greater recovery of taste sensation after treatment was concluded.[33]

Multivitamin-mineral

Many chemotherapy drugs can cause diarrhea, lack of appetite, vomiting, and damage to the gastrointestinal tract. Recent anti-nausea prescription medications are often effective. Nonetheless, nutritional deficiencies still occur.[34] It makes sense for people undergoing chemotherapy to take a high-potency multivitamin-mineral to protect against deficiencies.

Taurine

Taurine has been shown to be depleted in people taking chemotherapy.[35] It remains unclear how important this effect is or if people taking chemotherapy should take taurine supplements.

Thymus peptides

Peptides or short proteins derived from the thymus gland, an important immune organ, have been used in conjunction with chemotherapy drugs for people with cancer. One study using thymosin fraction V in combination with chemotherapy, compared with chemotherapy alone, found significantly longer survival times in the thymosin fraction V group.[36] A related substance, thymostimulin, decreased some side effects of chemotherapy and increased survival time compared with chemotherapy alone.[37] A third product, thymic extract TP1, was shown to improve immune function in people treated with chemotherapy compared with effects of chemotherapy alone.[38] Thymic peptides need to be administered by injection. People interested in their combined use with chemotherapy should consult a doctor.

Interactions with Herbs

Echinacea (Echinacea purpurea, Echinacea angustifolia)

Echinacea is a popular immune-boosting herb that has been investigated for use with chemotherapy. One study investigated the actions of cyclophosphamide, echinacea, and thymus gland extracts to treat advanced cancer patients. Although small and uncontrolled, this trial suggested that the combination modestly extended the life span of some patients with inoperable cancers.[39] Signs of restoration of immune function were seen in these patients.

Eleuthero (Eleutherococcus senticosus)

Russian research has looked at using eleuthero with chemotherapy. One study of patients with melanoma found that chemotherapy was less toxic when eleuthero was given simultaneously. Similarly, women with inoperable breast cancer given eleuthero were reported to tolerate more chemotherapy.[40] Eleuthero treatment was also associated with improved immune function in women with breast cancer treated with chemotherapy and radiation.[41]

Milk thistle (Silybum marianum)

Milk thistle's major flavonoids, known collectively as silymarin, have shown synergistic actions with the chemotherapy drugs **cisplatin** (page 64) and **doxoru-bicin** (page 100) (Adriamycin) in test tubes.[42] Silymarin also offsets the kidney toxicity of cisplatin in animals.[43] Silymarin has not yet been studied in humans treated with cisplatin. There is some evidence that silymarin may not interfere with some chemotherapy in humans with cancer.[44]

Ginger (Zingiber officinale)
Ginger can be helpful in alleviating nausea and vomiting caused by chemotherapy.[45, 46] Ginger, as tablets, capsules, or liquid herbal extracts, can be taken in 500 mg amounts every two or three hours, for a total of 1 gram per day.

German chamomile (Matricaria recutita)
A liquid preparation of German chamomile has been shown to reduce the incidence of mouth sores in people receiving radiation and systemic chemotherapy treatment in an uncontrolled study. [47]

PSK (Coriolus versicolor)
The mushroom *Coriolus versicolor* contains an immune-stimulating substance called polysaccharide krestin, or PSK. PSK has been shown in several studies to help cancer patients undergoing chemotherapy. One study involved women with estrogen receptor-negative breast cancer. PSK combined with chemotherapy significantly prolonged survival time compared with chemotherapy alone.[48] Another study followed women with breast cancer who were given chemotherapy with or without PSK. The PSK-plus-chemotherapy group had a 25% better chance of survival after ten years compared with those taking chemotherapy without PSK.[49] Another study investigated people who had surgically removed colon cancer. They were given chemotherapy with or without PSK. Those given PSK had a longer disease-free period and longer survival time.[50] Three grams of PSK were taken orally each day in these studies.

Although PSK is rarely available in the United States, hot-water extract products made from *Coriolus versicolor* mushrooms are available. These products may have activity related to that of PSK, but their use with chemotherapy has not been studied.

Interactions with Foods and Other Compounds
Food
It is recommended to take cyclophosphamide on an empty stomach. If this causes severe gastrointestinal (GI) upset, cyclophosphamide may be taken with food.[51] People with questions should ask their prescribing doctor or pharmacist.

Fruit drinks
Often, people who undergo chemotherapy develop aversions to certain foods, sometimes making it permanently difficult to eat those foods. Exposing people to what researchers have called a "scapegoat stimulus" just before the administration of chemotherapy can direct the food aversion to the "scapegoat" food instead of more important parts of the diet. In one trial, fruit drinks administered just before chemotherapy were most effective in protecting against aversions to other foods.[52]

CYCLO-PROGYNOVA

Contains the following ingredients:
Estradiol (page 108)
Levonorgestrel

CYCLOSERINE

Common names: Seromycin

Cycloserine is a broad-spectrum **antibiotic** (page 19) used to treat tuberculosis. It is used rarely for treating noninfectious diseases.

Summary of Interactions for Cycloserine
In some cases, an herb or supplement may appear in more than one category, which may seem contradictory. For clarification, read the full article for details about the summarized interactions.

✓ May be Beneficial: Depletion or interference	Calcium* Folic acid* Magnesium* Vitamin B$_{12}$* Vitamin B$_6$* Vitamin K
Side effect reduction/prevention	None known
Supportive interaction	None known
Reduced drug absorption/bioavailability	None known
Adverse interaction	None known

Interactions with Dietary Supplements

Calcium and magnesium

Cycloserine may interfere with calcium and magnesium absorption.[1] The clinical significance of these interactions is unclear.

Folic acid, vitamin B₆, vitamin B₁₂

Cycloserine may interfere with the absorption and/or activity of folic acid, vitamin B₆, and vitamin B₁₂.[2, 3] The clinical importance of this interaction is unclear.

Vitamin K

Many antibiotics taken by mouth, including cycloserine, may kill friendly bacteria in the large intestine that produce vitamin K.[4] With short-term (a few weeks or less) antibiotic use, the actions on vitamin K are usually mild and cause no problems. After antibiotic therapy is completed, vitamin K activity returns to normal.

Interactions with Foods and Other Compounds

Alcohol

Cycloserine may cause drowsiness.[5] Alcohol may intensify this drowsiness and increase the risk of accidents during activities requiring alertness. Seizures are a possible side effect of cycloserine therapy. Alcohol consumed during cycloserine therapy may increase the risk of seizures.[6] People should avoid alcohol-containing products during cycloserine therapy.

CYCLOSPORINE

Common names: Ciclosporin, Ciclosporine, Neoral, Sandimmune, Sandimmun, SangCya

Cyclosporine is a drug that suppresses the immune system. It is used in combination with other immune suppressive drugs to prevent rejection of transplanted organs by the immune system. There are two different forms of cyclosporine, Sandimmune and Neoral. These products differ in important ways and each is used in combination with different additional immunosuppressant drugs. Inadequate immune suppression may result in organ rejection and serious complications. People taking cyclosporine should follow their prescribing doctor's directions exactly and discuss with their doctor any changes in drug therapy, vitamins, supplements, herbal products, or any other substances before making the changes.

Summary of Interactions for Cyclosporine

In some cases, an herb or supplement may appear in more than one category, which may seem contradictory. For clarification, read the full article for details about the summarized interactions.

✓	May be Beneficial: Depletion or interference	Magnesium Red wine
✓	May be Beneficial: Side effect reduction/prevention	*Ginkgo biloba** Omega-3 fatty acids*
✓	May be Beneficial: Supportive interaction	Vitamin E*
⊘	Avoid: Reduced drug absorption/ bioavailability	Chinese scullcap St. John's wort*
ⓘ	Check: Other	Apple juice Grapefruit juice Milk Orange juice Quercetin
Adverse interaction		None known

Interactions with Dietary Supplements

Magnesium

Cyclosporine has been associated with low blood magnesium levels and undesirable side effects.[1, 2, 3] Some doctors suggest monitoring the level of magnesium in red blood cells, rather than in serum, as the red blood cell test may be more sensitive for evaluating magnesium status.

Potassium

Cyclosporine can cause excess retention of potassium, potentially leading to dangerous levels of the mineral in the blood (hyperkalemia).[4] Potassium supplements, potassium-containing salt substitutes (No Salt, Morton Salt Substitute, and others), and even high-potassium foods (primarily fruit) should be avoided by people taking cyclosporine, unless directed otherwise by their doctor.

Omega-3 fatty acids

Several studies have shown that in organ transplant patients treated with cyclosporine, addition of 4–6 grams per day of omega-3 fatty acids from fish oil helped reduce high blood pressure,[5, 6, 7] though not every study has found fish oil helpful.[8] It remains unclear to what extent fish oil supplementation will help people with high blood pressure taking cyclosporine following organ transplant.

Cyclosporine

Vitamin E

Twenty-six liver transplant patients (both adults and children) unable to achieve or maintain therapeutic cyclosporine blood levels during the early post-transplant period were given water-soluble vitamin E in the amount of 6.25 IU/2.2 pounds of body weight two times per day.[9] Addition of vitamin E in the early post-transplant period reduced the required amount of cyclosporine and the cost of cyclosporine therapy by 26%. These results imply that the addition of vitamin E to established cyclosporine therapy allows for a decrease in the amount of cyclosporine. Combining vitamin E and cyclosporine requires medical supervision to avoid cyclosporine toxicity.

Quercetin

In an animal study, oral administration of quercetin (50 mg per 2.2 pounds of body weight) at the same time as cyclosporine decreased the absorption of cyclosporine by 43%.[10] However, in a study of healthy human volunteers, supplementing with quercetin along with cyclosporine significantly increased blood levels of cyclosporine, when compared with administering cyclosporine alone.[11] Because the effect of quercetin supplementation on cyclosporine absorption or utilization appears to be unpredictable, individuals taking cyclosporine should not take quercetin without the supervision of a doctor.

Interactions with Herbs

Chinese scullcap

In a study in rats, oral administration of Chinese scullcap at the same time as cyclosporine significantly reduced the absorption of cyclosporine.[12] Chinese scullcap did not interfere with the availability of cyclosporine when cyclosporine was given intravenously. Because of the potential adverse interaction, people taking cyclosporine should not take Chinese scullcap.

Ginkgo biloba

Ginkgo was reported to protect liver cells from damage caused by cyclosporine in a test tube experiment.[13] A *Ginkgo biloba* extract partially reversed cyclosporine-induced reduced kidney function in a study of isolated rat kidneys.[14] Human trials have not studied the actions of ginkgo to prevent or reduce the side effects of cyclosporine.

St. John's wort (Hypericum perforatum)

Pharmacological research from Europe suggests that St. John's wort may reduce plasma levels of cyclosporine.[15]

Two case reports also describe heart transplant patients taking cyclosporine who showed signs of acute transplant rejection after taking St. John's wort extract.[16] In both cases, reduced plasma concentrations of cyclosporine were found. One report cites similar findings in three patients taking cyclosporine and St. John's wort together.[17] Finally, similar drops in cyclosporine blood levels were reported in 45 kidney or liver transplant patients who began taking St. John's wort.[18] Until more is known, people taking cyclosporine should avoid the use of St. John's wort.

Interactions with Foods and Other Compounds

Food

Food increases the absorption of cyclosporine.[19] A change in the timing of food and cyclosporine dosing may alter cyclosporine blood levels, requiring dose adjustment.

Grapefruit juice

In a randomized study of nine adults with cyclosporine-treated autoimmune diseases, grapefruit juice (5 ounces two times per day with cyclosporine, for ten days) caused a significant increase in cyclosporine blood levels compared with cyclosporine with water.[20] The rise in cyclosporine blood levels was associated with abdominal pain, lightheadedness, nausea, and tremor in one patient. Using grapefruit juice to reduce the amount of cyclosporine needed has not been sufficiently studied and cannot therefore be counted on to produce a predictable change in cyclosporine requirements. The same effects might be seen from eating grapefruit as from drinking its juice.

Red wine

Ingestion of red wine along with cyclosporine has been found to reduce blood levels of the drug.[21] Individuals taking cyclosporine should, therefore, not consume red wine at the same time as they take the drug. It is not known whether red wine consumed at a different time of the day would affect the availability of cyclosporine. Until more is known, it seems prudent for people taking cyclosporine to avoid red wine altogether.

Milk, apple juice, and orange juice

Mixing Sandimmune solution with room-temperature milk, chocolate milk, orange juice, or apple juice may improve its flavor.[22]

Mixing Neoral solution with room temperature orange or apple juice may improve its flavor, but combining it with milk makes an unpalatable mix.[23]

CYPROHEPTADINE

Common names: Periactin

Cyproheptadine is used to treat hay fever and skin rashes and eye inflammation caused by allergies. It is a type of drug called an antihistamine.

Summary of Interactions for Cyproheptadine

In some cases, an herb or supplement may appear in more than one category, which may seem contradictory. For clarification, read the full article for details about the summarized interactions.

Depletion or interference	None known
Side effect reduction/prevention	None known
Supportive interaction	None known
Reduced drug absorption/bioavailability	None known
Adverse interaction	None known

Interactions with Foods and Other Compounds
Alcohol
Drinking alcoholic beverages while taking cyproheptadine may enhance side effects common to both, such as drowsiness and dizziness.[1] Individuals taking cyproheptadine should avoid drinking alcohol, especially if staying alert is necessary.

DAKTACORT

Contains the following ingredients:
Hydrocortisone
Miconazole

DAPSONE

Common names: Avosulfon, DDS, Diaphenylsulfone

Dapsone is an **antibiotic** (page 19) effective against the bacteria that causes leprosy. It is an effective treatment for dermatitis herpetiformis, although it is unknown how dapsone helps with this disease. Dapsone is also used to prevent *Pneumocystis carinii* pneumonia in people infected with the human immunodeficiency virus (HIV).

Summary of Interactions for Dapsone

In some cases, an herb or supplement may appear in more than one category, which may seem contradictory. For clarification, read the full article for details about the summarized interactions.

✓	May be Beneficial: Depletion or interference	PABA* Vitamin K*
✓	May be Beneficial: Side effect reduction/prevention	*Bifidobacterium longum** *Lactobacillus acidophilus** *Lactobacillus casei** *Saccharomyces boulardii** *Saccharomyces cerevisiae** Vitamin C* Vitamin E* Vitamin K*
✓	May be Beneficial: Supportive interaction	*Saccharomyces boulardii**
	Reduced drug absorption/bioavailability	None known
	Adverse interaction	None known

Interactions with Dietary Supplements
PABA (para-aminobenzoic acid)
PABA is a compound found in foods that is considered by some to be a member of the B-vitamin family. PABA may interfere with the activity of dapsone.[1] Read supplement product labels for PABA content.

Probiotics
A common side effect of antibiotics is diarrhea, which may be caused by the elimination of beneficial bacteria normally found in the colon. Controlled studies have shown that taking probiotic microorganisms—such as *Lactobacillus casei*, *Lactobacillus acidophilus*, *Bifidobacterium longum*, or *Saccharomyces boulardii*—helps prevent antibiotic-induced diarrhea.[2]

The diarrhea experienced by some people who take antibiotics also might be due to an overgrowth of the bacterium *Clostridium difficile*, which causes a disease known as pseudomembranous colitis. Controlled studies have shown that supplementation with harmless yeast—such as *Saccharomyces boulardii*[3] or *Saccharomyces cerevisiae* (baker's or brewer's yeast)[4]—helps prevent recurrence of this infection. In one study, taking 500 mg of *Saccharomyces boulardii* twice daily enhanced the effectiveness of the antibiotic vancomycin in preventing recurrent clostridium infection.[5] Therefore, people taking antibiotics who later develop diarrhea might benefit from supplementing with saccharomyces organisms.

Treatment with antibiotics also commonly leads to an overgrowth of yeast *(Candida albicans)* in the vagina (candida vaginitis) and the intestines (sometimes referred to as "dysbiosis"). Controlled studies have shown that *Lactobacillus acidophilus* might prevent candida vaginitis.[6]

Vitamin E

In large amounts, dapsone causes oxidative damage to red blood cells. This damage may be reduced by using lower amounts of dapsone. Fifteen people who took dapsone for dermatitis herpetiformis were given 800 IU of vitamin E per day for four weeks, followed by four weeks with 1,000 mg of vitamin C per day, followed by four weeks of vitamin E and vitamin C together.[7] The authors reported only vitamin E therapy offered some protection against dapsone-induced hemolysis.

Vitamin K

Several cases of excessive bleeding have been reported in people who take antibiotics.[8, 9, 10, 11] This side effect may be the result of reduced vitamin K activity and/or reduced vitamin K production by bacteria in the colon. One study showed that people who had taken broad-spectrum antibiotics had lower liver concentrations of vitamin K_2 (menaquinone), though vitamin K_1 (phylloquinone) levels remained normal.[12] Several antibiotics appear to exert a strong effect on vitamin K activity, while others may not have any effect. Therefore, one should refer to a specific antibiotic for information on whether it interacts with vitamin K. Doctors of natural medicine sometimes recommend vitamin K supplementation to people taking antibiotics. Additional research is needed to determine whether the amount of vitamin K_1 found in some multivitamins is sufficient to prevent antibiotic-induced bleeding. Moreover, most multivitamins do not contain vitamin K.

DARVOCET N

Contains the following ingredients:
Acetaminophen (page 3)
Propoxyphene-N (page 224)

DARVON COMPOUND

Contains the following ingredients:
Aspirin (page 26)
Caffeine (page 44)
Propoxyphene (page 224)

DAYQUIL ALLERGY RELIEF

Contains the following ingredients:
Brompheniramine (page 43)
Phenylpropanolamine (page 218)

DEFEROXAMINE

Common names: Desferal

Deferoxamine is a drug that binds to some metals and carries them out of the body. It is used to treat acute iron intoxication, chronic iron overload, and aluminum accumulation in people with kidney failure.

Summary of Interactions for Deferoxamine
In some cases, an herb or supplement may appear in more than one category, which may seem contradictory. For clarification, read the full article for details about the summarized interactions.

⃠ Avoid: Adverse interaction	Iron
Depletion or interference	None known
Side effect reduction/prevention	None known
Supportive interaction	None known
Reduced drug absorption/bioavailability	None known

Interactions with Dietary Supplements
Iron
People treated with deferoxamine for dangerously high levels of iron should not take iron supplements, because iron exacerbates their condition, further increasing the need for the deferoxamine. They should read all labels carefully for iron content. All people treated with deferoxamine should consult their prescribing doctor before using any iron-containing products.

DERMOVATE-NN

Contains the following ingredients:
Clobetasol
Neomycin (page 187)
Nystatin (page 195)

DE WITT'S ANTACID POWDER

Contains the following ingredients:
Calcium
Kaolin
Magnesium
Peppermint oil
Sodium bicarbonate (page 240)

DE WITT'S ANTACID TABLETS

Contains the following ingredients:
Calcium
Magnesium
Peppermint oil

DETECLO

Contains the following ingredients:
Chlortetracycline
Demeclocycline
Tetracycline (page 253)

DEX-A-DIET PLUS VITAMIN C

Contains the following ingredients:
Phenylpropanolamine (page 218)
Vitamin C

DEXTROMETHORPHAN

Common names: Balminil DM, Benylin Non-drowsy for Dry Coughs, Broncho-Grippol-DM, Calmylin #1, Contac CoughCaps, Delsym, Koffex DM, Novahistex DM, Novahistine DM, Pertussin, Robitussin Dry Cough, Robitussin Cough Calmers, Robitussin Pediatric Cough, Sucrets Cough Control Formula, Triaminic DM, Vicks Vaposyrup Dry Cough, Vicks Formula 44

Combination drugs: Nyquil, Nyquil Hot Therapy Powder, Robitussin CF, Robitussin DM, Tylenol Cold, Tylenol Multi-Symptom Hot Medication

Dextromethorphan is a cough suppressant used for short-term treatment of nonproductive coughs. It is available in nonprescription products alone and in combination with other nonprescription drugs to treat symptoms of allergy, colds, and upper respiratory infections.

Summary of Interactions for Dextromethorphan
In some cases, an herb or supplement may appear in more than one category, which may seem contradictory. For clarification, read the full article for details about the summarized interactions.

Depletion or interference	None known
Side effect reduction/prevention	None known
Supportive interaction	None known
Reduced drug absorption/bioavailability	None known
Adverse interaction	None known

DIADEX GRAPEFRUIT DIET PLAN

Contains the following ingredients:
Grapefruit extract
Phenylpropanolamine (page 218)

DICLOFENAC

Common names: Acoflam, Apo-Diclo, Cataflam, Dexomon, Dicloflex, Diclomax, Diclotard MR, Diclotec, Diclovol, Diclozip, Digenac XL, Enzed, Flamatak MR, Flamrase, Flexotard MR, Isclofen, Lofensaid, Motifene, Novo-Difenac, Nu-Diclo, PMS-Diclofenac, Rhumalgan CR, Slofenac SR, Vifenal, Volraman, Volsaid Retard, Voltaren XR, Voltaren, Voltarol

Combination drug: Arthrotec

Diclofenac

Diclofenac is used in the treatment of osteoarthritis, rheumatoid arthritis, and ankylosing spondylitis. It is in a class of medications known as **nonsteroidal anti-inflammatory drugs** (page 193) (NSAIDs).

Summary of Interactions for Diclofenac

In some cases, an herb or supplement may appear in more than one category, which may seem contradictory. For clarification, read the full article for details about the summarized interactions.

✓	May be Beneficial: Depletion or interference	Calcium L-tryptophan* Lithium
✓	May be Beneficial: Supportive interaction	Stinging nettle
⊘	Avoid: Reduced drug absorption/ bioavailability	Trikatu Willow*
	Side effect reduction/prevention	None known
	Adverse interaction	None known

Interactions with Dietary Supplements

Calcium

Diclofenac decreases the amount of calcium lost in the urine,[1] which may help prevent bone loss in postmenopausal women.[2]

L-tryptophan

Diclofenac causes complex changes to L-tryptophan levels in the blood,[3] but the clinical implications of this are unknown. More research is needed to determine whether supplementation with L-tryptophan is a good idea for people taking diclofenac.

Lithium (page 157)

Lithium is a mineral that may be present in some supplements and is also used in large amounts to treat mood disorders such as manic-depression. Diclofenac may inhibit the excretion of lithium from the body, resulting in higher blood levels of the mineral.[4] Since minor changes in lithium blood levels can produce unwanted side effects, diclofenac should be used with caution in people taking lithium supplements.

Interactions with Herbs

Stinging nettle (Urtica dioica)

In a controlled human study, people who took stinging nettle with diclofenac obtained similar pain relief compared to people taking twice as much diclofenac with no stinging nettle.[5] More research is needed to deter-

mine whether people taking diclofenac might benefit from also taking stinging nettle.

Trikatu

Trikatu, an Ayurvedic herbal preparation that contains *Piper nigrum* (black pepper), *Piper longum* (Indian Long pepper), and *Zingiber officinale* (ginger), decreased both blood levels and the medicinal effect of diclofenac in a study in rabbits.[6]

Willow (Salix alba)

Willow bark contains salicin, which is related to **aspirin** (page 26). Both salicin and aspirin produce anti-inflammatory effects after they have been converted to salicylic acid in the body. The administration of aspirin to individuals taking diclofenac results in a significant reduction in blood levels of diclofenac.[7] Though there are no studies investigating interactions between willow bark and diclofenac, people taking the drug should avoid the herb until more information is available.

Interactions with Foods and Other Compounds

Food

Taking diclofenac with food may lower the maximum concentration of the drug in the blood and may delay, but not decrease, absorption.[8] NSAIDs such as diclofenac should be taken with a meal to reduce stomach irritation.

Smoking

Injury to the stomach caused by NSAIDs such as diclofenac can resolve naturally despite continued administration of the drug. However, the stomach lining of smokers is less likely to adapt to injury, leading to continued damage from the drug.[9]

Alcohol

Chronic consumption of alcohol can aggravate injury to the stomach and duodenal lining caused by diclofenac.[10] To prevent added injury, consumption of alcoholic beverages should be avoided in individuals taking diclofenac.

DICLOXACILLIN

Common names: Dycill, Dynapen

Dicloxacillin is used to treat infections of the lungs and skin caused by bacteria. It is in a class of **antibiotics** (page 19) known as penicillinase-resistant **penicillins** (page 211).

Summary of Interactions for Dicloxacillin

In some cases, an herb or supplement may appear in more than one category, which may seem contradictory. For clarification, read the full article for details about the summarized interactions.

✓ May be Beneficial: Depletion or interference	Vitamin K*
✓ May be Beneficial: Side effect reduction/prevention	Bifidobacterium longum* Lactobacillus acidophilus* Lactobacillus casei* Probiotics* Saccharomyces boulardii* Saccharomyces cerevisiae* Vitamin K*
✓ May be Beneficial: Supportive interaction	Saccharomyces boulardii*
Reduced drug absorption/bioavailability	None known
Adverse interaction	None known

Interactions with Dietary Supplements

Probiotics

A common side effect of antibiotics is diarrhea, which may be caused by the elimination of beneficial bacteria normally found in the colon. Controlled studies have shown that taking probiotic microorganisms—such as *Lactobacillus casei, Lactobacillus acidophilus, Bifidobacterium longum,* or *Saccharomyces boulardii*—helps prevent antibiotic-induced diarrhea.[1]

The diarrhea experienced by some people who take antibiotics also might be due to an overgrowth of the bacterium *Clostridium difficile,* which causes a disease known as pseudomembranous colitis. Controlled studies have shown that supplementation with harmless yeast—such as *Saccharomyces boulardii*[2] or *Saccharomyces cerevisiae* (baker's or brewer's yeast)[3]—helps prevent recurrence of this infection. In one study, taking 500 mg of *Saccharomyces boulardii* twice daily enhanced the effectiveness of the antibiotic vancomycin in preventing recurrent clostridium infection.[4] Therefore, people taking antibiotics who later develop diarrhea might benefit from supplementing with saccharomyces organisms.

Treatment with antibiotics also commonly leads to an overgrowth of yeast *(Candida albicans)* in the vagina (candida vaginitis) and the intestines (sometimes re-ferred to as "dysbiosis"). Controlled studies have shown that *Lactobacillus acidophilus* might prevent candida vaginitis.[5]

Vitamin K

Several cases of excessive bleeding have been reported in people who take antibiotics.[6, 7, 8, 9] This side effect may be the result of reduced vitamin K activity and/or reduced vitamin K production by bacteria in the colon. One study showed that people who had taken broad-spectrum antibiotics had lower liver concentrations of vitamin K_2 (menaquinone), though vitamin K_1 (phylloquinone) levels remained normal.[10] Several antibiotics appear to exert a strong effect on vitamin K activity, while others may not have any effect. Therefore, one should refer to a specific antibiotic for information on whether it interacts with vitamin K. Doctors of natural medicine sometimes recommend vitamin K supplementation to people taking antibiotics. Additional research is needed to determine whether the amount of vitamin K_1 found in some multivitamins is sufficient to prevent antibiotic-induced bleeding. Moreover, most multivitamins do not contain vitamin K.

Interactions with Foods and Other Compounds

Food

Taking dicloxacillin with food can reduce the absorption of the drug.[11] Therefore, dicloxacillin should be taken an hour before or two hours after a meal.

DICYCLOMINE

Common names: Antispas, Bemote, Bentylol, Bentyl, Bicyclomine, Di-Spaz, Dibent, Dicycloverine, Formulex, Lomine, Merbentyl, Spasmoject

Dicyclomine is an antispasmodic drug used to treat irritable bowel syndrome.

Summary of Interactions for Dicyclomine

In some cases, an herb or supplement may appear in more than one category, which may seem contradictory. For clarification, read the full article for details about the summarized interactions.

Depletion or interference	None known
Side effect reduction/prevention	None known
Supportive interaction	None known
Reduced drug absorption/bioavailability	None known
Adverse interaction	None known

Didanosine

DIDANOSINE

Common names: ddI, Dideoxyinosine, Videx

Didanosine is a drug that blocks reproduction of the human immunodeficiency virus (HIV). HIV is the virus that infects people causing acquired immunodeficiency syndrome (AIDS). Didanosine is used in combination with other drugs to treat HIV infection.

Summary of Interactions for Didanosine

In some cases, an herb or supplement may appear in more than one category, which may seem contradictory. For clarification, read the full article for details about the summarized interactions.

✓ May be Beneficial: Depletion or interference	Acetyl-L-carnitine
✓ May be Beneficial: Side effect reduction/prevention	Acetyl-L-carnitine Riboflavin
✓ May be Beneficial: Supportive interaction	Shiitake*
Reduced drug absorption/bioavailability	None known
Adverse interaction	None known

Interactions with Dietary Supplements

Riboflavin

Persons with AIDS have developed lactic acidosis and fatty liver while taking didanosine and other drugs in its class. Didanosine can inhibit crucial DNA-related riboflavin activity, which may be normalized by riboflavin supplementation. A 46-year-old woman with AIDS and lactic acidosis received a single dose of 50 mg of riboflavin, after which her laboratory tests returned to normal and her lactic acidosis was completely resolved.[1] More research is needed to confirm the value of riboflavin for preventing and treating this side effect.

Acetyl-L-carnitine

Severe peripheral neuropathy (painful sensations due to nerve damage in the hands and feet) often develops in people taking didanosine or other drugs in its class. People with peripheral neuropathy who were taking one of these drugs were found to be deficient in acetyl-L-carnitine.[2] In a preliminary trial, supplementation with 1,500 mg of acetyl-L-carnitine twice a day resulted in improvement in the neuropathy after six months in people taking didanosine or related drugs.[3]

Interactions with Herbs

Shiitake (Lentinas edodes)

Lentinan is a complex sugar found in shiitake mushrooms and is recognized as an immune modulator. In an early human trial, 88 HIV-infected people received didanosine (400 mg per day) plus a 2 mg lentinan injection per week.[4] Didanosine-lentinan combination therapy improved CD4 immune cell counts for a significantly longer period than didanosine alone. Lentinan is under investigation as an adjunct therapy to be used with didanosine for HIV infection.[5] Oral preparations of shiitake are available, but it is not known if they would be an effective treatment with didanosine for HIV infection.

Interactions with Foods and Other Compounds

Food

Didanosine should be taken on an empty stomach, one hour before or two hours after eating food.[6]

DIDRONEL PMO

Contains the following ingredients:
　　Calcium carbonate
　　Etidronate

DIGOXIN

Common names: Lanoxicaps, Lanoxin

Digoxin is a drug originally derived from the foxglove plant, *Digitalis lanata*. Digoxin is used primarily to improve the pumping ability of the heart in congestive heart failure (CHF). It is also used to help normalize some dysrhythmias (abnormal types of heartbeat).

Summary of Interactions for Digoxin

In some cases, an herb or supplement may appear in more than one category, which may seem contradictory. For clarification, read the full article for details about the summarized interactions.

✓ May be Beneficial: Depletion or interference	Magnesium Potassium (if levels are low)
✓ May be Beneficial: Side effect reduction/prevention	Magnesium Potassium

⊘ Avoid: Reduced drug absorption/ bioavailability	Senna* St. John's wort*
⊘ Avoid: Adverse interaction	Cascara* Digitalis Eleuthero* Licorice* Pleurisy root Sarsaparilla Senna*
ⓘ Check: Other	Alder buckthorn* Buckthorn* Hawthorn Potassium*
Supportive interaction	None known

Interactions with Dietary Supplements

Magnesium

People needing digoxin may have low levels of potassium or magnesium,[1] increasing the risk for digoxin toxicity. Digoxin therapy may increase magnesium elimination from the body.[2] People taking digoxin may benefit from magnesium supplementation.[3] Medical doctors do not commonly check magnesium status, and when they do, they typically use an insensitive indicator of magnesium status (serum or plasma levels). The red blood cell magnesium level may be a more sensitive indicator of magnesium status, although evidence is conflicting. It has been suggested that 300–500 mg of magnesium per day is a reasonable amount to supplement.[4]

Potassium

Medical doctors prescribing digoxin also check for potassium depletion and prescribe potassium supplements if needed. Potassium transport from the blood into cells is impaired by digoxin.[5] Although digoxin therapy does not usually lead to excess potassium in the blood (hyperkalemia), an overdose of digoxin could cause a potentially fatal hyperkalemia.[6] People taking digoxin should therefore avoid taking potassium supplements, or eating large quantities of fruit (e.g., bananas), unless directed to do so by their doctor. On the other hand, many people taking digoxin are also taking a **diuretic** (page 94); in these individuals, increased intake of potassium may be needed. These issues should be discussed with a doctor.

Interactions with Herbs

Alder buckthorn, buckthorn (Rhamnus catartica, Rhamnus frangula, Frangula alnus)

Use of buckthorn or alder buckthorn for more than ten days consecutively may cause a loss of electrolytes (espe-

cially the mineral potassium). Loss of potassium may increase the toxicity of digitalis-like medications with potentially fatal consequences.[7]

Cascara (Rhamnus purshiani cortex)

Loss of potassium due to cascara abuse could theoretically increase the effects of digoxin and other similar heart medications, with potentially fatal consequences. However, no cases of such an interaction have yet been reported.

Digitalis (Digitalis purpurea)

Digitalis refers to a group of plants commonly called foxglove that contain chemicals with actions and toxicities similar to digoxin. Digitalis was used as an herbal medicine to treat some heart conditions before the drug digoxin was available. Some doctors continue to use digitalis in the United States, and it is used as an herbal medicine in other countries as well. Due to the additive risk of toxicity, digitalis and digoxin should never be used together.

Eleuthero (Eleutherococcus senticosus)

People taking digoxin require regular monitoring of serum digoxin levels. In one report, addition of a product identified as Siberian ginseng to stable, therapeutic digoxin treatment was associated with dangerously high serum digoxin levels.[8] The patient never experienced symptoms of digoxin toxicity. Laboratory analysis found the product was free of digoxin-like compounds but the contents were not further identified. This report may reflect an interaction of eleuthero with the laboratory test to cause a falsely elevated reading, rather than actually increasing digoxin levels.

Hawthorn (Crataegus oxyacantha, Crataegus monogyna)

Hawthorn (leaf with flower) extract is approved in Germany to treat mild congestive heart failure.[9] Congestive heart failure is a serious medical condition that requires expert medical management rather than self-treatment. Due to the narrow safety index of digoxin, it makes sense for people taking digoxin for congestive heart failure to consult with their doctor before using hawthorn-containing products. Reports of hawthorn interacting with digitalis to enhance its effects have not been confirmed.

Licorice (Glycyrrhiza glabra)

Potassium deficiency increases the risk of digoxin toxicity. Excessive use of licorice plant or licorice plant products may cause the body to lose potassium.[10] Artificial licorice flavoring does not cause potassium loss. People taking digoxin should read product labels carefully for licorice plant ingredients.

Digoxin

Pleurisy root

As pleurisy root and other plants in the *Aesclepius* genus contain cardiac glycosides, it is best to avoid use of pleurisy root with heart medications such as digoxin.[11]

Sarsaparilla (Smilax spp.)

Sarsaparilla may increase the absorption of digitalis and bismuth, increasing the chance of toxicity.[12]

Senna (Cassia senna, Cassia angustifolia)

Bisacodyl (page 39), a laxative similar in action to senna, given with digoxin decreased serum digoxin levels in healthy volunteers compared with digoxin alone.[13] In patients taking digoxin, laxative use was also associated with decreased digoxin levels.[14] In addition, concern has been expressed that overuse or misuse of senna may deplete potassium levels and increase both digoxin activity and risk of toxicity.[15] However, overuse of senna could also decrease digoxin activity because, as noted, laxatives can decrease the levels of the drug.

St. John's wort (Hypericum perforatum)

One preliminary trial has suggested that St. John's wort may reduce blood levels of digoxin.[16] In this study, healthy volunteers took digoxin for five days, after which they added 900 mg per day of St. John's wort while continuing the daily digoxin. A normal blood level of digoxin was reached after five days of taking the drug, but this level dropped significantly when St. John's wort was added. This may have occurred because certain chemicals found in St. John's wort activate liver enzymes that are involved in the elimination of some drugs.[17, 18] Until more is known, people taking digoxin should avoid St. John's wort.

Interactions with Foods and Other Compounds

Food

Many foods may interfere with the absorption of digoxin. To avoid this problem, people should take digoxin one hour before or two hours after eating food.[19] People taking digoxin should consult their prescribing doctor or pharmacist if they have questions regarding this interaction.

DIJEX

Contains the following ingredients:
    Aluminium
    Magnesium

DILTIAZEM

Common names: Adizem-SR, Adizem-XL, Adizem, Alti-Diltiazem, Angiozem CR, Angiozem, Angitil SR, Angitil XL, Apo-Diltiaz, Calazem, Calcicard CR, Cardizem, Dilacor XR, Dilcardia SR, Diltia XT, Dilzem SR, Dilzem XL, Dilzem, Gen-Diltiazem, Novo-Diltiazem, Nu-Diltiaz, Optil SR, Optil XL, Optil, Slozem, Tiazac, Tildiem LA, Tildiem Retard, Tildiem, Tildiem, Viazem XL, Zemtard, Zemtard

Diltiazem is a **calcium-channel blocker** (page 46) used to treat angina pectoris, heart arrhythmias, and high blood pressure.

Summary of Interactions for Diltiazem

In some cases, an herb or supplement may appear in more than one category, which may seem contradictory. For clarification, read the full article for details about the summarized interactions.

⊘ Avoid: Reduced drug absorption/ bioavailability	DHEA
Depletion or interference	None known
Side effect reduction/prevention	None known
Supportive interaction	None known
Adverse interaction	None known

Interactions with Dietary Supplements

Dehydroepiandrosterone (DHEA)

Diltiazem has been shown to raise blood levels of DHEA and DHEA-sulfate in insulin-resistant, obese men with high blood pressure.[1]

Interactions with Herbs

Pleurisy root

As pleurisy root and other plants in the *Aesclepius* genus contain cardiac glycosides, it is best to avoid use of pleurisy root with heart medications such as calcium-channel blockers.[2]

Interactions with Foods and Other Compounds

Food

Diltiazem may be taken with or without food.[3] Sustained-release diltiazem products should be swallowed whole, without opening, crushing, or chewing.[4]

In a study of healthy volunteers, ingestion of grapefruit juice at the same time as diltiazem resulted in higher blood levels of the drug than when it was taken with water.[5] Studies with certain other medications suggest that grapefruit juice may affect drug availability, even if it is consumed at a different time of the day. Therefore, individuals taking diltiazem should probably avoid grapefruit and grapefruit juice.

DIMENHYDRINATE

Common names: Apo-Dimenhydrinate, Dramamine, Gravol, Hydrate, Marmine, Nico-Vert, Novo-Dimenate, PMS-Dimenhydrinate, Travamine, Travel Aid, Travel Tabs, Triptone

Dimenhydrinate is a combination of two drugs, diphenhydramine and chlorotheophylline. Dimenhydrinate is used to prevent and treat nausea, vomiting, dizziness, and motion sickness.

Summary of Interactions for Dimenhydrinate

In some cases, an herb or supplement may appear in more than one category, which may seem contradictory. For clarification, read the full article for details about the summarized interactions.

⊘ Avoid: Adverse interaction	Henbane*
Depletion or interference	None known
Side effect reduction/prevention	None known
Supportive interaction	None known
Reduced drug absorption/bioavailability	None known

Interactions with Herbs

Henbane (Hyoscyamus niger)

Antihistamines, including dimenhydrinate, can cause "anticholinergic" side effects such as dryness of mouth and heart palpitations. Henbane also has anticholinergic activity and side effects. Therefore, use with dimenhydrinate could increase the risk of anticholinergic side effects,[1] though apparently no interactions have yet been reported with dimenhydrinate and henbane. Henbane should not be taken except by prescription from a physician trained in its use, as it is extremely toxic.

Interactions with Foods and Other Compounds

Alcohol

Dimenhydrinate causes drowsiness.[2] Alcohol may intensify this effect and increase the risk of accidental injury.[3] To prevent problems, people taking dimenhydrinate or dimenhydrinate-containing products should avoid alcohol.

DIMETAPP

Contains the following ingredients:
  Brompheniramine (page 43)
  Phenylpropanolamine (page 218)

DIPHENHYDRAMINE

Common names: Allerdryl, Allernix, Banophen, Benadryl, Benylin, Calmex, Diphedryl, Insomal, Medinex, PMS-Diphenhydramine, Scheinpharm Diphenhydramine, Simply Sleep, Sleep Aid, Unisom

Combination drugs: Excedrin PM, Tylenol Allergy Sinus, Tylenol Flu NightTime Maximum Strength Powder, Tylenol PM

Diphenhydramine is an antihistamine used to relieve allergic rhinitis (seasonal allergy) symptoms including sneezing, runny nose, itching, and watery eyes and to relieve itching and swelling associated with uncomplicated allergic skin reactions. It is also used as a short-term sleep aid, to control coughs due to colds or allergy, and to prevent/treat motion sickness. Diphenhydramine is available in nonprescription products alone and in combination with other nonprescription drugs, to treat symptoms of allergy, colds, and upper respiratory infections.

Summary of Interactions for Diphenhydramine

In some cases, an herb or supplement may appear in more than one category, which may seem contradictory. For clarification, read the full article for details about the summarized interactions.

⊘ Avoid: Adverse interaction	Henbane*
Depletion or interference	None known
Side effect reduction/prevention	None known
Supportive interaction	None known
Reduced drug absorption/bioavailability	None known

Interactions with Herbs

Henbane (Hyoscyamus niger)

Antihistamines, including diphenhydramine, can cause "anticholinergic" side effects such as dryness of mouth and heart palpitations. Henbane also has anticholinergic activity and side effects. Therefore, use with diphenhydramine could increase the risk of anticholinergic side effects,[1] though apparently no interactions have yet been reported with diphenhydramine and henbane. Henbane should not be taken except by prescription from a physician trained in its use, as it is extremely toxic.

Interactions with Foods and Other Compounds
Alcohol
Diphenhydramine causes drowsiness.[2] Alcohol may intensify this effect and increase the risk of accidental injury.[3] To prevent problems, people taking diphenhydramine or diphenhydramine-containing products should avoid alcohol.

DIPROSALIC

Contains the following ingredients:
   Betamethasone
   Salicylic acid

DIPYRIDAMOLE

Common names: Apo-Dipyridamole FC, Cerebrovase, Modaplate, Novo-Dipiradol, Permole, Persantine, Persantin

Dipyridamole prevents platelet clumping and is used with **warfarin** (page 281) (Coumadin) to prevent blood clots from forming after heart valve replacement. It may be used alone or combined with **aspirin** (page 26) to prevent strokes.

Summary of Interactions for Dipyridamole
In some cases, an herb or supplement may appear in more than one category, which may seem contradictory. For clarification, read the full article for details about the summarized interactions.

✓ May be Beneficial: Depletion or interference	Iron*
✓ May be Beneficial: Supportive interaction	Garlic*
ⓘ Check: Other	**Caffeine** (page 44)
Side effect reduction/prevention	None known
Reduced drug absorption/bioavailability	None known
Adverse interaction	None known

Interactions with Dietary Supplements
Iron
Some studies suggest the taking of too much iron by individuals who are not iron deficient can result in tissue damage that may contribute to heart disease.[1] Test tube studies have shown dipyridamole blocks platelet clumping caused by iron,[2] which might reduce the damage caused by this mineral. Controlled human studies are needed to test this possibility.

Interactions with Herbs
Garlic (Allium sativa)
A test tube study has shown ajoene, a compound found in garlic that prevents platelet clumping, enhances the beneficial action of dipyridamole on human platelets.[3] Controlled research is needed to determine whether taking garlic supplements together with dipyridamole might enhance the effectiveness of either compound taken alone.

Interactions with Foods and Other Compounds
*Coffee and **caffeine** (page 44)*
Taking dipyridamole can cause a reduction in the amount of oxygen delivered to the heart, resulting in a rare side effect known as angina pectoris. Because dipyridamole has this effect, it has sometimes been used in heart stress tests. One person who consumed coffee prior to the test failed to experience the expected reduction in blood flow caused by dipyridamole.[4] Controlled studies are needed to determine whether consumption of beverages containing caffeine might reduce the likelihood of developing angina from the drug.

DISTALGESIC

Contains the following ingredients:
   Acetaminophen (page 3)
   Dextropropoxyphene

DIURETICS

Common names: Acetazolamide, Carbonic Anhydrase Inhibitors, Diamox, Mannitol, Methazolamide, Neptazane

Diuretics are a family of drugs that promote urination. They are used to reduce water accumulation or edema associated with heart failure, cirrhosis, and **corticosteroid** (page 77) therapy, as well as to treat high blood pressure. Diuretics are classified as "potassium-depleting" if they cause loss of potassium in the urine, or "potassium-sparing" if they cause retention of potassium.

Interactions involving diuretics in general are described on this page. For interactions involving a category of diuretics or a specific drug, refer to the highlighted items below.

Carbonic anhydrase inhibitors, Potassium-Depleting
- Acetazolamide (Diamox)
- Dichlorphenamide (Daranide)
- Methazolamide (Neptazane)

Thiazide Diuretics *(page 258), Potassium-Depleting*
- Bendroflumethiazide (Naturetin)
- Benzthiazide (Exna)
- Chlorothiazide (Diuril)
- Chlorthalidone (Hygroton)
- Hydrochlorothiazide (Esidrix, HydroDiuril, Microzide™)
- Hydroflumethiazide (Diucardin)
- Indapamide (Lozol)
- Methyclothiazide (Enduron)
- Metolazone (Zaroxolyn, Mykrox)
- Polythiazide (Renese)
- Quinethazone (Hydromox)
- Trichlormethiazide (Naqua)

Loop diuretics *(page 159), Potassium-Depleting*
- Bumetanide (Bumex)
- Ethacrynic acid (Edecrin)
- Furosemide (Lasix)
- Torsemide (Demadex)

Potassium-sparing
- **Amiloride** (page 11) (Midamor)
- Amiloride and Hydrochlorothiazide (Moduretic)
- **Spironolactone** (page 243) (Aldactone)
- Spironolactone and Hydrochlorothiazide (Aldactazide)
- **Triamterene** (page 268) (Dyrenium)
- Triamterene and Hydrochlorothiazide (Dyazide, Maxzide)

Summary of Interactions for Diuretics

In some cases, an herb or supplement may appear in more than one category, which may seem contradictory. For clarification, read the full article for details about the summarized interactions.

✓ May be Beneficial: Depletion or interference	Folic acid
⊘ Avoid: Adverse interaction	Alder buckthorn Buckthorn

Side effect reduction/prevention	None known
Supportive interaction	None known
Reduced drug absorption/bioavailability	None known

Interactions common to many, if not all, Diuretics are described in this article. Interactions reported for only one or several drugs in this class may not be listed in this article. Some drugs listed in this article are linked to articles specific to that respective drug; please refer to those individual drug articles. The information in this article may not necessarily apply to drugs in this class for which no separate article exists. If you are taking a Diuretic for which no separate article exists, talk with your doctor or pharmacist.

Interactions with Dietary Supplements
Folic acid
One study showed that people taking diuretics for more than six months had dramatically lower blood levels of folic acid and higher levels of homocysteine compared with individuals not taking diuretics.[1] Homocysteine, a toxic amino acid by-product, has been associated with atherosclerosis. Until further information is available, people taking diuretics for longer than six months should probably supplement with folic acid.

Interactions with Herbs
Alder buckthorn, buckthorn (Rhamnus catartica, Rhamnus frangula, Frangula alnus)
Use buckthorn or alder buckthorn for more than ten days consecutively may cause a loss of electrolytes (especially the mineral potassium). Medications that also cause potassium loss, such as some diuretics, should be used with caution when taking buckthorn or alder buckthorn.[2]

DOCETAXEL

Common names: Taxotere

Docetaxel is a semisynthetic **chemotherapy** (page 54) drug made from an extract of needles of the yew plant. It is used to treat people with some types of late-stage cancer.

Note: Many of the interactions described below, in the text and in the Summary of Interactions, have been reported only for specific chemotherapeutic drugs, and may not apply to other chemotherapeutic drugs. There are many unknowns concerning interactions of nutrients, herbs, and chemotherapy drugs. People receiving chemotherapy who wish to supplement with vitamins, minerals, herbs, or other natural substances should always consult a physician.

Summary of Interactions for Docetaxel

In some cases, an herb or supplement may appear in more than one category, which may seem contradictory. For clarification, read the full article for details about the summarized interactions.

✓ May be Beneficial: Side effect reduction/prevention	Beta-carotene* (mouth sores) Chamomile* (mouth sores) Eleuthero* (see text) Ginger* (nausea) Glutamine* (mouth sores) Melatonin* (see text) N-acetyl cysteine* (NAC) Spleen peptide extract* (see text) Thymus peptides* (see text) Vitamin B$_6$* Vitamin E*, topical (mouth sores) Zinc* (taste alterations)
ⓘ Check: Other	Echinacea* Multivitamin-mineral* Vitamin A* Vitamin C*
Depletion or interference	None known
Supportive interaction	None known
Reduced drug absorption/bioavailability	None known
Adverse interaction	None known

Interactions with Dietary Supplements

Antioxidants

Chemotherapy can injure cancer cells by creating oxidative damage. As a result, some oncologists recommend that patients avoid supplementing antioxidants if they are undergoing chemotherapy. Limited test tube research occasionally does support the idea that an antioxidant can interfere with oxidative damage to cancer

cells.[1] However, most scientific research does not support this supposition.

A modified form of vitamin A has been reported to work synergistically with chemotherapy in test tube research.[2] Vitamin C appears to increase the effectiveness of chemotherapy in animals[3] and with human breast cancer cells in test tube research.[4] In a double-blind study, Japanese researchers found that the combination of vitamin E, vitamin C, and N-acetyl cysteine (NAC)—all antioxidants—protected against chemotherapy-induced heart damage without interfering with the action of the chemotherapy.[5]

A comprehensive review of antioxidants and chemotherapy leaves open the question of whether supplemental antioxidants definitely help people with chemotherapy side effects, but it clearly shows that antioxidants need not be avoided for fear that the actions of chemotherapy are interfered with.[6] Although research remains incomplete, the idea that people taking chemotherapy should avoid antioxidants is not supported by scientific research.

A new formulation of selenium (Seleno-Kappacarrageenan) was found to reduce kidney damage and white blood cell–lowering effects of **cisplatin** (page 64) in one human study. However, the level used in this study (4,000 mcg per day) is potentially toxic and should only be used under the supervision of a doctor.[7]

Glutathione, the main antioxidant found within cells, is frequently depleted in individuals on chemotherapy and/or radiation. Preliminary studies have found that intravenously injected glutathione may decrease some of the adverse effects of chemotherapy and radiation, such as diarrhea.[8]

Glutamine

Though cancer cells use glutamine as a fuel source, studies in humans have not found that glutamine stimulates growth of cancers in people taking chemotherapy.[9, 10] In fact, animal studies show that glutamine may actually decrease tumor growth while increasing susceptibility of cancer cells to radiation and chemotherapy,[11, 12] though such effects have not yet been studied in humans.

Glutamine has successfully reduced chemotherapy-induced mouth sores. In one trial, people were given 4 grams of glutamine in an oral rinse, which was swished around the mouth and then swallowed twice per day.[13] Thirteen of fourteen people in the study had fewer days with mouth sores as a result. These excellent results have been duplicated in some,[14] but not all[15] double-blind research. In another study, patients receiving high-dose **paclitaxel** (page 205) and melphalan had significantly fewer episodes of oral ulcers and bleeding when they took 6 grams of glutamine four times daily along with the chemotherapy.[16]

One double-blind trial suggested that 6 grams of glutamine taken three times per day can decrease diarrhea caused by chemotherapy.[17] However, other studies using higher amounts or intravenous glutamine have not reported this effect.[18, 19]

Intravenous use of glutamine in people undergoing bone marrow transplants, a procedure sometimes used to allow very high amounts of chemotherapy to be used, has led to reduced hospital stays, leading to a savings of over $21,000 for each patient given glutamine.[20]

Melatonin

High amounts of melatonin have been combined with a variety of chemotherapy drugs to reduce their side effects or improve drug efficacy. One study gave melatonin at night in combination with the drug triptorelin to men with metastatic prostate cancer.[21] All of these men had previously become unresponsive to triptorelin. The combination decreased PSA levels—a marker of prostate cancer progression—in eight of fourteen patients, decreased some side effects of triptorelin, and helped nine of fourteen to live longer than one year. The outcome of this preliminary study suggests that melatonin may improve the efficacy of triptorelin even after the drug has apparently lost effectiveness.

N-acetyl cysteine (NAC)

NAC, an amino acid–like supplement that possesses antioxidant activity, has been used in four human studies to decrease the kidney and bladder toxicity of the chemotherapy drug ifosfamide.[22, 23, 24, 25] These studies used 1–2 grams NAC four times per day. There was no sign that NAC interfered with the efficacy of ifosfamide in any of these studies. Intakes of NAC over 4 grams per day may cause nausea and vomiting.

The newer anti-nausea drugs prescribed for people taking chemotherapy lead to greatly reduced nausea and vomiting for most people. Nonetheless, these drugs often do not totally eliminate all nausea. Natural substances used to reduce nausea should not be used instead of prescription anti-nausea drugs. Rather, under the guidance of a doctor, they should be added to those drugs if needed. At least one trial suggests that NAC, at 1,800 mg per day may reduce nausea and vomiting caused by chemotherapy.[26]

Spleen extract

Patients with inoperable head and neck cancer were treated with a spleen peptide preparation (Polyerga) in a double-blind trial during chemotherapy with cisplatin and 5-FU.[27] The spleen preparation had a significant stabilizing effect on certain white blood cells. People taking it also experienced stabilized body weight and a reduction in the fatigue and inertia that usually accompany this combination of chemotherapy agents.

Beta-carotene and vitamin E

Chemotherapy frequently causes mouth sores. In one trial, people were given approximately 400,000 IU of beta-carotene per day for three weeks and then 125,000 IU per day for an additional four weeks.[28] Those taking beta-carotene still suffered mouth sores, but the mouth sores developed later and tended to be less severe than mouth sores that formed in people receiving the same chemotherapy without beta-carotene.

In a study of chemotherapy-induced mouth sores, six of nine patients who applied vitamin E directly to their mouth sores had complete resolution of the sores compared with one of nine patients who applied placebo.[29] Others have confirmed the potential for vitamin E to help people with chemotherapy-induced mouth sores.[30] Applying vitamin E only once per day was helpful to only some groups of patients in another trial,[31] and not all studies have found vitamin E to be effective.[32] Until more is known, if vitamin E is used in an attempt to reduce chemotherapy-induced mouth sores, it should be applied topically twice per day and should probably be in the tocopherol (versus tocopheryl) form.

Vitamin A

A controlled French trial reported that when postmenopausal late-stage breast cancer patients were given very large amounts of vitamin A (350,000–500,000 IU per day) along with chemotherapy, remission rates were significantly better than when the chemotherapy was not accompanied by vitamin A.[33] Similar results were not found in premenopausal women. The large amounts of vitamin A used in the study are toxic and require clinical supervision.

Vitamin B$_6$

Docetaxel may cause a reddening, swelling, and pain in hands and feet. Two cases have been reported of people suffering these drug-induced symptoms and responding to 50 mg of vitamin B$_6$ given three times per day.[34] Symptoms began to resolve in 12 to 24 hours and continued to improve for several weeks.

Docetaxel

Zinc

Irradiation treatment, especially of head and neck cancers, frequently results in changes to normal taste sensation.[35, 36] Zinc supplementation may be protective against taste alterations caused or exacerbated by irradiation. A double-blind trial found that 45 mg of zinc sulfate three times daily reduced the alteration of taste sensation during radiation treatment and led to significantly greater recovery of taste sensation after treatment was concluded.[37]

Multivitamin-mineral

Many chemotherapy drugs can cause diarrhea, lack of appetite, vomiting, and damage to the gastrointestinal tract. Recent anti-nausea prescription medications are often effective. Nonetheless, nutritional deficiencies still occur.[38] It makes sense for people undergoing chemotherapy to take a high-potency multivitamin-mineral to protect against deficiencies.

Taurine

Taurine has been shown to be depleted in people taking chemotherapy.[39] It remains unclear how important this effect is or if people taking chemotherapy should take taurine supplements.

Thymus peptides

Peptides or short proteins derived from the thymus gland, an important immune organ, have been used in conjunction with chemotherapy drugs for people with cancer. One study using thymosin fraction V in combination with chemotherapy, compared with chemotherapy alone, found significantly longer survival times in the thymosin fraction V group.[40] A related substance, thymostimulin, decreased some side effects of chemotherapy and increased survival time compared with chemotherapy alone.[41] A third product, thymic extract TP1, was shown to improve immune function in people treated with chemotherapy compared with effects of chemotherapy alone.[42] Thymic peptides need to be administered by injection. People interested in their combined use with chemotherapy should consult a doctor.

Interactions with Herbs

Echinacea (Echinacea purpurea, Echinacea angustifolia)

Echinacea is a popular immune-boosting herb that has been investigated for use with chemotherapy. One study investigated the actions of **cyclophosphamide** (page 79), echinacea, and thymus gland extracts to treat advanced cancer patients. Although small and uncontrolled, this trial suggested that the combination modestly extended the life span of some patients with

inoperable cancers.[43] Signs of restoration of immune function were seen in these patients.

Eleuthero (Eleutherococcus senticosus)

Russian research has looked at using eleuthero with chemotherapy. One study of patients with melanoma found that chemotherapy was less toxic when eleuthero was given simultaneously. Similarly, women with inoperable breast cancer given eleuthero were reported to tolerate more chemotherapy.[44] Eleuthero treatment was also associated with improved immune function in women with breast cancer treated with chemotherapy and radiation.[45]

Milk thistle (Silybum marianum)

Milk thistle's major flavonoids, known collectively as silymarin, have shown synergistic actions with the chemotherapy drugs **cisplatin** (page 64) and **doxorubicin** (page 100) (Adriamycin) in test tubes.[46] Silymarin also offsets the kidney toxicity of cisplatin in animals.[47] Silymarin has not yet been studied in humans treated with cisplatin. There is some evidence that silymarin may not interfere with some chemotherapy in humans with cancer.[48]

Ginger (Zingiber officinale)

Ginger can be helpful in alleviating nausea and vomiting caused by chemotherapy.[49, 50] Ginger, as tablets, capsules, or liquid herbal extracts, can be taken in 500 mg amounts every two or three hours, for a total of 1 gram per day.

German chamomile (Matricaria recutita)

A liquid preparation of German chamomile has been shown to reduce the incidence of mouth sores in people receiving radiation and systemic chemotherapy treatment in an uncontrolled study. [51]

PSK (Coriolus versicolor)

The mushroom *Coriolus versicolor* contains an immune-stimulating substance called polysaccharide krestin, or PSK. PSK has been shown in several studies to help cancer patients undergoing chemotherapy. One study involved women with estrogen receptor-negative breast cancer. PSK combined with chemotherapy significantly prolonged survival time compared with chemotherapy alone.[52] Another study followed women with breast cancer who were given chemotherapy with or without PSK. The PSK-plus-chemotherapy group had a 25% better chance of survival after ten years compared with those taking chemotherapy without PSK.[53] Another study investigated people who had surgically removed colon cancer. They were given chemotherapy with or without PSK. Those given PSK had a longer disease-free period and longer survival time.[54] Three grams of PSK were taken orally each day in these studies.

Although PSK is rarely available in the United States, hot-water extract products made from *Coriolus versicolor* mushrooms are available. These products may have activity related to that of PSK, but their use with chemotherapy has not been studied.

Interactions with Foods and Other Compounds
Fruit drinks
Often, people who undergo chemotherapy develop aversions to certain foods, sometimes making it permanently difficult to eat those foods. Exposing people to what researchers have called a "scapegoat stimulus" just before the administration of chemotherapy can direct the food aversion to the "scapegoat" food instead of more important parts of the diet. In one trial, fruit drinks administered just before chemotherapy were most effective in protecting against aversions to other foods.[55]

DOCUSATE

Common names: Colace, Dioctyl Sodium Sulphosuccinate, Dioctyl, Docusol, PMS-Docusate Sodium, Selax, Soflax

Docusate, which is available without a prescription, is used to treat constipation and is in a class of laxatives known as stool softeners.

Summary of Interactions for Docusate
In some cases, an herb or supplement may appear in more than one category, which may seem contradictory. For clarification, read the full article for details about the summarized interactions.

✓ May be Beneficial: Depletion or interference	Magnesium* Potassium*
Side effect reduction/prevention	None known
Supportive interaction	None known
Reduced drug absorption/bioavailability	None known
Adverse interaction	None known

Interactions with Dietary Supplements
Magnesium
A woman and her newborn infant experienced low blood levels of magnesium, which was possibly due to chronic use of docusate throughout and after pregnancy.[1] Controlled research is necessary to determine whether people taking docusate for long periods of time need to supplement magnesium.

Potassium
Taking docusate increases the amount of potassium excreted from the body in the stool.[2] Whether people taking docusate for long periods of time need to increase their intake of potassium is unknown.

DONEPEZIL

Common names: Aricept

Donepezil is used to treat memory loss associated with Alzheimer's disease.

Summary of Interactions for Donepezil
In some cases, an herb or supplement may appear in more than one category, which may seem contradictory. For clarification, read the full article for details about the summarized interactions.

⊘ Avoid: Adverse interaction	Huperzine-A*
Depletion or interference	None known
Side effect reduction/prevention	None known
Supportive interaction	None known
Reduced drug absorption/bioavailability	None known

Interactions with Dietary Supplements
Huperzine-A
Further studies are needed to determine the long-term safety of huperizine A. Until more is known about it's actions in the body, it is best to avoid using it together with donepezil, which also prevents the breakdown of acetylcholine.

DORZOLAMIDE

Common names: Trusopt

Combination drug: Cosopt

Dorzolamide is a member of the carbonic anhydrase inhibitor family of drugs used to reduce pressure in the eyes of people with ocular hypertension or open-angle glaucoma. It is available in prescription eye drops alone a combination product.

Dorzolamide

Summary of Interactions for Dorzolamide

In some cases, an herb or supplement may appear in more than one category, which may seem contradictory. For clarification, read the full article for details about the summarized interactions.

Depletion or interference	None known
Side effect reduction/prevention	None known
Supportive interaction	None known
Reduced drug absorption/bioavailability	None known
Adverse interaction	None known

DOXAZOSIN

Common names: Cardura XL, Cardura

Doxazosin is a member of the alpha blocker family of drugs used to lower blood pressure in people with hypertension. Doxazosin is also used to treat symptoms of benign prostatic hyperplasia (BPH).

Summary of Interactions for Doxazosin

In some cases, an herb or supplement may appear in more than one category, which may seem contradictory. For clarification, read the full article for details about the summarized interactions.

Depletion or interference	None known
Side effect reduction/prevention	None known
Supportive interaction	None known
Reduced drug absorption/bioavailability	None known
Adverse interaction	None known

DOXORUBICIN

Common names: Adriamycin, Rubex

Doxorubicin is a **chemotherapy** (page 54) drug used primarily to treat people with cancer.

Summary of Interactions for Doxorubicin

In some cases, an herb or supplement may appear in more than one category, which may seem contradictory. For clarification, read the full article for details about the summarized interactions.

✓ May be Beneficial: Depletion or interference	Riboflavin*
✓ May be Beneficial: Side effect reduction/prevention	Carnitine* Coenzyme Q$_{10}$ Melatonin Vitamin C* Vitamin E*
✓ May be Beneficial: Supportive interaction	Melatonin
ⓘ Check: Other	N-acetyl cysteine (NAC)
Reduced drug absorption/bioavailability	None known
Adverse interaction	None known

Interactions with Dietary Supplements

Carnitine
Animal research suggests carnitine may prevent doxorubicin's toxicity.[1]

Coenzyme Q$_{10}$
Pretreating people with the antioxidant coenzyme Q$_{10}$ before administration of doxorubicin has reduced cardiac toxicity[2]—an action also reported in animals.[3] Some doctors recommend 100 mg per day.

Melatonin
Melatonin supplementation (20 mg per day) has decreased toxicity and improved effectiveness of chemotherapy with doxorubicin.[4]

N-acetyl cysteine (NAC)
The antioxidant supplement N-acetyl cysteine (NAC) has protected animals from the cardiotoxicity of doxorubicin,[5] although human research has not been able to confirm these results.[6] Most doctors do not yet suggest NAC for people taking doxorubicin.

Riboflavin
Animal research suggests doxorubicin may deplete riboflavin and that riboflavin deficiency promotes doxorubicin toxicity.[7]

Vitamin C
The antioxidant vitamin C has protected against cardiotoxicity (damage to the heart) of doxorubicin in an animal study.[8] In this trial, vitamin C significantly increased the life expectancy of mice and guinea pigs without interfering with anticancer action of the drug. Despite the lack of human data, some doctors recommend that patients taking doxorubicin supplement at least 1 gram of vitamin C per day.

Vitamin E

Animal studies show that the antioxidant activity of vitamin E protects against doxorubicin-induced cardiotoxicity.[9, 10] Test tube evidence suggests that vitamin E might also enhance the anticancer action of the drug.[11] Human trials exploring the cardioprotective action of vitamin E in people taking doxorubicin remain inconclusive; however, some evidence suggests that vitamin E may allow for higher drug doses without increasing toxicity.[12]

Anecdotal reports indicate that very high (1,600 IU) amounts of vitamin E may reduce the amount of hair loss accompanying use of doxorubicin.[13] However, while protection against hair loss was confirmed in a rabbit study, human research has not found this to be true.[14]

DOXYCYCLINE

Common names: Alti-Doxycycline, Apo-Doxy, Atridox, Cyclodox, Demix, Doryx, Doxycin, Doxylar, Doxytec, Doxy, Monodox, Novo-Doxylin, Nu-Doxycycline, Periostat, Ramysis, Vibramycin-D, Vibramycin

Doxycycline is a **tetracycline** (page 253)-like **antibiotic** (page 19). Doxycycline is used to treat a wide variety of infections and to prevent traveler's diarrhea.

Summary of Interactions for Doxycycline

In some cases, an herb or supplement may appear in more than one category, which may seem contradictory. For clarification, read the full article for details about the summarized interactions.

✓	May be Beneficial: Depletion or interference	Vitamin K*
✓	May be Beneficial: Side effect reduction/prevention	*Bifidobacterium longum** *Lactobacillus acidophilus** *Lactobacillus casei** Probiotics* *Saccharomyces boulardii** *Saccharomyces cerevisiae** Vitamin K*
✓	May be Beneficial: Supportive interaction	*Saccharomyces boulardii**
⊘	Avoid: Reduced drug absorption/ bioavailability	Minerals* (calcium, iron, magnesium, zinc)
⊘	Avoid: Adverse interaction	Milk or other dairy products
ⓘ	Check: Other	Berberine-containing herbs such as goldenseal, barberry, and Oregon grape

Interactions with Dietary Supplements

Berberine-containing herbs

Berberine is a chemical extracted from goldenseal *(Hydrastis canadensis)*, barberry *(Berberis vulgaris)*, and Oregon grape *(Berberis aquifolium)*, which has antibacterial activity. However, one double-blind study found that 100 mg berberine given with **tetracycline** (page 253) (a drug closely related to doxycycline) reduced the efficacy of tetracycline in people with cholera.[1] In that trial, berberine may have decreased tetracycline absorption. Another double-blind trial found that berberine neither improved nor interfered with tetracycline effectiveness in cholera patients.[2] Therefore, it remains unclear whether a significant interaction between berberine-containing herbs and doxycycline and related drugs exists.

Minerals

Many minerals can decrease the absorption and reduce effectiveness of doxycycline, including calcium, magnesium, iron, zinc, and others.[3] To avoid these interactions, doxycycline should be taken two hours before or two hours after dairy products (high in calcium) and mineral-containing **antacids** (page 18) or supplements.

Probiotics

A common side effect of antibiotics is diarrhea, which may be caused by the elimination of beneficial bacteria normally found in the colon. Controlled studies have shown that taking probiotic microorganisms—such as *Lactobacillus casei, Lactobacillus acidophilus, Bifidobacterium longum,* or *Saccharomyces boulardii*—helps prevent antibiotic-induced diarrhea.[4]

The diarrhea experienced by some people who take antibiotics also might be due to an overgrowth of the bacterium *Clostridium difficile*, which causes a disease known as pseudomembranous colitis. Controlled studies have shown that supplementation with harmless yeast—such as *Saccharomyces boulardii*[5] or *Saccharomyces cerevisiae* (baker's or brewer's yeast)[6]—helps prevent recurrence of this infection. In one study, taking 500 mg of *Saccharomyces boulardii* twice daily enhanced the effectiveness of the antibiotic vancomycin in preventing recurrent clostridium infection.[7] Therefore, people taking antibiotics who later develop diarrhea might benefit from supplementing with saccharomyces organisms.

Treatment with antibiotics also commonly leads to an overgrowth of yeast *(Candida albicans)* in the vagina (candida vaginitis) and the intestines (sometimes referred to as "dysbiosis"). Controlled studies have shown that *Lactobacillus acidophilus* might prevent candida vaginitis.[8]

Vitamin K

Several cases of excessive bleeding have been reported in people who take antibiotics.[9, 10, 11, 12] This side effect may be the result of reduced vitamin K activity and/or reduced vitamin K production by bacteria in the colon. One study showed that people who had taken broad-spectrum antibiotics had lower liver concentrations of vitamin K_2 (menaquinone), though vitamin K_1 (phylloquinone) levels remained normal.[13] Several antibiotics appear to exert a strong effect on vitamin K activity, while others may not have any effect. Therefore, one should refer to a specific antibiotic for information on whether it interacts with vitamin K. Doctors of natural medicine sometimes recommend vitamin K supplementation to people taking antibiotics. Additional research is needed to determine whether the amount of vitamin K_1 found in some multivitamins is sufficient to prevent antibiotic-induced bleeding. Moreover, most multivitamins do not contain vitamin K.

Interactions with Foods and Other Compounds
Food
Doxycycline may be taken with or without food and should be taken with a full glass of water.[14] However, doxycycline should not be taken with milk[15] or other dairy products.

DOXYLAMINE

Common names: Decapryn, Nighttime Sleep Aid, Sleep Aid, Unisom

Combination drugs: Nyquil, Nyquil Hot Therapy Powder

Doxylamine is an antihistamine used for short-term treatment of insomnia. Doxylamine is available alone in a nonprescription product for sleep and in combination with nonprescription drugs to treat symptoms of allergy, colds, and upper respiratory infections.

Summary of Interactions for Doxylamine
In some cases, an herb or supplement may appear in more than one category, which may seem contradictory.

For clarification, read the full article for details about the summarized interactions.

⊘ Avoid: Adverse interaction	Henbane*
Depletion or interference	None known
Side effect reduction/prevention	None known
Supportive interaction	None known
Reduced drug absorption/bioavailability	None known

Interactions with Herbs
Henbane (Hyoscyamus niger)
Antihistamines, including doxylamine, can cause "anticholinergic" side effects such as dryness of mouth and heart palpitations. Henbane also has anticholinergic activity and side effects. Therefore, use with doxylamine could increase the risk of anticholinergic side effects;[1] however, apparently no interactions have yet been reported with doxylamine and henbane. Henbane should not be taken except by prescription from a physician trained in its use, as it is extremely toxic.

Interactions with Foods and Other Compounds
Alcohol
Doxylamine causes drowsiness.[2] Alcohol may intensify this effect and increase the risk of accidental injury.[3] To prevent problems, people taking doxylamine or doxylamine-containing products should avoid alcohol.

DYAZIDE

Contains the following ingredients:
Hydrochlorothiazide
Triamterene (page 268)

DYNESE

Contains the following ingredients:
Aluminium
Magnesium

ECONACORT

Contains the following ingredients:
Econazole (page 103)
Hydrocortisone

ECONAZOLE

Common names: Ecostatin, Pevaryl, Spectazole

Combination drug: Econacort

Econazole is an antifungal cream used for topical (direct application to the skin) treatment of fungal skin infections. It is used most commonly to treat athlete's foot (fungal infection of the skin between the toes), jock itch (fungal infection of the skin in the groin region), and ringworm (fungal infection of nonhairy skin), and for external *Candida* infections. Econazole is for external use only.

Summary of Interactions for Econazole

In some cases, an herb or supplement may appear in more than one category, which may seem contradictory. For clarification, read the full article for details about the summarized interactions.

✓ May be Beneficial: Supportive interaction	Echinacea*
Depletion or interference	None known
Side effect reduction/prevention	None known
Reduced drug absorption/bioavailability	None known
Adverse interaction	None known

Interactions with Herbs

Echinacea (Echinacea purpurea, Echinacea angustifolia)
The combination of oral echinacea with a topical econazole nitrate cream reduced the recurrence of vaginal yeast infections in women compared to those using the cream alone.[1]

ELLESTE-DUET

Contains the following ingredients:
    Estradiol (page 108)
    Norethisterone

EMPIRIN WITH CODEINE

Contains the following ingredients:
    Aspirin (page 26)
    Codeine (page 75)

EMTRICITABINE

Common names: Emtriva

Emtricitabine is used in combination with other antiviral drugs to treat HIV infection. There are currently no reported nutrient or herb interactions involving emtricitabine.

ENALAPRIL

Common names: Ednyt, Enacard, Enalaprilat, Innovace, Pralenal, Vasotec

Combination drugs: Innozide, Vaseretic

Enalapril is a type of **angiotensin-converting enzyme (ACE) inhibitor** (page 17), a family of drugs used to treat high blood pressure and some types of heart failure. Enalapril is also used to slow the progression of kidney disease in people with diabetes.

Summary of Interactions for Enalapril

In some cases, an herb or supplement may appear in more than one category, which may seem contradictory. For clarification, read the full article for details about the summarized interactions.

✓ May be Beneficial: Side effect reduction/prevention	Iron
⊘ Avoid: Adverse interaction	High-potassium foods* Potassium supplements* Salt substitutes*
ⓘ Check: Other	Sodium
Depletion or interference	None known
Supportive interaction	None known
Reduced drug absorption/bioavailability	None known

Interactions with Dietary Supplements

Potassium
An uncommon yet potentially serious side effect of taking ACE inhibitors is increased blood potassium levels.[1, 2, 3] This problem is more likely to occur in people with advanced kidney disease. Taking potassium supplements,[4] potassium-containing salt substitutes (No

Salt, Morton Salt Substitute, and others),[5, 6, 7] or large amounts of high-potassium foods at the same time as ACE inhibitors could cause life-threatening problems.[8] Therefore, people should consult their healthcare practitioner before supplementing additional potassium and should have their blood levels of potassium checked periodically while taking ACE inhibitors.

Sodium

In a short-term study of nine overweight men, enalapril plus a low-salt diet reduced blood pressure more than a low-salt diet alone.[9] Additionally, enalapril plus a low-salt diet resulted in better **insulin** (page 144) response than the low-salt diet alone. The importance of this preliminary information for overweight people with high blood pressure is unclear.

Iron

In a double-blind study of patients who had developed a cough attributed to an ACE inhibitor, supplementation with iron (in the form of 256 mg of ferrous sulfate per day) for four weeks reduced the severity of the cough by a statistically significant 45%, compared with a nonsignificant 8% improvement in the placebo group.[10]

Interactions with Foods and Other Compounds

Food

Enalapril may be taken with or without food.[11]

ENDOCET

Contains the following ingredients:
   Acetaminophen (page 3)
   Oxycodone (page 205)

ENFUVIRTIDE

Enfuvirtide is used in combination with other antiviral drugs to treat HIV infection in those individuals who have not responded to prior therapy. There are currently no reported nutrient or herb interactions involving enfuvirtide.

ENTEX LA

Contains the following ingredients:
   Guaifenesin (page 133)
   Phenylpropanolamine (page 218)

EPHEDRINE AND PSEUDOEPHEDRINE

Common names: Balminil Decongestant, Boots Child Sugar Free Decongestant Syrup, Boots Decongestant Tablets, Bronalin Decongestant Elixir, CAM, Drixoral N.D., Eltor 120, Eltor, Galpseud, Novafed, Pretz-D, Pseudofrin, Sudafed, Vick's Vatronol

Combination drugs: Alka-Seltzer Plus, Allegra-D, Chlor-Trimeton 12 Hour, Claritin-D, Nyquil, Nyquil Hot Therapy Powder, Primatene Dual Action, Theraflu, Tylenol Allergy Sinus, Tylenol Cold, Tylenol Flu NightTime Maximum Strength Powder, Tylenol Multi-Symptom Hot Medication, Tylenol Sinus

Ephedrine and pseudoephedrine are closely related drugs with actions and side effects similar to the hormone **epinephrine** (page 105) (adrenaline). Ephedrine, available in prescription and nonprescription strengths, is sometimes used to dilate bronchi, making it easier for people with asthma to breathe. Nonprescription ephedrine nose drops and spray are used to relieve nasal congestion due to the flu or hay fever. Pseudoephedrine, a nonprescription drug taken by mouth, can also be used to relieve this symptom.

Summary of Interactions for Ephedrine and Pseudoephedrine

In some cases, an herb or supplement may appear in more than one category, which may seem contradictory. For clarification, read the full article for details about the summarized interactions.

✓ May be Beneficial: Supportive interaction	Coleus*
⊘ Avoid: Reduced drug absorption/ bioavailability	Tannin-containing herbs* such as green tea, black tea, uva ursi, black walnut, red raspberry, oak, and witch hazel
⊘ Avoid: Adverse interaction	**Caffeine** (page 44) Ephedra
ⓘ Check: Other	Vitamin C
Depletion or interference	None known
Side effect reduction/prevention	None known

Interactions with Herbs

Ephedra

Ephedra is the plant from which ephedrine was originally isolated. Until 2004, ephedra—also called ma huang—was used in many herbal products, including supplements promoted for weight loss. To prevent potentially serious interactions, people taking ephedrine or pseudoephedrine should avoid using ephedra-containing drug products and should read product labels carefully for ma huang or ephedra content. Native North American ephedra, sometimes called Mormon tea, contains no ephedrine.

Coleus

A test tube study demonstrated that the bronchodilating effects of salbutamol, a drug with similar actions in the lung to ephedrine, were significantly increased by the addition of forskolin, the active component of the herb *Coleus forskohlii*.[1] The results of this preliminary research suggest that the combination of forskolin and beta-agonists (like ephedrine) might provide an alternative to raising the doses of the beta-agonist drugs as they lose effectiveness. Until more is known, coleus should not be combined with ephedrine without the supervision of a doctor.

Tannin-containing herbs

Tannins are a group of unrelated chemicals that give plants an astringent taste. Herbs containing high amounts of tannins may interfere with the absorption of ephedrine or pseudoephedrine taken by mouth.[2] Herbs containing high levels of tannins include green tea, black tea, uva ursi (*Arctostaphylos uva-ursi*), black walnut (*Juglans nigra*), red raspberry (*Rubus idaeus*), oak (*Quercus* spp.), and witch hazel (*Hamamelis virginiana*).

Interactions with Foods and Other Compounds

Food

Foods that acidify the urine may increase the elimination of ephedrine from the body, potentially reducing the action of the drug.[3] Urine-acidifying foods include eggs, peanuts, meat, chicken, vitamin C (greater than 5 grams per day), wheat-containing foods, and others.

Foods that alkalinize the urine may slow the elimination of ephedrine from the body, potentially increasing the actions and side effects of the drug.[4] Urine-alkalinizing foods include dairy products, nuts, vegetables (except corn and lentils), most fruits, and others.

Caffeine (page 44)

Caffeine, which is found in coffee, tea, chocolate, guaraná (*Paullinia cupana*), and some nonprescription and supplement products, can amplify the side effects of ephedrine and pseudoephedrine. People should avoid combination products containing ephedrine/pseudoephedrine/ephedra and caffeine.

EPINASTINE

Common names: Elestat

Epinastine is used to prevent itching associated with redness of the eye caused by allergens. It belongs to a class of drugs called H1-receptor antagonists. There are currently no reported nutrient or herb interactions involving epinastine.

EPINEPHRINE

Common names: Adrenaline, Adrenalin, Ana-Gard, AsthmaHaler, AsthmaNefrin, Bronchaid, Bronkaid Mistometer, Bronkaid Mist, Brontin Mist, Epifin, Epinal, EpiPen, Epitrate, Eppy/N, Medihaler-Epi, Primatene Mist, S-2, Sus-Phrine

Epinephrine—also called adrenaline—is a synthetic human hormone available as an orally inhaled, nonprescription drug to relieve temporary shortness of breath, chest tightness, and wheezing due to bronchial asthma. Epinephrine is also available as a prescription drug used by injection in emergencies, including acute asthma attacks and severe allergic reactions.

Summary of Interactions for Epinephrine

In some cases, an herb or supplement may appear in more than one category, which may seem contradictory. For clarification, read the full article for details about the summarized interactions.

✓ May be Beneficial: Supportive interaction	Coleus*
⊘ Avoid: Adverse interaction	**Caffeine** (page 44)* Ephedra*
ⓘ Check: Other	Magnesium Potassium Vitamin C
Depletion or interference	None known
Side effect reduction/prevention	None known
Reduced drug absorption/bioavailability	None known

Epinephrine

Interactions with Dietary Supplements

Vitamins and minerals

Intravenous administration of epinephrine to human volunteers reduced plasma concentrations of vitamin C.[1] Epinephrine and other "stress hormones" may reduce intracellular concentrations of potassium and magnesium.[2] Although there are no clinical studies in humans, it seems reasonable that individuals using epinephrine should consume a diet high in vitamin C, potassium, and magnesium, or should consider supplementing with these nutrients.

Interactions with Herbs

Ephedra

Ephedra is the plant from which the drug ephedrine was originally isolated. Epinephrine and ephedrine have similar effects and side effects.[3] Until 2004, ephedra—also called ma huang—was used in many herbal products, including supplements promoted for weight loss. While interactions between epinephrine and ephedra have not been reported, it seems likely that such interactions could occur. To prevent potential problems, people should not be taking both epinephrine and ephedra/ephedrine-containing products.

Coleus

A test tube study demonstrated that the bronchodilating effects of salbutamol, a drug with similar actions in the lung to epinephrine, were significantly increased by the addition of forskolin, the active component of the herb *Coleus forskohlii*.[4] The results of this preliminary research suggest that the combination of forskolin and beta-agonists might provide an alternative to raising the doses of the beta-agonist drugs as they lose effectiveness. Until more is known, coleus should not be combined with epinephrine without the supervision of a doctor.

Interactions with Foods and Other Compounds

Caffeine (page 44)

Epinephrine can increase blood pressure and heart rate.[5] Caffeine, especially in large amounts, can also increase heart rate.[6] When given with **phenylpropanolamine** (page 218), a drug with effects similar to epinephrine, caffeine has been shown to produce an additive increase in blood pressure.[7] Caffeine is found in coffee, tea, soft drinks, chocolate, guaraná *(Paullinia cupana)*, nonprescription drugs, and supplements containing caffeine or guaraná. While no interactions have been reported between epinephrine and caffeine, people using epineph-

rine can minimize the potential for interactions by limiting or avoiding caffeine.

ERYTHROMYCIN

Common names: A/T/S, Akne-Mycin, Apo-Erythro, Arpimycin, Diomycin, E-Mycin, EES, Emgel, Ery-Tab, Erybid, Erycen, Erycette, Eryc, EryDerm, Erygel, Erymax, Eryped, Erythrocin, Erythromid, Erythroped A, Erythroped, Ilosone, Ilotycin, Novo-Rythro Encap, PCE, PMS-Erythromycin, Rommix Oral Suspension, Rommix, Staticin, T-Stat, Theramycin, Tiloryth

Erythromycin is a **macrolide antibiotic** (page 164) used to treat a wide variety of bacterial infections. Several chemical forms of erythromycin are available for oral use to treat infections in the body. Erythromycin-containing products are also available to treat eye and skin infections.

Summary of Interactions for Erythromycin

In some cases, an herb or supplement may appear in more than one category, which may seem contradictory. For clarification, read the full article for details about the summarized interactions.

✓ May be Beneficial: Depletion or interference	Multiple nutrients* (Magnesium, Vitamin B$_6$, Vitamin B$_{12}$) Vitamin K*
✓ May be Beneficial: Side effect reduction/prevention	Bifidobacterium *Bifidobacterium longum* Lactobacillus acidophilus* Lactobacillus casei* Saccharomyces boulardii* Saccharomyces cerevisiae* Vitamin K*
✓ May be Beneficial: Supportive interaction	Bromelain* Saccharomyces boulardii*
ⓘ Check: Other	Calcium Digitalis Folic acid
Reduced drug absorption/bioavailability	None known
Adverse interaction	None known

Interactions with Dietary Supplements

Probiotics

A common side effect of antibiotics is diarrhea, which may be caused by the elimination of beneficial bacteria normally found in the colon. Yogurt containing *Bifidobacterium longum* culture has decreased erythromycin-induced diarrhea in a single-blind study of ten healthy people.[1] Yogurt containing live cultures has also protected against other antibiotic-induced diarrhea.

Controlled studies have shown that taking probiotic microorganisms—such as *Lactobacillus casei*, *Lactobacillus acidophilus*, *Bifidobacterium longum*, or *Saccharomyces boulardii*—helps prevent antibiotic-induced diarrhea.[2]

The diarrhea experienced by some people who take antibiotics also might be due to an overgrowth of the bacterium *Clostridium difficile*, which causes a disease known as pseudomembranous colitis. Controlled studies have shown that supplementation with harmless yeast—such as *Saccharomyces boulardii*[3] or *Saccharomyces cerevisiae* (baker's or brewer's yeast)[4]—helps prevent recurrence of this infection. In one study, taking 500 mg of *Saccharomyces boulardii* twice daily enhanced the effectiveness of the antibiotic vancomycin in preventing recurrent clostridium infection.[5] Therefore, people taking antibiotics who later develop diarrhea might benefit from supplementing with saccharomyces organisms.

Treatment with antibiotics also commonly leads to an overgrowth of yeast *(Candida albicans)* in the vagina (candida vaginitis) and the intestines (sometimes referred to as "dysbiosis"). Controlled studies have shown that *Lactobacillus acidophilus* might prevent candida vaginitis.[6]

Bromelain

One report found bromelain improved the action of antibiotic drugs, including **penicillin** (page 211) and erythromycin, in treating a variety of infections. In that trial, 22 out of 23 people who had previously not responded to the antibiotics did so after adding bromelain four times per day.[7] Doctors will sometimes prescribe enough bromelain to equal 2,400 gelatin dissolving units (listed as GDU on labels) per day. This amount would equal approximately 3,600 MCU (milk clotting units), another common measure of bromelain activity.

Vitamin K

Several cases of excessive bleeding have been reported in people who take antibiotics.[8, 9, 10, 11] This side effect may be the result of reduced vitamin K activity and/or reduced vitamin K production by bacteria in the colon. One study showed that people who had taken broad-spectrum antibiotics had lower liver concentrations of vitamin K_2 (menaquinone), though vitamin K_1 (phylloquinone) levels remained normal.[12] Several antibiotics appear to exert a strong effect on vitamin K activity, while others may not have any effect. Therefore, one should refer to a specific antibiotic for information on whether it interacts with vitamin K. Doctors of natural medicine sometimes recommend vitamin K supplementation to people taking antibiotics. Additional research is needed to determine whether the amount of vitamin K_1 found in some multivitamins is sufficient to prevent antibiotic-induced bleeding. Moreover, most multivitamins do not contain vitamin K.

Other vitamins and minerals

Erythromycin may interfere with the absorption and/or activity of calcium, folic acid, magnesium, vitamin B_6 and vitamin B_{12},[13] which may cause problems, especially with long-term erythromycin treatment. Until more is known, it makes sense for people taking erythromycin for longer than two weeks to supplement with a daily multivitamin-multimineral.

Interactions with Herbs

Digitalis (Digitalis lanata, Digitalis purpurea)

Digitalis refers to a family of plants commonly called foxglove that contain digitalis glycosides, chemicals with actions and toxicities similar to the prescription drug **digoxin** (page 90).

Erythromycin can increase the serum level of digitalis glycosides, increasing the therapeutic effects and risk of side effects.[14] Erythromycin and digitalis-containing products should be used only under the direct supervision of a doctor trained in their use.

Interactions with Foods and Other Compounds

Food

Some forms of erythromycin are best absorbed when taken on an empty stomach, one hour before or two hours after food.[15] Individuals who experience stomach upset taking these forms of erythromycin on an empty stomach should use one of the other forms that can be taken with food.

Other forms of erythromycin may be taken with or without food.[16] People taking erythromycin should ask their pharmacist about the form of erythromycin they are taking and compatibility with or without food.

Erythromycin is best taken with water, rather than other beverages, to prevent degradation of the drug before it reaches the intestines.[17] Erythromycin tablets should be swallowed whole, without cutting, chewing, or crushing.[18]

ESSTRAPAK-50

Contains the following ingredients:
Estradiol (page 108)
Norethisterone

ESTRACOMBI

Contains the following ingredients:
Estradiol (page 108)
Norethisterone

ESTRADIOL

Common names: Adgyn Estro, Alora, Climara, Climaval, Dalergen, Delestrogen, Depo-Estradiol, Depogen, DepoGynogen, Dermestril-Septem, Dermestril, E-Cypionate, Elleste Solo, Elleste Solo MX, Escalim, Esclim, Estinyl, Estrace, Estraderm MX, Estraderm TTS, Estraderm, Estragyn LA 5, Estring, Estro-Cyp, Estro-L.A., Estrogel, Ethinyl Estradiol, Evorel, Fematrix, FemPatch, FemSeven, Gynodiol, Gynogen L.A., Harmonin, Menaval, Menorest, Noven, Oestradiol, Oestradiol Implants, Oestrogel, Progynova TS, Progynova, Sandrena, Vagifem, Vivelle, Zumenon

Combination drugs: Adgyn Combi, Climagest, Climesse, Cyclo-Progynova, Elleste-Duet, Esstrapak-50, Estracombi, Evorel, Femapak, Femostan, Indivina, Kliofem, Kliovance, Nuvelle TS, Nuvelle, Tridestra, Trisequens Forte, Trisequens

Estradiol is a semisynthetic human estrogenic hormone used to treat menopausal symptoms, to prevent osteoporosis in postmenopausal women, and as replacement therapy in other conditions of inadequate estrogen production.

Estradiol is available as an oral drug, a transdermal (skin) patch, and as a vaginal cream.

Summary of Interactions for Estradiol

In some cases, an herb or supplement may appear in more than one category, which may seem contradictory. For clarification, read the full article for details about the summarized interactions.

🚫 Avoid: Adverse interaction	Grapefruit* Quercetin*
ⓘ Check: Other	Vitamin D
Depletion or interference	None known
Side effect reduction/prevention	None known
Supportive interaction	None known
Reduced drug absorption/bioavailability	None known

Interactions with Dietary Supplements
Quercetin
Studies have shown that grapefruit juice significantly increases estradiol levels in the blood.[1, 2] One of the flavonoids found in grapefruit juice is quercetin. In a test tube study, quercetin was found to change estrogen metabolism in human liver cells in a way that increases estradiol levels and reduces other forms of estrogen.[3] This effect is likely to increase estrogen activity in the body. However, the levels of quercetin used to alter estrogen metabolism in the test tube were much higher than levels found in the body after supplementing with quercetin.

There is evidence from test tube stuudies that another flavonoid in grapefruit juice, naringenin, also has estrogenic activity.[4] It has yet to be shown that dietary or supplemental levels of quercetin (or naringenin) could create a significant problem.

Vitamin D
In controlled studies, the addition of 300 IU per day of vitamin D3 (cholecalciferol) did not improve the bone-preserving or fracture-preventing effects of hormone replacement with estradiol plus a progestin (a synthetic form of progesterone) in postmenopausal women without osteoporosis.[5, 6] However, in a controlled study of osteoporotic women, only those receiving both hormone replacement and vitamin D had increases in bone density of the hip; no improvement occurred in the hip with hormones alone.[7] More research is needed to determine conclusively when vitamin D is important to add to hormone replacement.

Interactions with Foods and Other Compounds
Grapefruit
In a small, controlled study of women with surgically removed ovaries, estradiol levels in the blood were significantly higher after estradiol was taken with grapefruit juice than when estradiol was taken alone.[8] These results have been independently confirmed,[9] suggesting that women taking oral estradiol should probably avoid grapefruit altogether.

ESTRATEST/ESTRATEST HS

Contains the following ingredients:
Esterified Estrogens (page 109)
Methyltestosterone (page 175)

ESTROGENS

Conjugated estrogens and esterified estrogens are both combinations of estrogenic hormones used to treat menopausal symptoms, to prevent osteoporosis in post-menopausal women, and as replacement therapy in other conditions of inadequate estrogen production. They are also used to treat some people with advanced breast and prostate cancers.

Drugs in this category include:
- **Conjugated estrogens** (page 109) (Premarin)
- **Esterified estrogens** (page 109) (Estratab, Menest) (conbinations Estratest)
- **Estropipate** (page 111) (Ogen, Ortho-Est)
- **Ethinyl estradiol** (page 108) (Estinyl)
- Diethylstilbestrol (Stilphostrol)
- Dienestrol (Ortho Dienestrol)
- Chlorotrianisene (Tace)
- **Estradiol cypionate** (page 108) (Depo-Estradiol, Depogen, Dura-Estrin, Estra-D, Estro-Cyp, Estroject-LA, Estronol-LA)
- **Estradiol** (page 108) (Estrace, Alora Transdermal, Climara Transdermal, Vivelle Transdermal)
- **Synthetic conjugated estrogens** (page 109) (Cenestin)

For interactions involving a specific Estrogen, see the individual drug article. For interactions involving an Estrogen for which no separate article exists, talk to your doctor or pharmacist.

ESTROGENS (COMBINED)

Common names: Cenestin, Conjugated Estrogens, Esterified Estrogens, Estratab, Menest, Premarin

Combination drugs: Estratest/Estratest HS, Premique, Prempak-C, Prempro

Conjugated estrogens and esterified estrogens are both combinations of estrogenic hormones used to treat menopausal symptoms, to prevent osteoporosis in post-menopausal women, and as replacement therapy in other conditions of inadequate estrogen production. They are also used to treat some people with advanced breast and prostate cancers. Conjugated estrogens are extracted and purified from the urine of pregnant horses. A synthetic conjugated estrogen product (Cenestin) is also available, as are combination products.

Combinations of estrogens with other hormones are also available. For example, Estratest is a combination of **methyltestosterone** (page 175) and esterified estrogens. Premarin is a combination of **estrogens** (page 109) and progestins.

The information in this article pertains to combined estrogens in general. The interactions reported here may not apply to all the Also Indexed As terms. Talk to your doctor or pharmacist if you are taking any of these drugs.

Summary of Interactions for Conjugated Estrogens

In some cases, an herb or supplement may appear in more than one category, which may seem contradictory. For clarification, read the full article for details about the summarized interactions.

✓ May be Beneficial: Depletion or interference	Vitamin B$_6$*
✓ May be Beneficial: Supportive interaction	Calcium Ipriflavone* Vitamin D* (increased bone density)
⊘ Avoid: Reduced drug absorption/ bioavailability	Herbal sources of isoflavone supplements (red clover*, soy*)
⊘ Avoid: Adverse interaction	Tobacco Vitamin D*
ⓘ Check: Other	Magnesium
ⓘ Check: Other	Zinc
Side effect reduction/prevention	None known

Interactions with Dietary Supplements
Calcium

Two months of conjugated estrogen therapy in women with surgically induced menopause decreased urinary calcium loss and increased serum vitamin D levels.[1] In a six-month placebo-controlled study of 21 women with postmenopausal osteoporosis, conjugated estrogens increased both calcium absorption and vitamin D blood levels.[2]

While estrogen may improve calcium absorption, it remains important for women taking estrogen to maintain adequate calcium intake through diet and supplementation. Many doctors recommend 800–1,200 mg of supplemental calcium in addition to the several hundred milligrams found in a typical daily diet.

Ipriflavone

Ipriflavone, a synthetic variation of isoflavones found in soy, is available as a supplement. In a controlled trial, ipriflavone (400 mg per day) plus conjugated estrogens increased vertebral bone density, while calcium (500 mg per day) plus conjugated estrogens could not prevent a decrease in bone density in postmenopausal women.[3] Similarly, a double-blind trial found ipriflavone (600 mg per day) plus conjugated estrogens and calcium (1 gram per day) increased bone density, while calcium with or without conjugated estrogens could not prevent bone loss.[4] While low doses of estrogens can counteract some menopausal symptoms, higher doses are required to prevent bone loss in postmenopausal women. However, the addition of ipriflavone to low-dose estrogen therapy has been shown in a controlled trial to preserve bone mass in postmenopausal women.[5]

Minerals

A preliminary trial found that osteoporotic postmenopausal women with elevated urinary zinc and magnesium excretion experienced reduced losses of these minerals after being treated with conjugated estrogens and **medroxyprogesterone** (page 167).[6] More research is needed to determine the significance of this finding.

Vitamin B6

A small preliminary trial found most women taking conjugated estrogens therapy without a progestin to have lower levels or a deficiency of vitamin B6.[7] Numerous studies have found negative effects of **oral contraceptives** (page 198) (OCs) on vitamin B6 status,[8, 9, 10] although some studies suggest that vitamin B6 deficiency does not occur when low-dose OCs are used.[11] While OCs contain different forms of estrogen than conjugated estrogens, there is a possibility of a similar problem when any form of estrogen is supplemented, but more research is needed.

Vitamin D

A controlled trial found two months of conjugated estrogens therapy in women with surgically induced menopause increased blood levels of vitamin D and de-

creased urinary calcium loss.[12] In a controlled study of women with postmenopausal osteoporosis, conjugated estrogens therapy was associated with increased blood levels of vitamin D and increased calcium absorption.[13] While conjugated estrogens appear to improve vitamin D metabolism, it remains important for women taking such hormones to consume adequate levels of vitamin D through diet and supplements.

One controlled study showed that taking 300 IU of vitamin D per day with **estradiol** (page 108), an estrogen related to conjugated estrogens, plus a progestin led to greater improvement in bone density compared with estradiol/progestin alone.[14] Further controlled studies are needed to determine whether taking conjugated estrogens and vitamin D together might also increase bone strength and prevent fractures. In contrast to the beneficial effects on bone, the study also revealed that supplementing vitamin D together with estradiol/progestin tended to reduce beneficial HDL cholesterol levels, unlike estradiol/progestin alone. These undesirable results were confirmed by two additional studies.[15, 16]

Additional research is needed to determine the degree to which supplemental vitamin D might exert a supportive or adverse effect on the actions of conjugated estrogens. Until more information is available, women taking hormone replacement therapy are advised to talk with a physician before combining vitamin D with conjugated estrogens.

Interactions with Herbs

Isoflavones

Herbal sources of isoflavones, such as red clover, may interfere with or even have an additive effect with conjugated estrogens.[17] Further studies are needed to establish the potential interaction of isoflavone supplements from red clover and soy with conjugated estrogens. Consult with your healthcare professional if you are currently taking estrogen replacement therapy and wish to take a supplement high in isoflavones.

Interactions with Foods and Other Compounds

Tobacco

Conjugated estrogens therapy in postmenopausal women has been reported to decrease LDL ("bad") cholesterol levels and to increase HDL ("good") cholesterol levels. However, despite the positive changes in blood levels of LDL and HDL cholesterol, there is evidence that conjugated estrogens do not reduce the risk of heart disease.[18] Nonetheless, smoking offsets the cholesterol changes induced by taking conjugated estrogens,[19] and this interference is likely to be detrimental.

Women taking conjugated estrogens who do not smoke should avoid starting, and those who do smoke should talk with their doctor about quitting.

ESTROPIPATE

Common names: Estraval- P.A., Estrone, Harmogen, Natural Estrogenic Substance, Ogen, Ortho-Est, Primestrin

Estropipate is used both to treat moderate to severe symptoms associated with menopause, including hot flashes and vaginal dryness, and to prevent osteoporosis. It is in a class of drugs known as estrogens.

There are currently no reported nutrient or herb interactions specifically involving estropipate; however, since it is an estrogen, estropipate might interact with similar compounds. For more information, refer to the **estrogen** (page 109) section.

Summary of Interactions for Estropipate

In some cases, an herb or supplement may appear in more than one category, which may seem contradictory. For clarification, read the full article for details about the summarized interactions.

Depletion or interference	None known
Side effect reduction/prevention	None known
Supportive interaction	None known
Reduced drug absorption/bioavailability	None known
Adverse interaction	None known

ETODOLAC

Common names: Apo-Etodolac, Lodine, Ultradol

Etodolac is a member of the **nonsteroidal anti-inflammatory drug** (page 193) (NSAIDs) family. NSAIDs reduce inflammation (swelling), pain, and temperature. Etodolac is used to treat mild to moderate pain, osteoarthritis, rheumatoid arthritis, ankylosing spondylitis, tendinitis, bursitis, and other conditions.

Summary of Interactions for Etodolac

In some cases, an herb or supplement may appear in more than one category, which may seem contradictory. For clarification, read the full article for details about the summarized interactions.

✓	May be Beneficial: Depletion or interference	Iron
✓	May be Beneficial: Side effect reduction/prevention	Copper* Licorice
✓	May be Beneficial: Supportive interaction	Copper*
🚫	Avoid: Adverse interaction	**Lithium** (page 157)* Sodium* White willow*
ⓘ	Check: Other	Potassium
	Reduced drug absorption/bioavailability	None known

Interactions with Dietary Supplements

Copper

Supplementation may enhance the anti-inflammatory effects of NSAIDs while reducing their ulcerogenic effects. One study found that when various anti-inflammatory drugs were chelated with copper, the anti-inflammatory activity was increased.[1] Animal models of inflammation have found that the copper chelate of **aspirin** (page 26) was active at one-eighth the effective amount of aspirin. These copper complexes are less toxic than the parent compounds, as well.

Iron

NSAIDs cause gastrointestinal (GI) irritation, bleeding, and iron loss.[2] Iron supplements can cause GI irritation.[3] However, iron supplementation is sometimes needed in people taking NSAIDs if those drugs have caused enough blood loss to lead to iron deficiency. If both iron and etodolac are prescribed, they should be taken with food to reduce GI irritation and bleeding risk.

Lithium (page 157)

Lithium is a mineral that may be present in some supplements and is also used in large amounts to treat mood disorders such as manic-depression (bipolar disorder). Most NSAIDs inhibit the excretion of lithium from the body, resulting in higher blood levels of the mineral, though **sulindac** (page 249) may have an opposite effect.[4] Since major changes in lithium blood levels can produce unwanted side effects or interfere with its efficacy, NSAIDs should be used with caution, and only under medical supervision, in people taking lithium supplements.

Potassium

NSAIDs have caused kidney dysfunction and increased blood potassium levels, especially in older people.[5] Peo-

Etodolac

ple taking NSAIDs, including etodolac, should not supplement potassium without consulting with their doctor.

Sodium
Etodolac may cause sodium and water retention.[6] It is healthful to reduce dietary salt intake by eliminating table salt and heavily salted foods.

Interactions with Herbs
Licorice (Glycyrrhiza glabra)
The flavonoids found in the extract of licorice known as DGL (deglycyrrhizinated licorice) are helpful for avoiding the irritating actions NSAIDs have on the stomach and intestines. One study found that 350 mg of chewable DGL taken together with each dose of aspirin reduced gastrointestinal bleeding caused by the aspirin.[7] DGL has been shown in controlled human research to be as effective as drug therapy (**cimetidine** [page 61]) in healing stomach ulcers.[8]

White willow bark (Salix alba)
White willow bark contains salicin, which is related to **aspirin** (page 26). Both salicin and aspirin produce anti-inflammatory effects after they have been converted to salicylic acid in the body. The administration of salicylates like aspirin to individuals taking oral NSAIDs may result in reduced blood levels of NSAIDs.[9] Though no studies have investigated interactions between white willow bark and NSAIDs, people taking NSAIDs should avoid the herb until more information is available.

Interactions with Foods and Other Compounds
Food
Etodolac should be taken with food to prevent gastrointestinal upset.[10]

Alcohol
Etodolac may cause drowsiness, dizziness, or blurred vision.[11] Alcohol may intensify these effects and increase the risk of accidental injury. Use of alcohol during etodolac therapy increases the risk of stomach irritation and bleeding. People taking etodolac should avoid alcohol.

EURAX HC

Contains the following ingredients:
Crotamiton
Hydrocortisone

EURAX-HYDROCORTISONE

Contains the following ingredients:
Crotamiton
Hydrocortisone

EVOREL

Contains the following ingredients:
Estradiol (page 108)
Norethisterone

EXCEDRIN PM

Contains the following ingredients:
Acetaminophen (page 3)
Diphenhydramine (page 93)

FAMOTIDINE

Common names: Apo-Famotidine, Boots Excess Acid Control, Gen-Famotidine, Maalox H2 Acid Controller, Mylanta-AR, Novo-Famotidine, Nu-Famotidine, Pepcid, Pepcid AC, Ulcidine

Famotidine is a member of the H-2 blocker (histamine blocker) family of drugs that prevents the release of acid into the stomach. Famotidine is used to treat stomach and duodenal ulcers, reflux of stomach acid into the esophagus, and Zollinger-Ellison syndrome. Famotidine is available as a prescription drug and as a nonprescription product for relief of heartburn, acid indigestion, and sour stomach.

Summary of Interactions for Famotidine
In some cases, an herb or supplement may appear in more than one category, which may seem contradictory. For clarification, read the full article for details about the summarized interactions.

✓	May be Beneficial: Depletion or interference	Iron* Vitamin B$_{12}$
⊘	Avoid: Adverse interaction	Tobacco
ⓘ	Check: Other	Copper Folic acid Magnesium
	Side effect reduction/prevention	None known
	Supportive interaction	None known
	Reduced drug absorption/bioavailability	None known

Interactions with Dietary Supplements

Iron

Stomach acid may increase absorption of iron from food. H-2 blocker drugs reduce stomach acid and are associated with decreased dietary iron absorption.[1] The iron found in supplements is available to the body without the need for stomach acid. People with ulcers may be iron deficient due to blood loss. If iron deficiency is present, iron supplementation may be beneficial. Iron levels in the blood can be checked with lab tests.

Magnesium-containing antacids

In healthy people, a **magnesium hydroxide** (page 166)/**aluminum hydroxide** (page 10) antacid, taken with famotidine, decreased famotidine absorption by 20–25%.[2] People can avoid this interaction by taking famotidine two hours before or after any aluminum/magnesium-containing antacids. Some magnesium supplements such as magnesium hydroxide are also antacids.

Vitamin B12

Stomach acid is needed for the vitamin B_{12} in food to be absorbed. H-2 blocker drugs reduce stomach acid and may therefore inhibit absorption of the vitamin B_{12} naturally present in food. However, the vitamin B_{12} found in supplements does not depend on stomach acid for absorption.[3] Lab tests can determine vitamin B_{12} levels in people.

Other vitamins and minerals

Some evidence indicates that other vitamins and minerals, such as folic acid[4] and copper,[5] require the presence of stomach acid for optimal absorption. Long-term use of H-2 blockers may therefore promote a deficiency of these nutrients. Individuals requiring long-term use of H-2 blockers may therefore benefit from a multiple vitamin/mineral supplement.

Interactions with Foods and Other Compounds

Food

Famotidine may be taken with or without food.[6] To prevent heartburn after meals, famotidine is best taken one hour before meals.[7]

Tobacco

In a study of 18 healthy people, cigarette smoking was found to decrease the acid blocking effects of famotidine.[8] A double-blind, randomized study of 594 patients with duodenal ulcers found that smoking inhibited the ulcer-healing effect of famotidine.[9]

FELODIPINE

Common names: Plendil, Renedil

Combination drug: Triapin

Felodipine is used to treat high blood pressure, Raynaud's syndrome, and congestive heart failure. It is in a class of drugs known as calcium-channel blockers.

Summary of Interactions for Felodipine

In some cases, an herb or supplement may appear in more than one category, which may seem contradictory. For clarification, read the full article for details about the summarized interactions.

✓ May be Beneficial: Depletion or interference	Calcium Magnesium Potassium
🚫 Avoid: Adverse interaction	Grapefruit juice Pleurisy root* Quercetin*
Side effect reduction/prevention	None known
Supportive interaction	None known
Reduced drug absorption/bioavailability	None known

Interactions with Dietary Supplements

Potassium

Felodipine can lead to increased excretion of potassium.[1] A potassium deficiency may result if potassium intake is not sufficient. People taking felodipine should eat a high-potassium diet and be checked regularly for low blood potassium by a doctor.

Magnesium

Increased magnesium excretion has been observed in studies of individuals taking felodipine.[2] Therefore, some physicians may recommend magnesium supplementation to their patients taking felodipine.

Calcium

A study of felodipine indicated that the drug caused increased excretion of calcium.[3] Whether this effect could lead to increased bone loss is unknown, but some health practitioners may recommend calcium supplementation to individuals taking felodipine. Although the effectiveness of some calcium channel blockers may be reduced with calcium supplementation,[4] this effect has not been observed in people taking felodipine.

Quercetin

Quercetin is a flavonoid found in grapefruit juice, tea, onions, and other foods; it is also available as a nutritional supplement. Quercetin has been shown in test tube studies to inhibit enzymes responsible for breaking down felodipine into an inactive form.[5] This interaction may result in increased blood levels of felodipine that could lead to unwanted side effects. Until more is known about this interaction, patients taking felodipine should avoid supplementing with quercetin.

Interactions with Herbs

Pleurisy root

As pleurisy root and other plants in the *Aesclepius* genus contain cardiac glycosides, it is best to avoid use of pleurisy root with heart medications such as calcium-channel blockers.[6]

Interactions with Foods and Other Compounds

Grapefruit

Regular consumption of grapefruit juice can increase the quantity of felodipine in the blood by reducing the breakdown of the drug.[7] The inhibitory effect of grapefruit juice lasts up to 24 hours after ingestion and can increase blood levels nearly three times the expected amount. In order to prevent side effects of the drug, individuals who are taking felodipine should avoid grapefruit and its juice.

Alcohol

Drinking alcoholic beverages while taking felodipine may enhance the blood pressure–lowering effect of the drug.[8] Those who combine alcoholic beverages with felodipine should be aware of possible adverse consequences, such as increased lightheadedness.

FEMAPAK

Contains the following ingredients:
Dydrogesterone
Estradiol (page 108)

FEMOSTAN

Contains the following ingredients:
Dydrogesterone
Estradiol (page 108)

FENOFIBRATE

Common names: Lipantil, Supralip, Tricor

Fenofibrate is used to lower elevated cholesterol and triglyceride levels when diet, exercise, and weight loss programs are ineffective. It is in a family of medications known as cholesterol-lowering drugs.

Summary of Interactions for Fenofibrate

In some cases, an herb or supplement may appear in more than one category, which may seem contradictory. For clarification, read the full article for details about the summarized interactions.

✓ May be Beneficial: Side effect reduction/prevention	Folic acid Vitamin B_{12} Vitamin B_6 Vitamin C Vitamin E
✓ May be Beneficial: Supportive interaction	Food
Depletion or interference	None known
Reduced drug absorption/bioavailability	None known
Adverse interaction	None known

Interactions with Dietary Supplements

Vitamin C and vitamin E

Several studies have shown that fenofibrate enhances the toxic effect of ultraviolet (UV) radiation from the sun, which might result in side effects such as skin rashes. One controlled study showed that taking 2 grams of vitamin C and 1,000 IU of vitamin E prior to ultraviolet exposure dramatically blocked UV-fenofibrate damage to red blood cells.[1] though further controlled studies are needed, people taking fenofibrate should probably supplement with vitamins C and E until more information is available.

Folic acid, vitamin B_6, and vitamin B_{12}

Increased blood levels of homocysteine are associated with increased risk of atherosclerosis and heart disease. One study revealed that fenofibrate dramatically increases blood homocysteine levels, though blood levels of vitamins were not reduced.[2] In one study, supplementation with 10 mg per day of folic acid prevented the increase in homocysteine levels resulting from fenofibrate therapy.[3] Further research is needed to determine whether supplemental vitamin B_6 and vitamin

B$_{12}$, which are also capable of lowering homocysteine levels, might lower fenofibrate-induced elevations in homocysteine levels.

Interactions with Foods and Other Compounds
Food
Taking fenofibrate together with food dramatically increases the absorption of the drug.[4] Therefore fenofibrate should be taken with a meal.

FENTANYL

Common names: Actiq oral lozenge, Duragesic, Durogesic patch

Fentanyl is used in surgery as a **general anesthetic** (page 129) and is available in a patch form to treat severe, chronic pain. It is in a class of drugs known as opioid analgesics.

Summary of Interactions for Fentanyl
In some cases, an herb or supplement may appear in more than one category, which may seem contradictory. For clarification, read the full article for details about the summarized interactions.

✓	May be Beneficial: Supportive interaction	Magnesium
⊘	Avoid: Reduced drug absorption/ bioavailability	Alcohol (chronic)
⊘	Avoid: Adverse interaction	Alcohol
	Depletion or interference	None known
	Side effect reduction/prevention	None known

Interactions with Dietary Supplements
Magnesium
One double-blind study showed that giving magnesium intravenously before surgery dramatically reduced the amount of fentanyl needed to control pain during and after an operation.[1] Further research is needed to determine whether people using fentanyl patches might benefit from supplementing with oral magnesium.

Interactions with Foods and Other Compounds
Alcohol
Drinking alcoholic beverages while using fentanyl patches increases the likelihood of side effect, such as drowsiness, dizziness, and poor coordination.[2] Therefore, people using fentanyl patches should avoid drinking alcohol, especially when they must stay alert. People who chronically consume alcohol require larger amounts of fentanyl to achieve adequate levels of anesthesia.[3] Further research is needed to determine whether chronic alcohol consumption increases the amount of fentanyl needed to relieve pain.

FEXOFENADINE

Common names: Allegra, Telfast

Combination drug: Allegra-D

Fexofenadine is a selective antihistamine used to relieve allergic rhinitis (seasonal allergy) symptoms including sneezing, runny nose, itching, and watery eyes. Fexofenadine is available alone and in a combination product.

Summary of Interactions for Fexofenadine
In some cases, an herb or supplement may appear in more than one category, which may seem contradictory. For clarification, read the full article for details about the summarized interactions.

ⓘ	Check: Other	St. John's wort
	Depletion or interference	None known
	Side effect reduction/prevention	None known
	Supportive interaction	None known
	Reduced drug absorption/bioavailability	None known
	Adverse interaction	None known

Interactions with Herbs
St. John's wort
In a study of healthy volunteers, administration of 900 mg of St. John's wort one hour prior to fexofenadine resulted in a significant increase in blood levels of fexofenadine, compared with the blood levels after taking fexofenadine alone.[1] On the other hand, long-term administration of St. John's wort (300 mg three times per day for two weeks) did not alter blood levels of fexofenadine. Until more is known, St. John's wort should not be combined with fexofenadine, except under the supervision of a doctor.

Interactions with Foods and Other Compounds
Food
Ingestion of grapefruit juice, orange juice, or apple juice along with fexofenadine decreases blood levels of the drug.[2]

Alcohol
Selective antihistamines, including fexofenadine, may cause drowsiness or dizziness; however, it is less likely than with nonselective antihistamines.[3] Alcohol can intensify drowsiness and dizziness, increasing the risk of accidental injury.

FINASTERIDE

Common names: Propecia, Proscar

Finasteride is used to improve symptoms of benign prostatic hyperplasia (BPH), as well as to reduce the need for surgery.

Summary of Interactions for Finasteride
In some cases, an herb or supplement may appear in more than one category, which may seem contradictory. For clarification, read the full article for details about the summarized interactions.

Depletion or interference	None known
Side effect reduction/prevention	None known
Supportive interaction	None known
Reduced drug absorption/bioavailability	None known
Adverse interaction	None known

FIORICET

Contains the following ingredients:
Acetaminophen (page 3)
Butalbital (page 44)
Caffeine (page 44)

FIORINAL

Contains the following ingredients:
Aspirin (page 26)
Butalbital (page 44)
Caffeine (page 44)
Codeine (page 75)

FLUCONAZOLE

Common names: Diflucan

Fluconazole is an antifungal drug used to treat *Candida* infections. Fluconazole is also used to treat onychomycosis (fungal infection) of the toenails or fingernails and meningitis caused by *Cryptococcus*.

Summary of Interactions for Fluconazole
In some cases, an herb or supplement may appear in more than one category, which may seem contradictory. For clarification, read the full article for details about the summarized interactions.

Depletion or interference	None known
Side effect reduction/prevention	None known
Supportive interaction	None known
Reduced drug absorption/bioavailability	None known
Adverse interaction	None known

Interactions with Foods and Other Compounds
Food
Fluconazole may be taken with or without food.[1]

FLUOROURACIL

Common names: 5-FU, Adrucil, Efudex, Efudix, Fluoroplex

Fluorouracil is a **chemotherapy** (page 54) drug given intravenously (iv) to treat colon, rectum, breast, stomach, and pancreas cancers. Fluorouracil is also available in creams and solutions for topical treatment of some skin cancers and genital warts.

Note: Many of the interactions described below, in the text and in the Summary of Interactions, have been reported only for specific chemotherapeutic drugs, and may not apply to other chemotherapeutic drugs. There are many unknowns concerning interactions of nutrients, herbs, and chemotherapy drugs. People receiving chemotherapy who wish to supplement with vitamins, minerals, herbs, or other natural substances should always consult a physician.

Summary of Interactions for Fluorouracil
In some cases, an herb or supplement may appear in more than one category, which may seem contradictory.

For clarification, read the full article for details about the summarized interactions.

✓ May be Beneficial: Depletion or interference	Multiple nutrients* (malabsorption) Taurine*
✓ May be Beneficial: Side effect reduction/prevention	Beta-carotene* (mouth sores) Chamomile* (mouth sores) Eleuthero* (see text) Ginger* (nausea) Glutamine (intestinal toxicity) Glutamine* (mouth sores) Melatonin N-acetyl cysteine* (NAC) Spleen peptide extract* (see text) Thymus peptides* (see text) Vitamin B$_6$ Vitamin E*, topical (mouth sores)
✓ May be Beneficial: Supportive interaction	Antioxidants* Melatonin Milk thistle* PSK*
ⓘ Check: Other	Echinacea* Multivitamin-mineral* Vitamin A* Vitamin C*
Reduced drug absorption/bioavailability	None known
Adverse interaction	None known

Interactions with Dietary Supplements

Antioxidants

Chemotherapy can injure cancer cells by creating oxidative damage. As a result, some oncologists recommend that patients avoid supplementing antioxidants if they are undergoing chemotherapy. Limited test tube research occasionally does support the idea that an antioxidant can interfere with oxidative damage to cancer cells.[1] However, most scientific research does not support this supposition.

A modified form of vitamin A has been reported to work synergistically with chemotherapy in test tube research.[2] Vitamin C appears to increase the effectiveness of chemotherapy in animals[3] and with human breast cancer cells in test tube research.[4] In a double-blind study, Japanese researchers found that the combination of vitamin E, vitamin C, and N-acetyl cysteine (NAC)—all antioxidants—protected against chemotherapy-induced heart damage without interfering with the action of the chemotherapy.[5]

A comprehensive review of antioxidants and chemotherapy leaves open the question of whether supplemental antioxidants definitely help people with chemotherapy side effects, but the article strongly suggests that antioxidants need not be avoided for fear that the actions of chemotherapy would be interfered with.[6]

A new formulation of selenium (Seleno-Kappacarrageenan) was found to reduce kidney damage and white blood cell–lowering effects of **cisplatin** (page 64) in one human study. However, the level used in this study (4,000 mcg per day) is potentially toxic and should only be used under the supervision of a doctor.[7]

Glutathione, the main antioxidant found within cells, is frequently depleted in individuals on chemotherapy and/or radiation. Preliminary studies have found that intravenously injected glutathione may decrease some of the adverse effects of chemotherapy and radiation, such as diarrhea.[8]

Glutamine

Though cancer cells use glutamine as a fuel source, studies in humans have not found that glutamine stimulates growth of cancers in people taking chemotherapy.[9, 10] In fact, animal studies show that glutamine may actually decrease tumor growth while increasing susceptibility of cancer cells to radiation and chemotherapy,[11, 12] though such effects have not yet been studied in humans.

Glutamine has successfully reduced chemotherapy-induced mouth sores. In one trial, people were given 4 grams of glutamine in an oral rinse, which was swished around the mouth and then swallowed twice per day.[13] Thirteen of fourteen people in the study had fewer days with mouth sores as a result. These excellent results have been duplicated in some,[14] but not all[15] double-blind research. In another study, patients receiving high-dose **paclitaxel** (page 205) and melphalan had significantly fewer episodes of oral ulcers and bleeding when they took 6 grams of glutamine four times daily along with the chemotherapy.[16]

One double-blind trial suggested that 6 grams of glutamine taken three times per day can decrease diarrhea caused by chemotherapy.[17] However, other studies using higher amounts or intravenous glutamine have not reported this effect.[18, 19]

Intravenous use of glutamine in people undergoing bone marrow transplants, a procedure sometimes used to allow very high amounts of chemotherapy to be used, has led to reduced hospital stays, leading to a savings of over $21,000 for each patient given glutamine.[20]

In a double-blind study, supplementation with 18 grams of glutamine per day for 15 days, starting five days before the beginning of 5-FU therapy, significantly reduced the severity of drug-induced intestinal toxicity.[21]

Intravenous use of glutamine in people undergoing bone marrow transplants, a procedure sometimes used to allow very high amounts of chemotherapy to be used, has led to reduced hospital stays, leading to a savings of over $21,000 for each patient given glutamine.[22]

Melatonin

Melatonin supplementation (20 mg per day) has decreased toxicity and improved effectiveness of chemotherapy with 5-FU plus folinic acid and 5-FU plus cisplatin.[23]

N-acetyl cysteine (NAC)

NAC, an amino acid–like supplement that possesses antioxidant activity, has been used in four human studies to decrease the kidney and bladder toxicity of the chemotherapy drug ifosfamide.[24, 25, 26, 27] These studies used 1–2 grams NAC four times per day. There was no sign that NAC interfered with the efficacy of ifosfamide in any of these studies. Intakes of NAC over 4 grams per day may cause nausea and vomiting.

The newer anti-nausea drugs prescribed for people taking chemotherapy lead to greatly reduced nausea and vomiting for most people. Nonetheless, these drugs often do not totally eliminate all nausea. Natural substances used to reduce nausea should not be used instead of prescription anti-nausea drugs. Rather, under the guidance of a doctor, they should be added to those drugs if needed. At least one trial suggests that NAC, at 1,800 mg per day, may reduce nausea and vomiting caused by chemotherapy.[28]

Spleen extract

Patients with inoperable head and neck cancer were treated with a spleen peptide preparation (Polyerga) in a double-blind trial during chemotherapy with cisplatin and 5-FU.[29] The spleen preparation had a significant stabilizing effect on certain white blood cells. People taking it also experienced stabilized body weight and a

reduction in the fatigue and inertia that usually accompany this combination of chemotherapy agents.

Beta-carotene and vitamin E

Chemotherapy frequently causes mouth sores. In one trial, people were given approximately 400,000 IU of beta-carotene per day for three weeks and then 125,000 IU per day for an additional four weeks.[30] Those taking beta-carotene still suffered mouth sores, but the mouth sores developed later and tended to be less severe than mouth sores that formed in people receiving the same chemotherapy without beta-carotene.

In a study of chemotherapy-induced mouth sores, six of nine patients who applied vitamin E directly to their mouth sores had complete resolution of the sores compared with one of nine patients who applied placebo.[31] Others have confirmed the potential for vitamin E to help people with chemotherapy-induced mouth sores.[32] Applying vitamin E only once per day was helpful to only some groups of patients in another trial,[33] and not all studies have found vitamin E to be effective.[34] Until more is known, if vitamin E is used in an attempt to reduce chemotherapy-induced mouth sores, it should be applied topically twice per day and should probably be in the tocopherol (versus tocopheryl) form.

Vitamin A

A controlled French trial reported that when postmenopausal late-stage breast cancer patients were given very large amounts of vitamin A (350,000–500,000 IU per day) along with chemotherapy, remission rates were significantly better than when the chemotherapy was not accompanied by vitamin A.[35] Similar results were not found in premenopausal women. The large amounts of vitamin A used in the study are toxic and require clinical supervision.

Multivitamin-mineral

Many chemotherapy drugs can cause diarrhea, lack of appetite, vomiting, and damage to the gastrointestinal tract. Recent anti-nausea prescription medications are often effective. Nonetheless, nutritional deficiencies still occur.[36] It makes sense for people undergoing chemotherapy to take a high-potency multivitamin-mineral to protect against deficiencies.

Taurine

Taurine has been shown to be depleted in people taking chemotherapy.[37] It remains unclear how important this effect is or if people taking chemotherapy should take taurine supplements.

Thymus peptides

Peptides or short proteins derived from the thymus gland, an important immune organ, have been used in conjunction with chemotherapy drugs for people with cancer. One study using thymosin fraction V in combination with chemotherapy, compared with chemotherapy alone, found significantly longer survival times in the thymosin fraction V group.[38] A related substance, thymostimulin, decreased some side effects of chemotherapy and increased survival time compared with chemotherapy alone.[39] A third product, thymic extract TP1, was shown to improve immune function in people treated with chemotherapy compared with effects of chemotherapy alone.[40] Thymic peptides need to be administered by injection. People interested in their combined use with chemotherapy should consult a doctor.

Vitamin B₆

Fluorouracil occasionally causes problems on the skin of the palms and soles. Preliminary reports have appeared showing that 100 mg per day of vitamin B_6 can sometimes eliminate the pain associated with this drug-induced condition.[41, 42]

Interactions with Herbs

Echinacea (Echinacea purpurea, Echinacea angustifolia)

Echinacea is a popular immune-boosting herb that has been investigated for use with chemotherapy. One study investigated the actions of **cyclophosphamide** (page 79), echinacea, and thymus gland extracts to treat advanced cancer patients. Although small and uncontrolled, this trial suggested that the combination modestly extended the life span of some patients with inoperable cancers.[43] Signs of restoration of immune function were seen in these patients.

Eleuthero (Eleutherococcus senticosus)

Russian research has looked at using eleuthero with chemotherapy. One study of patients with melanoma found that chemotherapy was less toxic when eleuthero was given simultaneously. Similarly, women with inoperable breast cancer given eleuthero were reported to tolerate more chemotherapy.[44] Eleuthero treatment was also associated with improved immune function in women with breast cancer treated with chemotherapy and radiation.[45]

Milk thistle (Silybum marianum)

Milk thistle's major flavonoids, known collectively as silymarin, have shown synergistic actions with the chemotherapy drugs **cisplatin** (page 64) and **doxoru-**

bicin (page 100) (Adriamycin) in test tubes.[46] Silymarin also offsets the kidney toxicity of cisplatin in animals.[47] Silymarin has not yet been studied in humans treated with cisplatin. There is some evidence that silymarin may not interfere with some chemotherapy in humans with cancer.[48]

Ginger (Zingiber officinale)

Ginger can be helpful in alleviating nausea and vomiting caused by chemotherapy.[49, 50] Ginger powder in tablets or capsules can be taken for nausea, in 500 mg amounts every two or three hours, for a total of 1 gram per day.

German chamomile (Matricaria recutita)

A liquid preparation of German chamomile has been shown to reduce the incidence of mouth sores in people receiving radiation and systemic chemotherapy treatment in an uncontrolled study. [51]

PSK (Coriolus versicolor)

The mushroom *Coriolus versicolor* contains an immune-stimulating substance called polysaccharide krestin, or PSK. PSK has been shown in several studies to help cancer patients undergoing chemotherapy. One study involved women with estrogen receptor-negative breast cancer. PSK combined with chemotherapy significantly prolonged survival time compared with chemotherapy alone.[52] Another study followed women with breast cancer who were given chemotherapy with or without PSK. The PSK-plus-chemotherapy group had a 25% better chance of survival after ten years compared with those taking chemotherapy without PSK.[53] Another study investigated people who had surgically removed colon cancer. They were given chemotherapy with or without PSK. Those given PSK had a longer disease-free period and longer survival time.[54] Three grams of PSK were taken orally each day in these studies.

Although PSK is rarely available in the United States, hot-water extract products made from *Coriolus versicolor* mushrooms are available. These products may have activity related to that of PSK, but their use with chemotherapy has not been studied.

Interactions with Foods and Other Compounds
Fruit drinks

Often, people who undergo chemotherapy develop aversions to certain foods, sometimes making it permanently difficult to eat those foods. Exposing people to what researchers have called a "scapegoat stimulus" just before the administration of chemotherapy can direct the food aversion to the "scapegoat" food instead of more important parts of the diet. In one trial, fruit drinks administered just before chemotherapy were most effective in protecting against aversions to other foods.[55]

FLUOXETINE

Common names: Apo-Fluoxetine, Novo-Fluoxetine, Nu-Fluoxetine, PMS-Fluoxetine, Prozac

Fluoxetine is a member of the selective serotonin reuptake inhibitor (SSRI) family of drugs. Fluoxetine is used to treat depression, bulimia (binge-eating and vomiting), obsessive-compulsive disorder, and others conditions.

Summary of Interactions for Fluoxetine

In some cases, an herb or supplement may appear in more than one category, which may seem contradictory. For clarification, read the full article for details about the summarized interactions.

✓ May be Beneficial: Depletion or interference	Melatonin*
✓ May be Beneficial: Side effect reduction/prevention	Ginkgo biloba
✓ May be Beneficial: Supportive interaction	DHEA* Folic acid*
⊘ Avoid: Adverse interaction	5-HTP Alcohol L-tryptophan St. John's wort
ⓘ Check: Other	Melatonin
Reduced drug absorption/bioavailability	None known

Interactions with Dietary Supplements
Folic acid
Low blood levels of folic acid have been correlated to poor response to fluoxetine.[1] Furthermore, the addition of folic acid to fluoxetine appears to enhance the effectiveness of the drug. A double-blind trial found that depressed women receiving 500 mcg of folic acid per day in addition to fluoxetine experienced significant improvement in their symptoms, as well as fewer side effects, compared with women receiving only fluoxetine.[2] Similar results were not observed in men; however, men appear to have a higher requirement for folic acid than do women, so a higher intake may be necessary.

Melatonin
Administration of fluoxetine for six weeks significantly lowered melatonin levels in people with seasonal affective disorder (SAD) and in healthy persons as well.[3] Further study is needed to determine if this might interfere with sleeping or whether melatonin supplementation might be appropriate.

L-tryptophan
L-tryptophan is an amino acid found in protein-rich foods. Foods rich in L-tryptophan are not believed to cause any problems during fluoxetine use. However, dietary supplements of L-tryptophan taken during fluoxetine treatment have been reported to cause headache, sweating, dizziness, agitation, restlessness, nausea, vomiting, and other symptoms.[4]

5-Hydroxytryptophan (5-HTP)
Fluoxetine works by increasing serotonin activity in the brain. 5-HTP is converted to serotonin in the brain, and taking it with fluoxetine may increase fluoxetine-induced side effects. Until more is known, 5-HTP should not be taken with any SSRI drug, including fluoxetine.

Dehydroepiandrosterone (DHEA)
DHEA supplementation (50 mg per day) has been shown to restore the response of beta-endorphin, a brain chemical involved in pain and pleasure sensations, to fluoxetine.[5] Further research is needed to determine if this drug combination is safe for long-term use.

Interactions with Herbs
Ginkgo biloba
Ginkgo biloba extract (GBE) may reduce the side effects experienced by some persons taking SSRIs such as fluoxetine or **sertraline** (page 237). An open-label study with elderly, depressed persons found that 200–240 mg of GBE daily was effective in alleviating sexual side effects in both men and women taking SSRIs.[6] One case study reported that 180–240 mg of GBE daily reduced genital anesthesia and sexual side effects secondary to fluoxetine use in a 37-year-old woman.[7]

St. John's wort (Hypericum perforatum)
There have been no published reports about negative consequences of combining St. John's wort and fluoxetine. One case has been reported of an interaction between St. John's wort and a weak serotonin reuptake inhibitor drug known as **trazodone** (page 267) that is vaguely similar to fluoxetine.[8] In another case, a patient experienced grogginess, lethargy, nausea, weakness, and

fatigue after taking one dose of **paroxetine** (page 208) (Paxil, another SSRI drug) after ten days of St. John's wort use.[9] Nevertheless, some doctors are concerned about the possibility of an interaction between St. John's wort and fluoxetine causing side effects (e.g., mental confusion, muscle twitching, sweating, flushing) known collectively as serotonin syndrome.[10, 11] Until more is known about interactions and adverse actions, people taking any SSRI drugs, including fluoxetine, should avoid St. John's wort, unless they are being closely monitored by a doctor.

Interactions with Foods and Other Compounds

Food
Fluoxetine may be taken with or without food.[12]

Alcohol
SSRI drugs, including fluoxetine, may cause dizziness or drowsiness.[13] Alcohol may intensify these actions and increase the risk of accidental injury. Alcohol should be avoided during fluoxetine therapy. Fluoxetine has been reported to decrease the desire to drink alcohol in a group of alcoholics.[14]

FLURBIPROFEN

Common names: Ansaid, Froben SR, Froben

Flurbiprofen is used to treat pain caused by rheumatoid arthritis and osteoarthritis, and is in a family of medications known as **nonsteroidal anti-inflammatory drugs** (page 193) (NSAIDs).

Summary of Interactions for Flurbiprofen

In some cases, an herb or supplement may appear in more than one category, which may seem contradictory. For clarification, read the full article for details about the summarized interactions.

✓ May be Beneficial: Depletion or interference	Calcium* Vitamin D*
✓ May be Beneficial: Side effect reduction/prevention	N-acetyl cysteine
⊘ Avoid: Reduced drug absorption/ bioavailability	Food
⊘ Avoid: Adverse interaction	**Lithium** (page 157)* White willow*
Supportive interaction	None known

Interactions with Dietary Supplements

Calcium and vitamin D
Elevated calcium and vitamin D blood levels are commonly found in people with sarcoidosis. In one individual with sarcoidosis, taking flubiprofen lowered elevated blood calcium levels, but did not alter the concentration of vitamin D.[1] One controlled study showed that flurbiprofen reduced blood levels of vitamin D in people with frequent calcium kidney stones.[2] Further research is needed to determine whether flurbiprofen reduces blood calcium and vitamin D levels in healthy people.

Lithium (page 157)
Lithium is a mineral that may be present in some supplements and is also used in large amounts to treat mood disorders such as manic-depression (bipolar disorder). Most NSAIDs inhibit the excretion of lithium from the body, resulting in higher blood levels of the mineral, though **sulindac** (page 249) may have an opposite effect.[3] Since major changes in lithium blood levels can produce unwanted side effects or interfere with its efficacy, NSAIDs should be used with caution, and only under medical supervision, in people taking lithium supplements.

N-acetyl cysteine (NAC)
Nonsteroidal anti-inflammatory drugs commonly cause damage to stomach and intestinal tissue. Though the mechanism by which NSAIDs cause this side effect is unknown, some researchers believe that free-radical damage is involved. A test tube study showed that flurbiprofen increases free-radical activity in stomach cells, which is blocked by the antioxidant N-acetyl cysteine.[4] Additional research is needed to determine whether people taking flurbiprofen together with N-acetyl cysteine might experience fewer gastrointestinal side effects.

Interactions with Herbs

White willow bark (Salix alba)
White willow bark contains salicin, which is related to **aspirin** (page 26). Both salicin and aspirin produce anti-inflammatory effects after they have been converted to salicylic acid in the body. The administration of salicylates like aspirin to individuals taking oral NSAIDs may result in reduced blood levels of NSAIDs.[5] Though no studies have investigated interactions between white willow bark and NSAIDs, people taking NSAIDs should avoid the herb until more information is available.

Interactions with Foods and Other Compounds
Food

Taking NSAIDs with food may reduce stomach and intestinal side effects.[6] Although taking flurbiprofen with food reduces the rate at which the drug is absorbed, it does not reduce the total amount that is absorbed.[7] Therefore, to avoid possible side effects, people on long-term flurbiprofen therapy should take the drug with meals.

FLUVASTATIN

Common names: Lescol

Fluvastatin is a member of the HMG-CoA reductase inhibitor family of drugs that blocks the body's production of cholesterol. Fluvastatin is used to lower elevated cholesterol and to slow or prevent hardening of the arteries.

Summary of Interactions for Fluvastatin

In some cases, an herb or supplement may appear in more than one category, which may seem contradictory. For clarification, read the full article for details about the summarized interactions.

✓ May be Beneficial: Depletion or interference	Coenzyme Q10
⊘ Avoid: Adverse interaction	Vitamin A*
ⓘ Check: Other	Niacin
Side effect reduction/prevention	None known
Supportive interaction	None known
Reduced drug absorption/bioavailability	None known

Interactions with Dietary Supplements
Coenzyme Q10

In a randomized, double-blind trial, blood levels of coenzyme Q_{10} (CoQ_{10}) were measured in 45 people with high cholesterol treated with **lovastatin** (page 163) or **pravastatin** (page 220) (drugs related to fluvastatin) for 18 weeks.[1] A significant decline in blood levels of CoQ_{10} occurred with either drug. One study found that supplementation with 100 mg of CoQ_{10} prevented declines in CoQ_{10} when taken with **simvastatin** (page 239) (another HMG-CoA reductase inhibitor drug).[2] Many doctors recommend that people taking HMG-CoA reductase inhibitor drugs such as fluvastatin also supplement with approximately 100 mg

CoQ_{10} per day, although lower amounts, such as 10–30 mg per day, might conceivably be effective in preventing the decline in CoQ_{10} levels.

Niacin

Niacin is the form of vitamin B_3 used to lower cholesterol. Fluvastatin and niacin used together have been shown to be more effective than either substance alone.[3] Ingestion of large amounts of niacin along with HMG-CoA reductase inhibitors such as fluvastatin may cause muscle disorders (myopathy) that can become serious (rhabdomyolysis).[4, 5] Such problems appear to be uncommon.[6, 7] Nonetheless, individuals taking fluvastatin should consult with their doctor before taking niacin.

Vitamin A

A study of 37 people with high cholesterol treated with diet and HMG-CoA reductase inhibitors found blood vitamin A levels increased during two years of therapy.[8] Until more is known, people taking HMG-CoA reductase inhibitors, including fluvastatin, should have blood levels of vitamin A monitored if they intend to supplement vitamin A.

Interactions with Foods and Other Compounds
Food

Fluvastatin is equally effective taken with or without food in the evening.[9]

Alcohol

In a study of 31 people with primary hypercholesterolemia treated with fluvastatin, six weeks of daily, moderate alcohol consumption slowed the absorption and metabolism of fluvastatin but did not interfere with its effectiveness.[10]

FLUVOXAMINE

Common names: Alti-Fluvoxamine, Apo-Fluvoxamine, Faurin, Faverin, Luvox

Fluvoxamine is a selective serotonin reuptake inhibitor (SSRI) drug, related to Prozac. It is used primarily to treat obsessive-compulsive disorder and is under investigation to treat depression.

Summary of Interactions for Fluvoxamine

In some cases, an herb or supplement may appear in more than one category, which may seem contradictory.

For clarification, read the full article for details about the summarized interactions.

✓ May be Beneficial: Side effect reduction/prevention	*Ginkgo biloba*
✓ May be Beneficial: Supportive interaction	Yohimbe*
⃠ Avoid: Adverse interaction	5-HTP Grapefruit/ grapefruit juice L-tryptophan St. John's wort* Tobacco
ⓘ Check: Other	Melatonin
Depletion or interference	None known
Reduced drug absorption/bioavailability	None known

Interactions with Dietary Supplements

5-Hydroxytryptophan (5-HTP) and L-tryptophan
Fluvoxamine works by increasing serotonin activity in the brain. 5-HTP and L-tryptophan are converted to serotonin in the brain, and taking them with fluvoxamine may increase fluvoxamine-induced side effects. Until more is known, 5-HTP and L-tryptophan should not be taken with any SSRI drug, including fluvoxamine.

Melatonin
Fluvoxamine has been shown to significantly raise the amount of melatonin in the blood after oral administration.[1] Researchers suggest that fluvoxamine may inhibit elimination of melatonin, but the clinical significance of this finding is as yet unclear.

Interactions with Herbs

Ginkgo biloba
Ginkgo biloba extract (GBE) may reduce the side effects experienced by some persons taking SSRIs such as **fluoxetine** (page 120) or **sertraline** (page 237). An open-label study with elderly, depressed persons found that 200–240 mg of GBE daily was effective in alleviating sexual side effects in both men and women taking SSRIs.[2]

One case study reported that 180–240 mg of GBE daily reduced genital anesthesia and sexual side effects secondary to fluoxetine use in a 37-year-old woman.[3]

St. John's wort (Hypericum perforatum)
One report describes a case of serotonin syndrome in a patient who took St. John's wort and **trazodone** (page 267), a weak SSRI drug.[4] The patient experienced mental confusion, muscle twitching, sweating, flushing, and ataxia. In another case, a patient experienced groggi-

ness, lethargy, nausea, weakness, and fatigue after taking one dose of **paroxetine** (page 208) (Paxil, an SSRI drug related to fluvoxamine) after ten days of St. John's wort.[5] Until more is known about interactions and adverse actions, people taking any SSRI drugs, including fluvoxamine, should avoid St. John's wort, unless they are being closely monitored by a doctor.

Yohimbe (Pausinystalia yohimbe)
The alkaloid yohimbine from the African yohimbe tree affects the nervous system in a way that may complement fluvoxamine. One report studied depressed people who had not responded to fluvoxamine. When 5 mg of yohimbine was added three times each day, there was significant improvement. Some people required higher amounts of yohimbine before their depression improved. Because yohimbine can have side effects, it should only be taken under a doctor's supervision. Yohimbine is a prescription drug, but standardized extracts of yohimbe that contain yohimbine are available as a supplement.

Interactions with Foods and Other Compounds

Alcohol
SSRI drugs, including fluvoxamine, may cause dizziness or drowsiness.[6] Alcohol may intensify the drowsiness and increase the risk of accidental injury. People should avoid alcohol-containing products during fluvoxamine treatment.

Grapefruit
In a study of healthy volunteers, ingestion of 250 ml (approximately 8 ounces) of grapefruit juice along with fluvoxamine increased the blood level of fluvoxamine by 60%, compared with ingestion of fluvoxamine with water.[7] Because a higher concentration of the drug could increase its adverse effects, individuals should not consume grapefruit or grapefruit juice around the same time they take fluvoxamine.

Tobacco (Nicotiana species)
Smoking increases the metabolism of fluvoxamine, which may reduce effectiveness.[8] People should avoid smoking while taking fluvoxamine.

FOLIC ACID

Though supplements containing 0.8 mg of folic acid are available over-the-counter, tablets and injectable forms that contain more than 1 mg of folic acid are available only with a prescription. The vitamin is used to treat anemia caused by folic acid deficiency, which may result from poor absorption, a dietary deficiency, or pregnancy.

Summary of Interactions for Folic Acid

In some cases, an herb or supplement may appear in more than one category, which may seem contradictory. For clarification, read the full article for details about the summarized interactions.

✓ May be Beneficial: Depletion or interference	Zinc
✓ May be Beneficial: Supportive interaction	Vitamin B$_6$
⊘ Avoid: Reduced drug absorption/ bioavailability	Alcohol **Antacids** (page 18) Beans Food Smoking Vitamin B$_6$
Side effect reduction/prevention	None known
Adverse interaction	None known

Interactions with Dietary Supplements
Vitamin B$_6$
Folic acid and vitamin B$_6$ have been used to reduce elevated blood levels of homocysteine, which has been associated with atherosclerosis. One controlled study showed that taking 0.3 mg of folic acid together with 120 mg of vitamin B$_6$ reduced homocysteine levels more than taking either vitamin alone. The study also revealed that long-term supplementation with vitamin B$_6$ alone might reduce blood folic acid levels.[1] Therefore, people with elevated blood homocysteine levels should supplement with both folic acid and vitamin B$_6$.

Zinc
Though some studies indicate that supplementing with folic acid reduces blood levels of zinc, most show no interaction between the two nutrients when folic acid is taken at moderate levels.[2] Therefore, until more convincing evidence is available, people taking moderate amounts of folic acid do not need to supplement with zinc. Zinc supplementation is recommended when folic acid intake is high. A doctor should be consulted to determine the appropriate time to add zinc supplementation to folic acid therapy.

Interactions with Foods and Other Compounds
Food
Studies have shown that taking folic acid with different foods can alter the absorption of the vitamin. One study showed that taking folic acid supplements with wheat bran fiber increased, while beans reduced absorption of the vitamin.[3] Though it is unlikely that either food will clinically affect folic acid absorption from a mixed diet, people should probably avoid taking the vitamin with a meal consisting primarily of beans. Another study revealed that folic acid is better absorbed on an empty stomach, though a light meal only slightly reduced absorption.[4]

Alcohol
One study showed that the majority of individuals who chronically consume alcohol have below-normal red blood cell levels of folic acid.[5] Though lower intake of foods containing folic acid may be involved, some researchers believe that alcohol may directly reduce blood levels of nutrients.[6] Animal studies have shown that chronic alcohol consumption might reduce absorption[7] or increase elimination of folic acid.[8] Studies involving acute consumption of alcohol in humans have shown that alcohol may increase urinary elimination of folic acid.[9] Additional studies are needed to determine whether heavy drinkers taking folic acid might require larger-than-normal amounts of the vitamin to treat anemia.

Antacids (page 18)
One controlled study showed that taking folic acid together with an antacid containing **aluminum** (page 10) and **magnesium hydroxide** (page 166) reduced the absorption of the vitamin.[10] Therefore, individuals should take folic acid one hour before or two hours after taking antacids containing aluminum and magnesium hydroxide.

Smoking
A study of individuals aged 65 and older revealed that people who smoke cigarettes have lower red cell and blood folic acid levels compared with those who do not smoke.[11] Lower intake of folic acid through food only partly explained the reduced blood levels observed in smokers. Additional research is needed to determine whether smokers taking folic acid might need to take larger-than-normal amounts of the vitamin to treat anemia.

FOSAMPRENAVIR

Common names: Lexiva

Fosamprenavir is used in combination with other antiviral drugs to treat HIV infection.

Summary of Interactions for Fosamprenavir

In some cases, an herb or supplement may appear in more than one category, which may seem contradictory. For clarification, read the full article for details about the summarized interactions.

⊘ Avoid: Reduced drug absorption/ bioavailability	St. John's wort
Depletion or interference	None known
Side effect reduction/prevention	None known
Supportive interaction	None known
Adverse interaction	None known

Interactions with Herbs

St. John's wort (Hypericum perforatum)

Taking St. John's wort when taking fosamprenavir might result in reduced blood levels of the drug, which could lead to reduced effectiveness and eventual resistance. Individuals taking fosamprenavir should avoid taking St. John's wort at the same time.

FUCIBET

Contains the following ingredients:
Betamethasone
Fusidic acid

FUCIDIN H

Contains the following ingredients:
Fusidic acid
Hydrocortisone

GABAPENTIN

Common names: Neurontin

Gabapentin is a drug used to treat or prevent seizures in people with seizure disorders.

Summary of Interactions for Gabapentin

In some cases, an herb or supplement may appear in more than one category, which may seem contradictory. For clarification, read the full article for details about the summarized interactions.

✓ May be Beneficial: Depletion or interference	Biotin* Calcium* Folic acid* L-carnitine* Vitamin A* Vitamin B$_{12}$* Vitamin B$_6$* Vitamin D* Vitamin K*
✓ May be Beneficial: Side effect reduction/prevention	Folic acid* L-carnitine* Vitamin B$_{12}$* Vitamin D* Vitamin K*
✓ May be Beneficial: Supportive interaction	Folic acid*
⊘ Avoid: Adverse interaction	Folic acid*
Reduced drug absorption/bioavailability	None known

Interactions with Dietary Supplements

Biotin

Several controlled studies have shown that long-term anticonvulsant treatment decreases blood levels of biotin.[1, 2, 3, 4] In children, a deficiency of biotin can lead to withdrawn behavior and a delay in mental development. Adults with low biotin levels might experience a loss of appetite, feelings of discomfort or uneasiness, mental depression, or hallucinations. To avoid side effects, individuals taking anticonvulsants should supplement with biotin either alone or as part of a multivitamin.

Calcium

Individuals on long-term multiple anticonvulsant therapy may develop below-normal blood levels of calcium, which may be related to drug-induced vitamin D deficiency.[5] Two infants born to women taking high doses of phenytoin and **phenobarbital** (page 215) while pregnant developed jitteriness and tetany (a syndrome characterized by muscle twitches) cramps, and spasm during the first two weeks of life.[6] Controlled research is needed to determine whether pregnant women who are taking anticonvulsant medications should supplement with additional amounts of calcium and vitamin D.

Gabapentin

L-carnitine

Several controlled and preliminary studies showed that multiple drug therapy for seizures results in dramatic reductions in blood carnitine levels.[7, 8, 9] Further controlled research is needed to determine whether children taking anticonvulsants might benefit by supplementing with L-carnitine, since current studies yield conflicting results. For example, one controlled study indicated that children taking **valproic acid** (page 275) and carbamazepine received no benefit from supplementing with L-carnitine.[10] However, another small study revealed that children taking valproic acid experienced less fatigue and excessive sleepiness following L-carnitine supplementation.[11] Despite the lack of well-controlled studies, individuals who are taking anticonvulsants and experiencing side effects might benefit from supplementing with L-carnitine.

Folic acid

Several studies have shown that multiple anticonvulsant therapy reduces blood levels of folic acid and dramatically increases homocysteine levels.[12, 13, 14] Homocysteine, a potential marker for folic acid deficiency, is a compound used experimentally to induce seizures and is associated with atherosclerosis.

One preliminary study showed that pregnant women who use anticonvulsant drugs without folic acid supplementation have an increased risk of having a child with birth defects, such as heart defects, cleft lip and palate, neural tube defects, and skeletal abnormalities. However, supplementation with folic acid greatly reduces the risk.[15] Consequently, some healthcare practitioners recommend that women taking multiple anticonvulsant drugs supplement with 5 mg of folic acid daily, for three months prior to conception and during the first trimester, to prevent folic acid deficiency-induced birth defects.[16] Other practitioners suggest that 1mg or less of folic acid each day is sufficient to prevent deficiency during pregnancy.[17]

One well-controlled study showed that adding folic acid to multiple anticonvulsant therapy resulted in reduced seizure frequency.[18] In addition, three infants with seizures who were unresponsive to medication experienced immediate relief following supplementation with the active form of folic acid.[19]

Despite the apparent beneficial effects, some studies have indicated that as little as 0.8 mg of folic acid taken daily can increase the frequency and/or severity of seizures.[20, 21, 22, 23] However, a recent controlled study showed that both healthy and epileptic women taking less than 1 mg of folic acid per day had no increased risk for seizures.[24] Until more is known about the risks and benefits of folic acid, individuals taking multiple anticonvulsant drugs should consult with their healthcare practitioner before supplementing with folic acid. In addition, pregnant women or women who might become pregnant while taking anticonvulsant drugs should discuss folic acid supplementation with their practitioner.

Vitamin A

Anticonvulsant drugs can occasionally cause birth defects when taken by pregnant women, and their toxicity might be related to low blood levels of vitamin A. One controlled study showed that taking multiple anticonvulsant drugs results in dramatic changes in the way the body utilizes vitamin A.[25] Further controlled research is needed to determine whether supplemental vitamin A might prevent birth defects in children born to women on multiple anticonvulsant therapy. Other research suggests that ingestion of large amounts of vitamin A may promote the development of birth defects, although the studies are conflicting.

Vitamin B6

One controlled study revealed that taking anticonvulsant drugs dramatically reduces blood levels of vitamin B6.[26] A nutritional deficiency of vitamin B6 can lead to an increase in homocysteine blood levels, which has been associated with atherosclerosis. Vitamin B6 deficiency is also associated with symptoms such as dizziness, fatigue, mental depression, and seizures. On the other hand, supplementation with large amounts of vitamin B6 (80–200 mg per day) has been reported to reduce blood levels of some anticonvulsant drugs, which could theoretically trigger seizures. People taking multiple anticonvulsant drugs should discuss with their doctor whether supplementing with vitamin B6 is advisable.

Vitamin B12

Anemia is an uncommon side effect experienced by people taking anticonvulsant drugs. Though many researchers believe that low blood levels of folic acid are involved, the effects might be caused by a vitamin B12 deficiency. Deficiencies of folic acid and vitamin B12 can lead to nerve and mental problems. One study revealed that individuals on long-term anticonvulsant therapy, despite having no laboratory signs of anemia, had dramatically lower levels of vitamin B12 in their cerebrospinal fluid (the fluid that bathes the brain) when compared with people who were not taking seizure medications. Improvement in mental status and nerve function was observed in a majority of symptomatic individuals after taking 30 mcg of vitamin B_{12} daily for a few days.[27] Another study found that long-term anticonvulsant therapy had no effect on blood levels of vitamin B_{12}.[28] The results of these two studies indicate that people taking anticonvulsant drugs might experience side effects of vitamin B_{12} deficiency, and that the deficiency is not easily detected by the usual blood tests. Therefore, individuals taking anticonvulsant drugs for several months or years might prevent nerve and mental problems by supplementing with vitamin B_{12}.

Vitamin D

Though research results vary, long-term use of anticonvulsant drugs appears to interfere with vitamin D activity, which might lead to softening of bones (osteomalacia). One study showed that blood levels of vitamin D in males taking anticonvulsants were lower than those found in men who were not taking seizure medication.[29] In a controlled study, bone strength improved in children taking anticonvulsant drugs who were supplemented with the activated form of vitamin D and 500 mg per day of calcium for nine months.[30] Some research suggests that differences in exposure to sunlight—which normally increases blood levels of vitamin D—might explain why some studies have failed to find a beneficial effect of vitamin D supplementation. In one controlled study, blood vitamin D levels in children taking anticonvulsants were dramatically lower in winter months than in summer months.[31] Another study of 450 people in Florida taking anticonvulsants found that few had drug-induced bone disease.[32] Consequently, people taking anticonvulsant drugs who do not receive adequate sunlight should supplement with 400 IU of vitamin D each day to help prevent osteomalacia.

Vitamin E

Two studies showed that individuals taking phenytoin and **phenobarbital** (page 215) had lower blood vitamin E levels than those who received no treatment for seizures.[33, 34] Though the consequences of lower blood levels of vitamin E are unknown, people taking multiple anticonvulsant drugs should probably supplement with 100 to 200 IU of vitamin E daily to prevent a deficiency.

Vitamin K

Some studies have shown that babies born to women taking anticonvulsant drugs have low blood levels of vitamin K, which might cause bleeding in the infant.[35] Though some researchers recommend vitamin K supplementation prior to delivery,[36, 37] not all agree that supplementation for women taking anticonvulsant drugs is necessary.[38] Until more information is available, pregnant women or women who might become pregnant while taking anticonvulsant drugs should discuss vitamin K supplementation with their healthcare practitioner.

Interactions with Foods and Other Compounds

Alcohol

Gabapentin may cause dizziness or sleepiness.[39] Alcohol may intensify these effects and increase the risk of accidental injury. To prevent problems, people taking gabapentin should avoid alcohol.

GAVISCON 250 TABLETS

Contains the following ingredients:
  Alginic acid
  Aluminium
  Magnesium
  Sodium bicarbonate (page 240)

GELUSIL

Contains the following ingredients:
  Aluminium
  Magnesium

GEMFIBROZIL

Common names: Apo-Gemfibrozil, Emfib, Gen-Fibro, Lopid, Novo-Gemfibrozil, Nu-Gemfibrozil, PMS-Gemfibrozil

Gemfibrozil is a drug used to lower cholesterol and triglycerides in people with high cholesterol. Other drugs, especially members of the HMG-CoA reductase inhibitor drug family, are more commonly used.

Summary of Interactions for Gemfibrozil

In some cases, an herb or supplement may appear in more than one category, which may seem contradictory.

For clarification, read the full article for details about the summarized interactions.

✓	May be Beneficial: Depletion or interference	Coenzyme Q₁₀* Vitamin E*
✓	May be Beneficial: Supportive interaction	Vitamin B₃ (niacin)
🚫	Avoid: Adverse interaction	Red yeast rice*
	Side effect reduction/prevention	None known
	Reduced drug absorption/bioavailability	None known

Interactions with Dietary Supplements

Coenzyme Q₁₀
In a randomized study of 21 men with combined hyperlipidemia, ten to twelve weeks of gemfibrozil therapy reduced coenzyme Q_{10} blood levels to the levels seen in healthy men.[1] The clinical significance of this finding is unknown.

Vitamin E
In a randomized study of 21 men with combined hyperlipidemia, ten to twelve weeks of gemfibrozil therapy reduced alpha- and gamma-tocopherol blood levels to the levels seen in healthy men.[2] The clinical significance of this finding is unknown and may reflect a normal physiological response to a reduction in serum cholesterol levels.

Vitamin B₃ (Niacin)
Niacin (not niacinamide) and gemfibrozil have successfully raised HDL (good) cholesterol levels, both alone and in combination.[3]

Interactions with Herbs

Red yeast rice (Monascus purpureus)
Monascus purpureus, a form of red yeast, is fermented with rice to produce a dietary supplement, Cholestin, that contains low levels of **lovastatin** (page 163), a drug otherwise available only by prescription. Gemfibrozil taken with the prescription drug lovastatin has been reported to cause rhabdomyolysis, a potentially life-threatening muscle disease.[4] People taking gemfibrozil should avoid lovastatin-containing products, including Cholestin, until more is known. The levels of lovastatin in Cholestin are significantly lower than those given of the drug as a single agent. Cholestin also contains numerous other compounds that may alter the interaction of lovastatin and gemfibrozil.

Interactions with Foods and Other Compounds

Food
Gemfibrozil should be taken 30 minutes before meals.[5]

Alcohol
Gemfibrozil may cause dizziness or blurred vision.[6] Alcohol may intensify these effects, increasing the risk for accidental injury. People taking gemfibrozil should avoid alcohol.

GEMIFLOXACIN

Common names: Factive

Gemifloxacin is used to treat bacterial infections, such as chronic bronchitis and mild to moderate pneumonia.

Summary of Interactions for Gemifloxacin
In some cases, an herb or supplement may appear in more than one category, which may seem contradictory. For clarification, read the full article for details about the summarized interactions.

🚫	Avoid: Reduced drug absorption/ bioavailability	Calcium Iron Magnesium
	Depletion or interference	None known
	Side effect reduction/prevention	None known
	Supportive interaction	None known
	Adverse interaction	None known

Interactions with Dietary Supplements

Calcium
A recent study showed that taking calcium carbonate and gemifloxacin at the same time results in a significant reduction in blood levels of the drug.[1] Consequently, gemifloxacin and calcium supplements should not be taken at the same time.

Iron
A review of interactions involving quinolone antibiotics indicated that supplements containing iron, when taken at the same time as gemifloxacin, might reduce absorption of the drug up to 50%.[2] Consequently, gemifloxacin and supplements containing iron should not be taken at the same time.

Magnesium
One study showed that taking an antacid containing magnesium and aluminum ten minutes before gemi-

floxacin results in an 85% reduction in the absorption of the drug.[3] Consequently, gemifloxacin and supplements containing magnesium should not be taken at the same time.

GENERAL ANESTHETICS

Common names: Amidate, Desflurane, Dipravin, Droperidol, Enflurane, Ethrane, Etomidate, Forane, Halothane, Inapsine, Isoflurane, Ketalar, Ketamine, Methoxyflurane, Penthrane, Propofol, Sevoflurane, Suprane, Ultane

General anesthetics are used to produce unconsciousness during surgery. Unlike local anesthetics that are used in dentistry and minor surgery, general anesthetics circulate throughout the body, which results in a stronger action on the nervous system and a greater potential for side effects. Medications used as general anesthetics come from many different drug classifications, including barbiturates and benzodiazepines.

The interactions described below pertain to anesthetics in general. For specific interactions, refer to the individual drugs.

- Desflurane (Suprane)
- Droperidol (Inapsine)
- Enflurane (Ethrane)
- Etomidate (Amidate)
- Halothane
- Isoflurane (Forane)
- Ketamine (Ketalar)
- Methohexital (Brevital)
- Methoxyflurane (Penthrane)
- Midazolam (Versed)
- **Nitrous oxide** (page 191)
- Propofol (Diprivan)
- Sevoflurane (Ultane)
- Thiopental (Pentothal)

Summary of Interactions for General Anesthetics

In some cases, an herb or supplement may appear in more than one category, which may seem contradictory. For clarification, read the full article for details about the summarized interactions.

✓	May be Beneficial: Side effect reduction/prevention	Catechin* Ginger* Milk thistle
	Depletion or interference	None known
	Supportive interaction	None known

Reduced drug absorption/bioavailability	None known
Adverse interaction	None known

Interactions common to many, if not all, General Anesthetics are described in this article. Interactions reported for only one or several drugs in this class may not be listed in this article. Some drugs listed in this article are linked to articles specific to that respective drug; please refer to those individual drug articles. The information in this article may not necessarily apply to drugs in this class for which no separate article exists. If you are taking a General Anesthetic for which no separate article exists, talk with your doctor or pharmacist.

Interactions with Dietary Supplements
Catechin
Some general anesthetic drugs have infrequently caused liver damage. One animal study showed that taking catechin (a bioflavonoid) prior to halothane exposure reduced the amount of liver damage caused by the drug.[1] Additional research is needed to determine whether this protective effect occurs in humans and with other general anesthetics.

Interactions with Herbs
Ginger (Zingiber officinale)
General anesthetics commonly cause nausea upon waking. In a double-blind study, taking 1 gram of ginger one hour before surgery was as effective at reducing nausea and vomiting as the anti-nausea drug **metoclopramide** (page 175).[2] Individuals taking ginger in order to avoid side effects should disclose this to their doctor prior to surgery, since the herb might affect blood clotting.

Milk thistle (Silybum marianum)
Some general anesthetic drugs have infrequently caused liver damage. One animal study showed that taking silybine, an active compound found in milk thistle, prior to halothane exposure reduced the amount of liver damage caused by the drug.[3] Though controlled research in humans is necessary, some doctors of natural medicine currently suggest taking milk thistle standardized to contain 140 mg of silymarin three times a day, beginning a week before surgery and continuing for at least one week after surgery.

GENTAMICIN

Common names: Alcomicin, Cidomycin, Diogent, Garamycin, Garatec, Gentacidin, Genticin, Minims Gentamicin, Scheinpharm Gentamicin

Gentamicin

Gentamicin is an **aminoglycoside antibiotic** (page 11) used to treat infections caused by many different types of bacteria. Gentamicin is usually administered by intravenous (IV) infusion or intramuscular injection. There are special gentamicin-containing drug products to treat eye and skin infections.

Summary of Interactions for Gentamicin

In some cases, an herb or supplement may appear in more than one category, which may seem contradictory. For clarification, read the full article for details about the summarized interactions.

✓ May be Beneficial: Depletion or interference	Calcium* Magnesium Potassium* Vitamin K*
✓ May be Beneficial: Side effect reduction/prevention	*Bifidobacterium longum* * *Lactobacillus acidophilus* * *Lactobacillus casei* * N-acetyl cysteine* *Saccharomyces boulardii* * *Saccharomyces cerevisiae* * Vitamin B₁₂* Vitamin K*
✓ May be Beneficial: Supportive interaction	*Saccharomyces boulardii* *
ⓘ Check: Other	Vitamin B₆
Reduced drug absorption/bioavailability	None known
Adverse interaction	None known

Interactions with Dietary Supplements
Calcium

Gentamicin has been associated with hypocalcemia (low calcium levels) in humans.[1] In a study using rats, authors reported oral calcium supplementation reduced gentamicin-induced kidney damage.[2] The implications of this report for humans are unclear. People receiving gentamicin should ask their doctor about monitoring calcium levels and calcium supplementation.

Magnesium

Gentamicin has been associated with urinary loss of magnesium, resulting in hypomagnesemia (low magnesium levels) in humans.[3, 4]

Potassium

Gentamicin has been associated with hypokalemia (low potassium levels) in humans.[5]

Probiotics

A common side effect of antibiotics is diarrhea, which may be caused by the elimination of beneficial bacteria normally found in the colon. Controlled studies have shown that taking probiotic microorganisms—such as *Lactobacillus casei, Lactobacillus acidophilus, Bifidobacterium longum,* or *Saccharomyces boulardii*—helps prevent antibiotic-induced diarrhea.[6]

The diarrhea experienced by some people who take antibiotics also might be due to an overgrowth of the bacterium *Clostridium difficile,* which causes a disease known as pseudomembranous colitis. Controlled studies have shown that supplementation with harmless yeast, such as *Saccharomyces boulardii*[7] or *Saccharomyces cerevisiae* (baker's or brewer's yeast),[8] helps prevent recurrence of this infection. In one study, taking 500 mg of *Saccharomyces boulardii* twice daily enhanced the effectiveness of the antibiotic vancomycin in preventing recurrent clostridium infection.[9] Therefore, people taking antibiotics who later develop diarrhea might benefit from supplementing with saccharomyces organisms.

Treatment with antibiotics also commonly leads to an overgrowth of yeast *(Candida albicans)* in the vagina (candida vaginitis) and the intestines (sometimes referred to as "dysbiosis"). Controlled studies have shown that *Lactobacillus acidophilus* might prevent candida vaginitis.[10]

Vitamin B₆

Gentamicin administration has been associated with vitamin B₆ depletion in rabbits.[11] The authors of this study mention early evidence that vitamin B₆ administration may protect against gentamicin-induced kidney damage.

Vitamin K

Several cases of excessive bleeding have been reported in people who take antibiotics.[12, 13, 14, 15] This side effect may be the result of reduced vitamin K activity and/or reduced vitamin K production by bacteria in the colon. One study showed that people who had taken broad-spectrum antibiotics had lower liver concentrations of vitamin K₂ (menaquinone), though vitamin K₁ (phylloquinone) levels remained normal.[16] Several antibiotics appear to exert a strong effect on vitamin K activity, while others may not have any effect. Therefore, one should refer to a specific antibiotic for information on whether it interacts with vitamin K. Doctors of natural medicine sometimes recommend vitamin K supplementation to people taking antibiotics. Additional research is needed to determine whether the amount of vitamin K_1 found in some multivitamins is sufficient to prevent antibiotic-induced bleeding. Moreover, most multivitamins do not contain vitamin K.

In a study of guinea pigs, a single intramuscular injection of methylcobalamin (a form of vitamin B_{12}), in the amount of 125 mg per 2.2 pounds of body weight, given immediately after administration of gentamicin, prevented damage to the inner ear, which is a common side effect of gentamicin therapy.[17] No studies have been done to determine whether the same protective effect would occur in humans.

In another animal study, injections of N-Acetyl cysteine (10 mg per 2.2 pounds of body weight per day for five days) reduced the severity of kidney damage resulting from administration of gentamicin.[18]

GLIMEPIRIDE

Common names: Amaryl

Glimepiride is used to treat type 2, or non-insulin dependent, diabetes when diet and exercise alone have been ineffective. It is a type of drug called a sulfonylurea.

Summary of Interactions for Glimepiride
In some cases, an herb or supplement may appear in more than one category, which may seem contradictory. For clarification, read the full article for details about the summarized interactions.

✓ May be Beneficial: Supportive interaction	**Lithium** (page 157)* Magnesium*
⊘ Avoid: Adverse interaction	*Ginkgo biloba* Vitamin B_3* (niacin)
Depletion or interference	None known
Side effect reduction/prevention	None known
Reduced drug absorption/bioavailability	None known

Interactions with Dietary Supplements
Vitamin B_3 (Niacin)
Vitamin B_3 can raise blood sugar levels, which makes diabetes difficult to control.[1] Use of niacin along with

glimepiride may increase requirements for the drug. On the other hand, individuals who stop taking niacin while on glimepiride should monitor their blood for lower-than-usual glucose levels.

Magnesium
Supplementing magnesium may enhance the blood-sugar-lowering effects of sulfonylurea drugs.[2] Though no current studies have investigated whether glimepiride increases the risk of developing hypoglycemia, individuals should closely monitor their blood glucose while taking glimepiride together with magnesium supplements.

Lithium *(page 157)*
Lithium is a mineral that may be present in some supplements and is also used in large amounts to treat mood disorders such as manic-depression. Taking lithium and sulfonylurea drugs together may increase the risk of developing hypoglycemia.[3] Consequently, people taking glimepiride and lithium together should frequently monitor themselves for low blood glucose.

Ginkgo biloba
In a preliminary trial, administration of *Ginkgo biloba* extract (120 mg per day) for three months to patients with type 2 diabetes who were taking oral anti-diabetes medication resulted in a significant worsening of glucose tolerance. Ginkgo did not impair glucose tolerance in individuals whose diabetes was controlled by diet.[4] Individuals taking oral anti-diabetes medication should consult a doctor before taking *Ginkgo biloba*.

Interactions with Food and Other Compounds
Food
The ingestion of food with glimepiride can lower the overall blood levels of the drug by nearly 10%.[5] Though this is a minor reduction, maximum effectiveness would be achieved if glimepiride were taken on an empty stomach.

GLIPIZIDE

Common names: Glibenese, Glucotrol, Minodiab

Glipizide is a sulfonylurea drug used to lower blood sugar levels in people with type 2 (non-insulin-dependent) diabetes.

Summary of Interactions for Glipizide
In some cases, an herb or supplement may appear in more than one category, which may seem contradictory.

Glipizide

For clarification, read the full article for details about the summarized interactions.

⊘ Avoid: Adverse interaction	Fenugreek* *Ginkgo biloba* *Gymnema sylvestre**
ⓘ Check: Other	Magnesium
Depletion or interference	None known
Side effect reduction/prevention	None known
Supportive interaction	None known
Reduced drug absorption/bioavailability	None known

Interactions with Dietary Supplements

Magnesium

In a study of people with poorly controlled type 2 diabetes and low blood levels of magnesium, treatment with glipizide was associated with a significant rise in magnesium levels.[1] In a randomized trial with eight healthy people, 850 mg **magnesium hydroxide** (page 166) increased glipizide absorption and activity.[2] In theory, such changes could be therapeutic or detrimental under varying circumstances. Therefore, people taking glipizide should consult with their doctor before taking magnesium supplements.

Interactions with Herbs

Fenugreek (Trigonella foenum-graecum)

In a randomized study of 15 patients with type 1 (insulin-dependent) diabetes, fenugreek (100 grams per day for ten days) was reported to reduce blood sugar, urinary sugar excretion, serum cholesterol, and triglycerides, with no change in insulin levels, compared with ten days of placebo.[3] In a study of 60 people with type 2 diabetes, fenugreek (25 grams per day for 24 weeks) was reported to significantly reduce blood glucose levels.[4] People using glipizide should talk with their doctor before making any therapy changes.

Ginkgo biloba

In a preliminary trial, administration of *Ginkgo biloba* who were taking oral anti-diabetes medication resulted in a significant worsening of glucose tolerance. Ginkgo did not impair glucose tolerance in individuals whose diabetes was controlled by diet.[5] Individuals taking oral anti-diabetes medication should consult a doctor before taking *Ginkgo biloba*.

Gymnema sylvestre

Herbs such as *Gymnema sylvestre* will often improve blood-sugar control in diabetics.

Interactions with Foods and Other Compounds

Food

Glipizide works best when taken 30 minutes before meals.[6] Effective treatment of type 2 diabetes with glipizide includes adherence to recommended dietary guidelines.

GLYBURIDE

Common names: Albert Glyburide, Apo-Glyburide, Calabren, Daonil, Diabetamide, Diabeta, Euglucon, Gen-Glybe, Glibenclamide, Gliken, Glynase Prestab, Glynase, Libanil, Malix, Micronase, Novo-Glyburide, Nu-Glyburide, PMS-Glyburide, Pres Tab, Semi-Daonil

Glyburide is a sulfonylurea drug used to lower blood sugar levels in people with type 2 (non-insulin-dependent) diabetes. Maintaining normal blood sugar levels helps reduce health problems associated with diabetes. People with diabetes should consult with their doctor before starting or stopping any form of treatment including drug therapy, herbal products, supplements, and others.

Consumption of a high-fiber diet and/or supplementation with nutrients such as chromium, biotin, vitamin E, and others or herbs such as *Gymnema sylvestre* will often improve blood-sugar control in diabetics. In such cases, the amount of blood sugar-lowering drugs may need to be reduced in order to avoid a hypoglycemic reaction. Anyone taking medication for diabetes should consult the prescribing physician before making dietary changes or taking nutrients or herbs that are designed to lower blood-sugar levels.

Summary of Interactions for Glyburide

In some cases, an herb or supplement may appear in more than one category, which may seem contradictory. For clarification, read the full article for details about the summarized interactions.

✓ May be Beneficial: Supportive interaction	*Aloe vera**
⊘ Avoid: Adverse interaction	Chromium* *Ginkgo biloba*
ⓘ Check: Other	Biotin *Gymnema sylvestre* Vitamin E
Depletion or interference	None known
Side effect reduction/prevention	None known
Reduced drug absorption/bioavailability	None known

Interactions with Herbs

Aloe (Aloe vera)

One single-blind study in Thailand reported that combining 1 Tbsp (15 ml) of aloe juice twice daily with glyburide significantly improved blood sugar and lipid levels in people with diabetes, compared with placebo.[1] Previously, glyburide by itself had not effectively controlled the diabetes in the people in this study.

Ginkgo biloba

In a preliminary trial, administration of Ginkgo biloba extract (120 mg per day) for three months to patients with type 2 diabetes who were taking oral anti-diabetes medication resulted in a significant worsening of glucose tolerance. Ginkgo did not impair glucose tolerance in individuals whose diabetes was controlled by diet.[2] Individuals taking oral anti-diabetes medication should consult a doctor before taking Ginkgo biloba.

Interactions with Foods and Other Compounds

Food

Glyburide may be taken with food to avoid gastrointestinal (GI) upset.[3] Effective treatment of type 2 diabetes with glyburide includes adherence to recommended dietary guidelines.

Alcohol

Alcohol consumption may interfere with blood-sugar control during glyburide therapy.[4] Alcohol may interact with glyburide, causing facial flushing, headache, lightheadedness, nausea, breathlessness, and other symptoms.[5] People taking glyburide should avoid alcohol.

GREGODERM

Contains the following ingredients:
Hydrocortisone
Neomycin (page 187)
Nystatin (page 195)
Polymyxin B

GRISEOFULVIN

Common names: Fulcin, Fulvicin, Grifulvin, Gris-PEG, Grisactin, Grisovin, Gristatin

Griseofulvin is an antifungal drug used to treat ringworm infections of the skin, hair, and nails caused by specific fungi.

Summary of Interactions for Griseofulvin

In some cases, an herb or supplement may appear in more than one category, which may seem contradictory. For clarification, read the full article for details about the summarized interactions.

✓ May be Beneficial: Supportive interaction	Vitamin E*
Depletion or interference	None known
Side effect reduction/prevention	None known
Reduced drug absorption/bioavailability	None known
Adverse interaction	None known

Interactions with Dietary Supplements

Vitamin E

Adding 50 IU of vitamin E per day was reported to increase blood levels of this drug within four weeks in children, allowing the drug dose to be cut in half. Reducing the amount of griseofulvin should decrease the likelihood of side effects. This evidence is preliminary, so people taking griseofulvin should not supplement vitamin E on their own but may wish to discuss this matter with their doctor.[1]

Interactions with Foods and Other Compounds

Food

Food, especially with high fat content, increases griseofulvin absorption.[2] It is recommended to take griseofulvin with food to maximize absorption of the drug. People on low-fat diets who are taking griseofulvin should talk with their doctor or pharmacist.

Alcohol

Alcohol may interact with griseofulvin causing a reaction marked by facial flushing, headache, light-headedness, nausea, and breathlessness.[3] To prevent unwanted reactions, people should avoid alcohol-containing products during griseofulvin therapy.

GUAIFENESIN

Common names: Balminil Expectorant, Benylin Children's Chesty Coughs, Benylin E, Boots Child Sugar Free Chesty Cough Syrup, Breonesin, Calmylin Expectorant, Do-Do Expectorant, Famel Expectorant, Fenesin, GG-Sen, Guaiphenesin, Guiatuss, Humibid, Jackson's All Fours, Junior Meltus Expectorant, Lemsip Chesty Cough, Liqufruta Garlic, Meltus Expectorant, Meltus Honey and Lemon, Methoxypropanediol, Methphenoxydiol, Muco-Fen, Nirolex Chesty Cough Linctus, Nurse Sykes Balsam, Organidin NR,

Phanasin, Robitussin Chesty Cough, Robitussin, Tixylix Chesty Cough, Venos Expectorant, Venos For Dry Coughs, Vicks Vaposyrup Chesty Cough

Combination drugs: Ami-Tex LA, Entex LA, Primatene Dual Action, Robitussin AC, Robitussin CF, Robitussin DM

Guaifenesin is a drug that reduces the thickness and stickiness of mucus. It is used for short-term relief of dry, nonproductive cough and mucus in the breathing passages. Guaifenesin is available in prescription products, nonprescription products alone, and in combination with other nonprescription drugs, to treat symptoms of allergy, colds, and upper respiratory infections.

Summary of Interactions for Guaifenesin

In some cases, an herb or supplement may appear in more than one category, which may seem contradictory. For clarification, read the full article for details about the summarized interactions.

Depletion or interference	None known
Side effect reduction/prevention	None known
Supportive interaction	None known
Reduced drug absorption/bioavailability	None known
Adverse interaction	None known

GUANFACINE

Common names: Tenex

Guanfacine is used to treat high blood pressure and is in a class of drugs known as centrally acting antihypertensives.

Summary of Interactions for Guanfacine

In some cases, an herb or supplement may appear in more than one category, which may seem contradictory. For clarification, read the full article for details about the summarized interactions.

Depletion or interference	None known
Side effect reduction/prevention	None known
Supportive interaction	None known
Reduced drug absorption/bioavailability	None known
Adverse interaction	None known

HALOPERIDOL

Common names: Apo-Haloperidol, Dozic, Haldol, Novo-Peridol, Peridol, PMS-Haloperidol, Rho-Haloperidol, Serenace

Haloperidol is a drug used to treat people with psychotic disorders, including schizophrenia.

Summary of Interactions for Haloperidol

In some cases, an herb or supplement may appear in more than one category, which may seem contradictory. For clarification, read the full article for details about the summarized interactions.

✓	May be Beneficial: Depletion or interference	Iron* Sodium*
✓	May be Beneficial: Side effect reduction/prevention	Ginkgo biloba Milk thistle* Vitamin E
✓	May be Beneficial: Supportive interaction	Glycine
🚫	Avoid: Reduced drug absorption/bioavailability	Coffee and tea*
ⓘ	Check: Other	Potassium
	Adverse interaction	None known

Interactions with Dietary Supplements
Glycine

Two double-blind studies have found that 0.4–0.8 mg/kg body weight per day of glycine can reduce the so-called negative symptoms of schizophrenia when combined with haloperidol and related drugs.[1, 2] Negative symptoms include reduced emotional expression or general activity. The action of glycine in combination with the drugs was greater than the drugs alone, suggesting a synergistic action. Another double-blind study using approximately half the amount in the positive studies could not find any benefit from adding glycine to antipsychotic drug therapy.[3] Patients with low blood levels of glycine appeared to improve the most when given glycine in addition to their antipsychotic drugs.[4] No side effects were noticed in these studies, even when more than 30 grams of glycine were given daily.

Iron

Haloperidol may cause decreased blood levels of iron.[5] The importance of this interaction remains unclear. Iron should not be supplemented unless a deficiency is diagnosed.

Potassium

Haloperidol may cause hyperkalemia (high blood levels of potassium) or hypokalemia (low blood levels of potassium).[6] The incidence and severity of these changes remains unclear. Serum potassium can be measured by any doctor.

Vitamin E

Haloperidol and related antipsychotic drugs can cause a movement disorder called tardive dyskinesia. Several double-blind studies suggest that vitamin E may be beneficial for treatment of tardive dyskinesia.[7] Taking the large amount of 1,600 IU per day of vitamin E simultaneously with antipsychotic drugs has also been shown to lessen symptoms of tardive dyskinesia.[8] It is unknown if combining vitamin E with haloperidol could prevent tardive dyskinesia.

Sodium

Haloperidol may cause hyponatremia (low blood levels of sodium).[9] The incidence and severity of these changes remains unclear.

Interactions with Herbs

Milk thistle (Silybum marianum)

Haloperidol may cause liver damage. A double-blind study in 60 women treated with drugs such as haloperidol were given 800 mg per day silymarin extract made from milk thistle.[10] Test subjects who were given silymarin experienced a significant decrease in free radical levels, unlike those given placebo.

Ginkgo biloba

In a double-blind trial, supplementation of schizophrenic patients with Ginkgo biloba extract, in the amount of 250 mg per 2.2 pounds of body weight per day for 12 weeks, enhanced the effectiveness of haloperidol and also reduced the side effects of the drug.[11]

Interactions with Foods and Other Compounds

Coffee and tea

Cofee and tea are reported to cause precipitation of haloperidol in the test tube.[12] If this interaction happens in people, it would reduce the amount of haloperidol absorbed and the effectiveness of therapy. People taking haloperidol may avoid this possible interaction by taking haloperidol one hour before or two hours after drinking coffee or tea.

Alcohol

Haloperidol may cause drowsiness.[13] Alcohol may compound this drowsiness and increase the risk of accidents during activities requiring alertness. People should avoid alcohol-containing products during haloperidol therapy.

HELIDAC

Contains the following ingredients:
Bismuth subsalicylate (page 40)
Metronidazole (page 177)
Tetracycline (page 253)

HEPARIN

Common names: Calciparine, Hepalean, Heparin Leo, Minihep Calcium, Minihep, Monoparin Calcium, Monoparin, Multiparin, Pump-Hep, Unihep, Uniparin Calcium, Uniparin Forte

Heparin is a natural product, available by prescription, which is used as an anticoagulant (slows the rate of blood clot formation). Blood clots can cause severe and life-threatening problems. Heparin is used to prevent formation of blood clots (after surgery and in other settings) and in circumstances to help dissolve blood clots already formed (deep vein thrombosis, pulmonary embolism, and other situations involving excessive blood clotting).

Summary of Interactions for Heparin

In some cases, an herb or supplement may appear in more than one category, which may seem contradictory. For clarification, read the full article for details about the summarized interactions.

✓ May be Beneficial: Depletion or interference	Vitamin D
⊘ Avoid: Adverse interaction	Digitalis* Dong quai* Fenugreek* Ginger* Ginkgo biloba* Horse chestnut* Red clover* Reishi Sweet clover* Sweet woodruff*
ⓘ Check: Other	Potassium
Side effect reduction/prevention	None known
Supportive interaction	None known
Reduced drug absorption/bioavailability	None known

Heparin

Interactions with Dietary Supplements

Potassium

Heparin therapy may cause hyperkalemia (abnormally high potassium levels).[1, 2] Potassium supplements, potassium-containing salt substitutes (No Salt, Morton Salt Substitute, and others), and even high-potassium foods (primarily fruit) should be avoided by persons on heparin therapy, unless directed otherwise by their doctor.

Vitamin D

Heparin may interfere with activation of vitamin D in the body.[3] Osteoporosis (thinning of the bone) has been reported in patients who received high amounts of heparin for several months.[4] Osteopenia (decreased bone density) has been reported in women who received heparin therapy during pregnancy.[5, 6]

Interactions with Herbs

Digitalis (Digitalis purpurea)

Digitalis refers to a group of plants commonly called foxglove, which contains chemicals related to the drug **digoxin** (page 90). Digitalis may interfere with the anticoagulant action of heparin, reducing its action.[7] Digitalis should only be used under the direct supervision of a doctor trained in its use.

Ginger

Ginger has been shown to reduce platelet stickiness in test tubes. Although there are no reports of interactions with anticoagulant drugs, people should consult a healthcare professional if they are taking an anticoagulant and wish to use ginger.[8]

Ginkgo biloba

Ginkgo extracts may reduce the ability of platelets to stick together, possibly increasing the tendency toward bleeding.[9] Standardized extracts of ginkgo have been associated with two cases of spontaneous bleeding, although the ginkgo extracts were not definitively shown to be the cause of the problem.[10, 11] People taking heparin should consult with a physician knowledgeable about botanical medicines if they are considering taking ginkgo.

Herbs containing coumarin-derivatives

Although there are no specific studies demonstrating interactions with anticoagulants, the following herbs contain coumarin-like substances that may interact with heparin and could conceivably cause bleeding.[12] These herbs include dong quai, fenugreek, horse chestnut, red clover, sweet clover, and sweet woodruff. People should consult a healthcare professional if they're taking an anticoagulant and wish to use one of these herbs.

Reishi (Ganoderma lucidum)

As it may increase bleeding time, reishi is not recommended for those taking anticoagulant (blood-thinning) medications.[13]

Interactions with Foods and Other Compounds

Alcohol

Alcohol consumption during heparin therapy may increase the risk of serious bleeding.[14] It is important for people receiving heparin to avoid alcohol during the entire course of heparin therapy.

HYDRALAZINE

Common names: Apo-Hydralazine, Apresoline, Novo-Hylazin, Nu-Hydral

Combination drug: Apresazide

Hydralazine is a drug used to lower blood pressure in people with hypertension. Hydralazine relaxes the muscles that control the diameter of blood vessels. This relaxation allows the blood vessels to dilate (open wider), lowering blood pressure.

Summary of Interactions for Hydralazine

In some cases, an herb or supplement may appear in more than one category, which may seem contradictory. For clarification, read the full article for details about the summarized interactions.

✓ May be Beneficial: Depletion or interference	Vitamin B$_6$
Side effect reduction/prevention	None known
Supportive interaction	None known
Reduced drug absorption/bioavailability	None known
Adverse interaction	None known

Interactions with Dietary Supplements

Vitamin B$_6$

Vitamin B$_6$ can bind to hydralazine to form a complex that is excreted in the urine, increasing vitamin B$_6$ loss.[1] This may lead to vitamin B$_6$ deficiency.[2] People taking hydralazine should consult with their doctor to discuss the possibility of vitamin B$_6$ supplementation.

Interactions with Foods and Other Compounds
Food

Taking hydralazine with food improves the absorption of the drug.[3] People with questions should ask their prescribing doctor or pharmacist.

Alcohol

Alcohol causes blood vessels to dilate, lowering blood pressure. This action may add to the blood pressure-lowering effect of hydralazine and increase the risk of dizziness, fainting, or accidental falls. People taking hydralazine should avoid alcohol and should read all product labels carefully for alcohol content.

HYDROCODONE

Combination drugs:
- **Lortab** (page 162)
- **Tussionex** (page 275)
- **Vicodin** (page 280)
- **Vicoprofen** (page 280)

Hydrocodone is a narcotic analgesic used in combination products to relieve mild to moderate pain and an antitussive agent to relieve cough and upper respiratory symptoms associated with allergy or cold.

Summary of Interactions for Hydrocodone

In some cases, an herb or supplement may appear in more than one category, which may seem contradictory. For clarification, read the full article for details about the summarized interactions.

Depletion or interference	None known
Side effect reduction/prevention	None known
Supportive interaction	None known
Reduced drug absorption/bioavailability	None known
Adverse interaction	None known

Interactions with Foods and Other Compounds
Food

Hydrocodone may cause gastrointestinal (GI) upset. Hydrocodone-containing products may be taken with food to reduce or prevent GI upset.[1] A common side effect of narcotic analgesics is constipation.[2] Increasing dietary fiber (especially vegetables and whole-grain foods) and water intake can ease constipation.

Alcohol

Hydrocodone may cause drowsiness, dizziness, or blurred vision. Alcohol may intensify these effects and increase the risk of accidental injury.[3] To prevent problems, people taking hydrocodone should avoid alcohol.

HYDROXYCHLOROQUINE

Common names: Plaquenil

Hydroxychloroquine is used to prevent and treat acute attacks of malaria and to treat both acute and chronic rheumatoid arthritis and lupus. It is in a class of drugs known as antimalarials.

Summary of Interactions for Hydroxychloroquine

In some cases, an herb or supplement may appear in more than one category, which may seem contradictory. For clarification, read the full article for details about the summarized interactions.

✓ May be Beneficial: Depletion or interference	Calcium* Vitamin D*
✓ May be Beneficial: Supportive interaction	Vitamin B6*
⊘ Avoid: Reduced drug absorption/ bioavailability	Magnesium*
Side effect reduction/prevention	None known
Adverse interaction	None known

Interactions with Dietary Supplements
Calcium and vitamin D

Normally, the active form of vitamin D increases the absorption of calcium into the body. In a 45-year-old woman with sarcoidosis, taking hydroxychloroquine blocked the formation of active vitamin D, which helped normalize elevated blood levels of calcium in this case.[1] Whether hydroxychloroquine has this effect in people who don't have sarcoidosis or elevated calcium is unknown. Until controlled research explores this interaction more thoroughly, people taking hydroxychloroquine might consider having their vitamin D and/or calcium status monitored by a health practitioner.

Vitamin B6

An individual who took hydroxychloroquine and vitamin B6 together for nine years experienced a complete

Hydroxychloroquine

disappearance of skin nodules caused by rheumatoid arthritis.[2] Controlled study is needed to determine whether taking vitamin B_6 with or without hydroxychloroquine might help eliminate nodules in people with rheumatoid arthritis.

Magnesium
Magnesium supplementation may reduce blood levels of chloroquine, a compound similar to hydroxychloroquine, and decrease its effectiveness.[3] Until more is known, people taking hydroxychloroquine for arthritis who are also using magnesium supplements and are not experiencing relief might try avoiding the supplements or taking them at separate times.

Interaction with Foods and Other Compounds
Hydroxychloroquine should be taken with food to avoid possible stomach upset.[4]

HYDROXYZINE

Common names: Apo-Hydroxyzine, Atarax, Atazine, Dovaril, Hypam, Multipax, Novo-Hydroxyzin, PMS-Hydroxyzine, Ucerax, Vistacot, Vistaril, Vistawin

Hydroxyzine is used to treat itching due to hives, eczema, and allergic reactions, as well as to treat anxiety and tension. It is in a class of drugs known as antihistamines.

Summary of Interactions for Hydroxyzine
In some cases, an herb or supplement may appear in more than one category, which may seem contradictory. For clarification, read the full article for details about the summarized interactions.

Depletion or interference	None known
Side effect reduction/prevention	None known
Supportive interaction	None known
Reduced drug absorption/bioavailability	None known
Adverse interaction	None known

Interactions with Foods and Other Compounds
Alcohol
Alcohol's effects on human functioning may increase when it is consumed at the same time as hydroxyzine. Therefore, alcohol consumption should be avoided while taking hydroxyzine.[1]

HYOSCYAMINE

Common names: Anaspaz, Colidrops Liquid Pediatric, Cystospaz, Donnamar, ED-Spaz, Hyco Elixir, Hyosol, Hyospaz, Hyosyne, Levbid, Levsinex, Levsin, Losamine, Medispaz, Spacol, Spasdel, Symax

Hyoscyamine is used in the treatment of peptic ulcers and of Parkinson's disease to reduce stiffness, tremors, and excess sweating. It acts as a drying agent in the treatment of hay fever and is also used to treat spasm and increased movement of both the intestines in irritable bowel syndrome and the bladder in urinary tract infections. Hyoscyamine is a belladonna alkaloid in a class of drugs known as anticholinergic antispasmodics.

Summary of Interactions for Hyoscyamine
In some cases, an herb or supplement may appear in more than one category, which may seem contradictory. For clarification, read the full article for details about the summarized interactions.

✓	May be Beneficial: Depletion or interference	Iron
🚫	Avoid: Adverse interaction	*Anisodus tanguticus**
	Side effect reduction/prevention	None known
	Supportive interaction	None known
	Reduced drug absorption/bioavailability	None known

Interactions with Dietary Supplements
Iron
Absorption of ferrous citrate, an iron compound that is usually well absorbed, is reduced in individuals taking hyoscyamine;[1] therefore, these two substances should not be taken at the same time.

Interactions with Herbs
Anisodus tanguticus
The herb *Anisodus tanguticus* contains a chemical that has effects similar to **atropine** (page 30), a compound related to hyoscyamine.[2] Though no human studies have investigated a possible adverse interaction between hyoscyamine and anisodus, individuals should avoid the combination until more is known.

Interactions with Foods and Other Compounds
Alcohol
Drinking alcohol interferes with the stomach acid–blocking action of **atropine** (page 30),[3] a drug similar

to hyoscyamine. Alcohol may reduce the effectiveness of hyoscyamine for this reason, and should therefore be avoided by people taking hyoscyamine.

HYZAAR

Contains the following ingredients:
Hydrochlorothiazide
Losartan (page 162)

IBUPROFEN

Common names: Actiprofen, Advil, Alti-Ibuprofen, Anadin Ibuprofen, Apo-Ibuprofen, Arthrofen, Boots Fever & Pain Relief, Brufen Retard, Brufen, Cuprofen, Ebufac, Excedrin IB, Fenbid, Froben (flurbiprofen), Galprofen, Hedex Ibuprofen, Ibrufhalal, Ibufem, Inoven, Isisfen, Junifen, Librofem, Lidifen, Migrafen, Motrin, Motrin IB, Novaprin, Novo-Profen, Nu-Ibuprofen, Nuprin, Nurofen, Pacifene, Pedia Care Fever Drops, PhorPain, Proflex, Provel, Reclofen, Rimafen, Rufen

Combination drug: Vicoprofen

Ibuprofen is a member of the **nonsteroidal anti-inflammatory drug** (page 193) (NSAIDs) family. NSAIDs reduce inflammation (swelling), pain, and temperature. Ibuprofen is used to treat mild to moderate pain, fever, osteoarthritis, rheumatoid arthritis, primary dysmenorrhea, and other conditions. Ibuprofen is available in prescription and nonprescription strengths.

Summary of Interactions for Ibuprofen

In some cases, an herb or supplement may appear in more than one category, which may seem contradictory. For clarification, read the full article for details about the summarized interactions.

✓	May be Beneficial: Depletion or interference	Iron
✓	May be Beneficial: Side effect reduction/prevention	Copper* Licorice
✓	May be Beneficial: Supportive interaction	Copper*
⊘	Avoid: Adverse interaction	**Lithium** (page 157)* Sodium* White willow*
ⓘ	Check: Other	Potassium
	Reduced drug absorption/bioavailability	None known

Interactions with Dietary Supplements

Copper

Supplementation may enhance the anti-inflammatory effects of NSAIDs while reducing their ulcerogenic effects. One study found that when various anti-inflammatory drugs were chelated with copper, the anti-inflammatory activity was increased.[1] Animal models of inflammation have found that the copper chelate of **aspirin** (page 26) was active at one-eighth the effective amount of aspirin. These copper complexes are less toxic than the parent compounds as well.

Iron

NSAIDs cause gastrointestinal (GI) irritation, bleeding, and iron loss.[2] Iron supplements can cause GI irritation.[3] However, iron supplementation is sometimes needed in people taking NSAIDs if those drugs have caused enough blood loss to lead to iron deficiency. If both iron and ibuprofen are prescribed, they should be taken with food to reduce GI irritation and bleeding risk.

Lithium (page 157)

Lithium is a mineral that may be present in some supplements and is also used in large amounts to treat mood disorders such as manic-depression (bipolar disorder). Most NSAIDs inhibit the excretion of lithium from the body, resulting in higher blood levels of the mineral, though **sulindac** (page 249) may have an opposite effect.[4] Since major changes in lithium blood levels can produce unwanted side effects or interfere with its efficacy, NSAIDs should be used with caution, and only under medical supervision, in people taking lithium supplements.

Potassium

Ibuprofen has caused kidney dysfunction and increased blood potassium levels, especially in older people.[5] People taking ibuprofen should not supplement potassium without consulting with their doctor.

Sodium

Ibuprofen may cause sodium and water retention.[6] It is healthful to reduce dietary salt intake by eliminating table salt and heavily salted foods.

Interactions with Herbs

Licorice (Glycyrrhiza glabra)

The flavonoids found in the extract of licorice known as DGL (deglycyrrhizinated licorice) are helpful for avoiding the irritating actions NSAIDs have on the stomach and intestines. One study found that 350 mg of chewable DGL taken together with each dose of aspirin reduced gastrointestinal bleeding caused by the aspirin.[7] DGL has been shown in controlled human research to be as effective as drug therapy (**cimetidine** [page 61]) in healing stomach ulcers.[8]

White willow bark (Salix alba)

White willow bark contains salicin, which is related to **aspirin** (page 26). Both salicin and aspirin produce anti-inflammatory effects after they have been converted to salicylic acid in the body. The administration of salicylates like aspirin to individuals taking oral NSAIDs may result in reduced blood levels of NSAIDs.[9] Though no studies have investigated interactions between white willow bark and NSAIDs, people taking NSAIDs should avoid the herb until more information is available.

Interactions with Foods and Other Compounds

Food

Ibuprofen should be taken with food to prevent gastrointestinal upset.[10]

Alcohol

Ibuprofen may cause drowsiness, dizziness, or blurred vision.[11] Alcohol may intensify these effects and increase the risk of accidental injury. Use of alcohol during ibuprofen therapy increases the risk of stomach irritation and bleeding. People taking ibuprofen should avoid alcohol.

IMAZIN XL

Contains the following ingredients:
    Aspirin (page 26)
    Isosorbide mononitrate (page 148)

IMAZIN XL FORTE

Contains the following ingredients:
    Aspirin (page 26)
    Isosorbide mononitrate (page 148)

INDAPAMIDE

Common names: Apo-Indapamide, Gen-Indapamide, Lozide, Lozol, Natramid, Natrilix SR, Natrilix, Nindaxa 2.5, Novo-Indapamide, Nu-Indapamide, Opumide

Indapamide is a thiazide-like diuretic used, either alone or in combination with other drugs, to treat high blood pressure and to prevent salt and fluid retention associated with heart failure. Indapamide may interact with nutrients and herbs in ways similar to interactions described for **thiazide diuretics** (page 258), such as hydrochlorothiazide. However, research has not investigated these interactions specifically for indapamide.

Summary of Interactions for Indapamide

In some cases, an herb or supplement may appear in more than one category, which may seem contradictory. For clarification, read the full article for details about the summarized interactions.

✓	May be Beneficial: Depletion or interference	Calcium **Lithium** (page 157) Potassium Sodium Vitamin D*
	Side effect reduction/prevention	None known
	Supportive interaction	None known
	Reduced drug absorption/bioavailability	None known
	Adverse interaction	None known

Interactions with Dietary Supplements

Potassium and sodium

Taking indapamide may result in sodium and potassium loss, which may cause dry mouth, thirst, fatigue, drowsiness, or muscle cramps.[1] Doctors may suggest supplements or foods high in potassium to prevent unwanted side effects.

Calcium

Slight increases in blood calcium levels may occur in people taking indapamide, which could be aggravated by calcium supplementation.[2] Therefore, people taking both calcium supplements and indapamide should have their blood calcium levels monitored by their healthcare practitioner, and it may be necessary to avoid calcium supplementation.

Lithium (page 157)

Lithium is a mineral that may be present in some supplements and is also used in large amounts to treat mood disorders such as manic-depression. Taking indapamide may elevate blood levels of lithium, resulting in unwanted side effects such as diarrhea, nausea, and drowsiness.[3] It is unknown whether people taking small amounts of supplemental lithium will experience adverse reactions.

Vitamin D
Thiazide diuretics (page 258) enhance the actions of vitamin D;[4] however, it is unknown whether indapamide has the same effect. Until more is known, people taking indapamide should supplement vitamin D only under the supervision of a health practitioner.

INDERETIC

Contains the following ingredients:
Bendroflumethiazide
Propranolol (page 224)

INDEREX

Contains the following ingredients:
Bendroflumethiazide
Propranolol (page 224)

INDERIDE

Contains the following ingredients:
Hydrochlorothiazide
Propranolol (page 224)

INDINAVIR

Common names: Crixivan

Indinavir is an antiviral drug used to treat HIV infection, and is in a class of medications known as protease inhibitors.

Summary of Interactions for Indinavir

In some cases, an herb or supplement may appear in more than one category, which may seem contradictory. For clarification, read the full article for details about the summarized interactions.

⊘ Avoid: Reduced drug absorption/ bioavailability	Food St. John's wort
Depletion or interference	None known
Side effect reduction/prevention	None known
Supportive interaction	None known
Adverse interaction	None known

Interactions with Herbs
St. John's wort (Hypericum perforatum)
Studies have shown that taking indinavir together with St. John's wort results in increased breakdown and dramatically reduced blood levels of indinavir.[1, 2] Therefore, people taking indinavir should not take St. John's wort.

Indinavir is a protease inhibitor used to treat people with HIV infection. A pharmacological study gave indinavir to healthy volunteers for two days.[3] On day 3, volunteers added 900 mg of St. John's wort extract per day. At the end of the study, it was found that St. John's wort led to a significant reduction in serum levels of indinavir. Until more is known, people taking indinavir or other antiretroviral drugs for HIV infection should avoid using St. John's wort.

Interactions with Foods and Other Compounds
Food
Taking indinavir with a meal high in calories, protein, and fat dramatically reduces the absorption of the drug.[4] One controlled trial showed that taking indinavir with a high-fat breakfast greatly reduced blood levels of the drug, while two types of low-fat meals had no effect.[5] Therefore, indinavir should be taken either with a low-fat meal or on an empty stomach.

INDIVINA

Contains the following ingredients:
Estradiol (page 108)
Medroxyprogesterone (page 167)

INDOMETHACIN

Common names: Apo-Indomethacin, Flexin Continuous, Imbrilon, Indocid-R, Indocid, Indocin, Indolar SR, Indomax 75 SR, Indomax, Indometacin, Indomod, Indotard, Indotec, Novo-Methacin, Nu-Indo, Pardelprin, Rheumacin LA, Rhodacine, Rimacid, Slo-Indo

Indomethacin is a member of the **nonsteroidal anti-inflammatory drug** (page 193) (NSAIDs) family of drugs. NSAIDs reduce inflammation (swelling), pain, and temperature. Indomethacin is used to reduce pain/swelling involved in osteoarthritis, rheumatoid arthritis, bursitis, tendinitis, gout, ankylosing spondylitis, and headaches.

Summary of Interactions for Indomethacin

In some cases, an herb or supplement may appear in more than one category, which may seem contradictory. For clarification, read the full article for details about the summarized interactions.

✓ May be Beneficial: Depletion or interference	Calcium* Folic acid Vitamin C
🚫 Avoid: Adverse interaction	**Lithium** (page 157)* Potassium Sodium White willow*
ⓘ Check: Other	Iron
Side effect reduction/prevention	None known
Supportive interaction	None known
Reduced drug absorption/bioavailability	None known

Interactions with Dietary Supplements

Iron

Iron supplements can cause stomach irritation. Use of iron supplements with indomethacin increases the risk of stomach irritation and bleeding.[1] However, stomach bleeding causes iron loss. If both iron and indomethacin are prescribed, they should be taken with food to reduce stomach irritation and bleeding risk.

Lithium (page 157)

Lithium is a mineral that may be present in some supplements and is also used in large amounts to treat mood disorders such as manic-depression (bipolar disorder). Most NSAIDs inhibit the excretion of lithium from the body, resulting in higher blood levels of the mineral, though **sulindac** (page 249) may have an opposite effect.[2] Since major changes in lithium blood levels can produce unwanted side effects or interfere with its efficacy, NSAIDs should be used with caution, and only under medical supervision, in people taking lithium supplements.

Potassium

Indomethacin may cause elevated blood potassium levels in people with normal and abnormal kidney function.[3, 4, 5, 6] Until more is known, people taking indomethacin should not supplement potassium without medical supervision.

Vitamins and minerals

Indomethacin has been reported to decrease absorption of folic acid and vitamin C.[7] Under certain circumstances, indomethacin may interfere with the actions of vitamin C.[8] Calcium and phosphate levels may also be reduced with indomethacin therapy.[9] It remains unclear whether people taking this drug need to supplement any of these nutrients.

Sodium

Indomethacin may cause sodium and water retention.[10] It is healthful to reduce dietary salt intake by decreasing the use of table salt and avoiding heavily salted foods.

Interactions with Herbs

White willow bark (Salix alba)

White willow bark contains salicin, which is related to **aspirin** (page 26). Both salicin and aspirin produce anti-inflammatory effects after they have been converted to salicylic acid in the body. The administration of salicylates like aspirin to individuals taking oral NSAIDs may result in reduced blood levels of NSAIDs.[11] Though no studies have investigated interactions between white willow bark and NSAIDs, people taking NSAIDs should avoid the herb until more information is available.

Interactions with Foods and Other Compounds

Food

Indomethacin should be taken with food to prevent stomach irritation.[12] However, applesauce, high-protein foods, and high-fat foods have been reported to interfere with indomethacin absorption and/or activity.[13]

Alcohol

Indomethacin may cause drowsiness or dizziness.[14] Alcohol may amplify these actions. Use of alcohol during indomethacin therapy increases the risk of stomach irritation and bleeding.[15] People taking indomethacin should avoid alcohol.

INFLUENZA VIRUS VACCINE

Common names: Begrivac, Fluarix, Fluogen, FluShield, Fluviral S/F, Fluvirin, Fluzone, Inactivated Influenza Vaccine, Influvac Sub-unit, Vaxigrip

The influenza vaccine is given by injection to help prevent influenza (flu), particularly in people with compromised immune systems. The vaccine is altered yearly to correspond to mutations in the flu virus.

Summary of Interactions for Influenza Vaccine

In some cases, an herb or supplement may appear in more than one category, which may seem contradictory. For clarification, read the full article for details about the summarized interactions.

✓	May be Beneficial: Side effect reduction/prevention	Eleuthero*
✓	May be Beneficial: Supportive interaction	Asian ginseng*
	Depletion or interference	None known
	Reduced drug absorption/bioavailability	None known
	Adverse interaction	None known

Interactions with Herbs

Asian ginseng (Panax ginseng)

In a randomized, double-blind study, 227 people received influenza vaccine plus 100 mg of standardized extract of Asian ginseng or placebo two times per day for four weeks before and eight weeks after influenza vaccination.[1] Compared with placebo, Asian ginseng extract was reported to prevent colds and flu, improve immune cell activity, and increase antibody levels after vaccination.

Eleuthero

Some Russian studies suggest that eleuthero (Siberian ginseng) may reduce the risk of postvaccination reactions.[2]

INHALED CORTICOSTEROIDS

Common names: AeroBec Forte, AeroBec, AeroBid Inhaled, Asmabec, Azmacort Inhaled, Beclazone, Becloforte, Beclomethasone Inhaled, Beclovent Inhaled, Becodisks, Beconase AQ Inhaled, Beconase Inhaled, Becotide Rotocaps, Becotide, Budesonide Inhaled, Cutivate Inhaled, Decadron Phosphate Turbinaire or Respihaler, Dexamethasone Inhaled, Filair Forte, Flixotide, Flonase Inhaled, Flovent Inhaled, Flunisolide Inhaled, Fluticasone Inhaled, Levalbuterol Inhaled, Mometasone Inhaled, Nasacort AQ Inhaled, Nasacort Inhaled, Nasalide Inhaled, Nasonex Inhaled, Proventil Inhaled, Pulmicort, Pulmicort Inhaled, Qvar, Rhinocort Inhaled, Triamcinolone Inhaled, Vancenase AQ Inhaled, Vancenase Inhaled, Vanceril Inhaled, Ventolin Inhaled, Volmax Inhaled, Xopenex™

Combination drug: Viskaldix

Corticosteroids are inhaled by mouth to treat and prevent asthma, as well as other inflammatory conditions of the lungs that restrict breathing. They are inhaled into the nose to treat and prevent symptoms of hay fever and other allergies. In addition, some agents may be used to prevent recurrence of nasal polyps following surgical removal.

The information in this article pertains to inhaled corticosteroids in general. The interactions reported here may not apply to all the Also Indexed As terms. Talk to your doctor or pharmacist if you are taking any of these drugs.

Summary of Interactions for Inhaled Corticosteroids

In some cases, an herb or supplement may appear in more than one category, which may seem contradictory. For clarification, read the full article for details about the summarized interactions.

✓	May be Beneficial: Depletion or interference	Calcium Dehydroepiandrosterone (DHEA)*
	Side effect reduction/prevention	None known
	Supportive interaction	None known
	Reduced drug absorption/bioavailability	None known
	Adverse interaction	None known

Interactions with Dietary Supplements

Calcium

Most of an inhaled dose of beclomethasone is actually swallowed, which may lead to reduced absorption of calcium.[1] Health practitioners may recommend calcium supplementation to individuals using beclomethasone inhalers.

Dehydroepiandrosterone (DHEA)

A group of women with asthma who had been taking inhaled beclomethasone were shown to have low levels of DHEA compared to women with asthma who were not taking beclomethasone.[2] The authors speculated that this effect may partially explain how corticosteroids can cause osteoporosis. However, more research is needed to confirm these suspicions and to evaluate whether supplemental DHEA is beneficial to patients taking inhaled corticosteroids.

INNOZIDE

Contains the following ingredients:
Enalapril (page 103)
Hydrochlorothiazide

Insulin

INSULIN

Common names: Animal-Source Insulin: Iletin, Humalog Mix25, Humalog Mix50, Human Actarapid, Human Analog Insulin: Humanlog, Human Insulin (Humulin, Novolin), Human Mixtard, Human Monotard, Human Ultratard, Hypurin, Isulatard, Lentard MC, Novolin ge, NovoRapid, Oralin, Pork Mixtard

Insulin is a natural protein made by the pancreas that helps the body use sugar. Insulin is injected by all people with type 1 (insulin-dependent) diabetes mellitus and by some people with type 2 (non-insulin-dependent) diabetes mellitus to help control blood sugar levels.

Any substance (dietary, supplemental, herbal, and others) that affects blood sugar levels will directly or indirectly affect the amount of insulin required by a person with diabetes. For example, consumption of a high-fiber diet and/or supplementation with nutrients such as chromium, biotin, vitamin E, or herbs such as *Gymnema sylvestre* will often improve blood sugar control in diabetics. In such cases, the amount of insulin may need to be reduced in order to avoid a hypoglycemic reaction. Anyone taking insulin should consult the prescribing physician before making dietary changes or taking nutrients or herbs that are designed to lower blood sugar levels.

Summary of Interactions for Insulin

In some cases, an herb or supplement may appear in more than one category, which may seem contradictory. For clarification, read the full article for details about the summarized interactions.

✓	May be Beneficial: Depletion or interference	DHEA
✓	May be Beneficial: Supportive interaction	Biotin Chromium Fenugreek *Gymnema sylvestre** Vitamin E
🚫	Avoid: Adverse interaction	Chromium* *Gymnema sylvestre** Tobacco
	Side effect reduction/prevention	None known
	Reduced drug absorption/bioavailability	None known

Interactions with Dietary Supplements
Dehydroepiandrosterone (DHEA)
Insulin has been shown to decrease the levels of DHEA and DHEA-sulfate in the blood.[1] More research is

needed to determine the significance of this finding.

Interactions with Herbs
Fenugreek (Trigonella foenum-graecum)
In a controlled study of patients with type 1 diabetes, fenugreek (100 grams per day for ten days) was reported to reduce blood sugar, urinary sugar excretion, serum cholesterol, and triglycerides, with no change in insulin levels.[2] In a controlled study of people with type 2 diabetes, fenugreek (25 grams per day for 24 weeks) was reported to significantly reduce blood glucose levels.[3] People using insulin should talk with their prescribing doctor before incorporating large amounts of fenugreek into their diet.

Gymnema sylvestre
Although no interactions have been reported, gymnema may decrease the required daily dose of insulin.[4] Therefore, people currently using insulin for the treatment of diabetes should discuss the use of this herb with their healthcare professional.

Interactions with Foods and Other Compound
Food
Diet is an important factor in effective diabetes prevention and treatment. People using insulin should monitor their blood sugar carefully and talk with their doctor about the role of diet in diabetes control.

Alcohol
Alcohol may increase the action of insulin, leading to hypoglycemia (low blood sugar).[5] People using insulin should avoid alcohol.

Tobacco (Nicotiana species)
Smoking may decrease insulin activity,[6] and it compounds the health problems associated with diabetes. People using insulin are cautioned to avoid smoking.

INTERFERON

Common names: Actimmune, Alferon N, Avonex, Betaferon, Betaseron, Immukin, Immune Interferon, Infergen, Intron, Rebif, Rebif (interferon beta), Roferon-A, Viraferon (interferon alfa), Wellferon

Interferons are proteins made by the human immune system for fighting viral infections and regulating cell function. Three types of interferons are used as drugs: interferon alpha, interferon beta, and interferon gamma. They are used by injection to treat viral infections, hepatitis, multiple sclerosis, some cancers, and other diseases.

The information in this article pertains to interferon in general. The interactions reported here may not apply to all the Also Indexed As terms. Talk to your doctor or pharmacist if you are taking any of these drugs.

Summary of Interactions for Interferon

In some cases, an herb or supplement may appear in more than one category, which may seem contradictory. For clarification, read the full article for details about the summarized interactions.

✓	May be Beneficial: Side effect reduction/prevention	Thymus peptides*
✓	May be Beneficial: Supportive interaction	Licorice* N-acetyl cysteine (NAC)* Thymus peptides*
⊘	Avoid: Reduced drug absorption/ bioavailability	Thymus peptides*
⊘	Avoid: Adverse interaction	Bupleurum
	Depletion or interference	None known

Interactions with Dietary Supplements

N-acetyl cysteine (NAC)

One preliminary trial found that adding 600 mg NAC three times per day to interferon therapy for people with chronic hepatitis C led to improvement in their conditions not seen with interferon alone.[1] However, other preliminary[2, 3] and double-blind trials[4, 5] have failed to confirm the efficacy of this approach. At the present time, sufficient evidence is lacking to support the use of this drug-nutrient combination in persons with hepatitis.

Thymus peptides

Peptides or short proteins derived from the immune organ known as the thymus gland have been investigated in combination with interferon therapy for people with hepatitis B and C. One study found that adding thymus humoral factor-gamma 2 to interferon therapy prevented decreases in white blood cell counts sometimes seen with interferon alone, and also seemed to improve the efficacy of interferon against hepatitis B.[6] Thymus humoral factor-gamma 2 must be administered by injection, requiring consultation with a doctor. It is not known whether orally administered thymus extracts would be useful in combination with interferon.

Interactions with Herbs

Bupleurum (Bupleurum chinense)

Bupleurum is the major constituent of a Japanese Kampo (herbal) medicine formula called sho-saiko-to. This formula has been used alone or with interferon to treat hepatitis. Eighty or more cases of drug-induced pneumonitis (inflammation of the lungs) have been associated with the use of sho-saiko-to alone or with interferon.[7, 8, 9, 10] Until more is known, sho-saiko-to should not be combined with interferon.

Licorice (Glycyrrhiza glabra)

Injections of the licorice compound glycyrrhizin are commonly used to treat hepatitis in Japan. The combination of glycyrrhizin and interferon may be more effective than interferon alone.[11, 12] Injectable glycyrrhizin is available from some physicians. So far, human studies have not used *orally* administered licorice extracts in conjunction with interferon.

IPECAC

Common names: Ipecacuanha Emetic Mixture

Ipecac syrup is a drug used to induce vomiting in the treatment of drug overdoses and in certain poisonings. In addition, people with eating disorders, such as bulimia and anorexia nervosa, occasionally abuse ipecac to avoid weight gain. In emergency situations, a local poison control center should be contacted before ipecac is given.

Summary of Interactions for Ipecac

In some cases, an herb or supplement may appear in more than one category, which may seem contradictory. For clarification, read the full article for details about the summarized interactions.

✓	May be Beneficial: Side effect reduction/prevention	Potassium
⊘	Avoid: Reduced drug absorption/ bioavailability	Activated charcoal Carbonated beverages Milk
	Depletion or interference	None known
	Supportive interaction	None known
	Adverse interaction	None known

Ipecac

Interactions with Dietary Supplements
Potassium
In order to lose weight, some individuals who are overly zealous, as well as those with eating disorders, occasionally induce vomiting with ipecac. However, chronic abuse of ipecac can result in low blood levels of potassium,[1] which might result in an irregular heart rhythm. Though avoidance of this behavior is the best form of prevention, individuals who abuse ipecac should supplement with potassium or high-potassium foods to prevent potassium deficiency.

Interactions with Foods and Other Compounds
Milk and carbonated beverages
Some references have suggested that taking ipecac along with milk or carbonated beverages might reduce the effectiveness of the drug.[2] However, controlled studies have shown that drinking neither milk[3] nor carbonated beverages[4] inhibits the action of ipecac. Consequently, ipecac can be given with or without milk or carbonated beverages.

Activated charcoal
In the treatment of certain poisonings, activated charcoal is used to reduce the amount of poison absorbed into the body. Some references have suggested that people avoid giving ipecac and activated charcoal together.[5] However, controlled studies have shown that activated charcoal may not completely block the effects of ipecac,[6] and that the combination is effective when activated charcoal is given ten minutes after ipecac treatment.[7] Until more information is available, individuals should probably wait to give activated charcoal until after the ipecac-induced vomiting stops.

IPRATROPIUM BROMIDE

Common names: Alti-Ipratropium, Apo-Ipravent, Atrovent, Ipratropium Steri-Neb, Novo-Ipramide, Nu-Ipratropium, PMS-Ipratropium, Respontin, Rinatec

Combination drug: Combivent

Ipratropium bromide is a drug used by oral inhalation to keep breathing passages open in chronic obstructive pulmonary diseases, including chronic bronchitis and emphysema. Ipratropium bromide for oral inhalation is available alone and in a combination product. It is also available as a nasal spray to relieve runny nose associated with allergies and common colds.

Summary of Interactions for Ipratropium Bromide
In some cases, an herb or supplement may appear in more than one category, which may seem contradictory. For clarification, read the full article for details about the summarized interactions.

ⓘ Check: Other	Soy
Depletion or interference	None known
Side effect reduction/prevention	None known
Supportive interaction	None known
Reduced drug absorption/bioavailability	None known
Adverse interaction	None known

Interactions with Foods and Other Compounds
Food
Atrovent and Combivent for oral inhalation contain soy lecithin. Rarely, people very sensitive to soy have reacted to these drugs,[1] and life-threatening anaphylactic reaction is possible, though extremely rare. Ipratropium bromide nasal spray and solution for inhalation contain no soy lecithin.

IRBESARTAN

Common names: Aprovel, Avapro

Combination drug: CoAprovel

Irbesartan is an angiotensin II receptor antagonist used to treat high blood pressure.

Summary of Interactions for Irbesartan
In some cases, an herb or supplement may appear in more than one category, which may seem contradictory. For clarification, read the full article for details about the summarized interactions.

Depletion or interference	None known
Side effect reduction/prevention	None known
Supportive interaction	None known
Reduced drug absorption/bioavailability	None known
Adverse interaction	None known

ISONIAZID

Common names: INH, Isotamine, Laniazid, Nydrazid, PMS-Isoniazid

Combination drugs: Rifamate, Rimactane

Isoniazid is an **antibiotic** (page 19) used to prevent and treat tuberculosis. To prevent development of resistant tuberculosis bacteria, people with tuberculosis are treated with long courses of combination drug therapy, most commonly isoniazid, rifampin, and pyrazinamide.

Summary of Interactions for Isoniazid

In some cases, an herb or supplement may appear in more than one category, which may seem contradictory. For clarification, read the full article for details about the summarized interactions.

✓ May be Beneficial: Depletion or interference	Calcium* Folic acid* Magnesium* Vitamin B₁₂ Vitamin B₃ (niacin) Vitamin D* Vitamin E* Vitamin K
✓ May be Beneficial: Side effect reduction/prevention	Picrorhiza*
✓ May be Beneficial: Supportive interaction	Licorice*
ⓘ Check: Other	Vitamin B₆
Reduced drug absorption/bioavailability	None known
Adverse interaction	None known

Interactions with Dietary Supplements

Vitamin B₃

Isoniazid is capable of causing vitamin B_3 (niacin) deficiency, most likely due to its ability to interfere with cell-repair enzymes made from niacin. Significant niacin deficiency, also known as pellagra, features dermatitis, diarrhea, and dementia (impaired intellectual function). Supplementation with vitamin B_6 is thought to reduce this risk, although small amounts (e.g. 10 mg daily) has been noted to be inadequate in some cases.[1]

Vitamin B₆

Isoniazid can interfere with the activity of vitamin B_6.[2] Vitamin B_6 supplementation is recommended, especially in people with poor nutritional status, to prevent development of isoniazid-induced peripheral neuritis (inflamed nerves).[3] One case is reported in which injectable vitamin B_6 reversed isoniazid-induced coma.[4] In another case, however, 10 mg per day of vitamin B_6 failed to reverse isoniazid-induced psychosis. The author suggested that higher amounts (e.g., 50 mg per day) may be needed.[5] Although the optimal amount remains unknown, some doctors suggest that adults tak-

ing isoniazid supplement with 100 mg of vitamin B_6 per day to prevent side effects. However, as animal studies suggest that very large amounts of vitamin B_6 can interfere with the effect of isoniazid,[6] people taking isoniazid should consult their doctor to determine the appropriate amount of vitamin B_6 to take.

Vitamin K

Many antibiotics taken by mouth, including isoniazid, may kill friendly bacteria in the large intestine that produce vitamin K.[7] Vitamin K_1 (phylloquinone) is now found in some multivitamins.

Other nutrient interactions

Isoniazid may interfere with the activity of other nutrients, including vitamin B_3 (niacin), vitamin B_{12}, vitamin D, and vitamin E, folic acid, calcium, and magnesium.[8, 9] Supplementation with vitamin B_6 is thought to help prevent isoniazid-induced niacin deficiency; however, small amounts of vitamin B_6 (e.g. 10 mg per day) appear to be inadequate in some cases.[10] People should consider using a daily multivitamin-mineral supplement during isoniazid therapy.

Interactions with Herbs

Licorice (Glycyrrhiza glabra)

The potent anti-inflammatory substance known as glycyrrhizin from licorice has been combined with isoniazid for treatment of tuberculosis. An older study found a benefit from combining the two compared to using isoniazid alone.[11] Glycyrrhizin was given by injection, so it is not certain if licorice extracts containing glycyrrhizin would be as effective given by mouth. The treatment required at least three months of administration.

Picrorhiza (Picrorhiza kurroa)

Picrorhiza is an herb from India with well-established anti-inflammatory and liver protective actions.[12] Use of a combination formula known as Liv.100 that contains picrorhiza protected animal livers against damage caused by isoniazid and other antituberculosis antibiotics.[13]

Interactions with Foods and Other Compounds

Food

Food decreases absorption of isoniazid. Isoniazid should be taken one hour before or two hours after eating. However, people may take isoniazid with food to decrease stomach upset.[14]

Isoniazid has some monoamine oxidase inhibitor (MAOI) activity.[15] Isoniazid can alter metabolism of tyramine-containing foods, leading to reactions associated with MAOI drugs (diarrhea, flushing, sweating, pounding chest, dangerous changes in blood pressure, and other symptoms).[16] People taking isoniazid should avoid tyramine-containing foods. Isoniazid can also alter metabolism of histamine-containing foods, leading to headaches, sweating, pounding chest, flushing, diarrhea, low blood pressure, and itching.[17] People taking isoniazid should avoid histamine-containing foods (such as tuna, sauerkraut juice, or yeast extract).

Alcohol
Daily alcohol intake increases the risk of isoniazid-related hepatitis.[18] Alcohol may interact with isoniazid, causing facial flushing, headache, light-headedness, nausea, breathlessness, and other symptoms.[19] To prevent unwanted reactions, people taking isoniazid should avoid alcohol-containing products.

ISOSORBIDE DINITRATE

Common names: Angitak, Cedocard Retard, Isocard, Isoket Retard, Isordil, Sorbid SA, Sorbitrate

Isosorbide dinitrate (ISDN) is used primarily to prevent and treat angina, and in the treatment of acute heart attacks and heart failure.

Summary of Interactions for Isosorbide Dinitrate
In some cases, an herb or supplement may appear in more than one category, which may seem contradictory. For clarification, read the full article for details about the summarized interactions.

✓ May be Beneficial: Supportive interaction	High-fat meals N-acetyl cysteine
⊘ Avoid: Adverse interaction	Alcohol
Depletion or interference	None known
Side effect reduction/prevention	None known
Reduced drug absorption/bioavailability	None known

Interactions with Dietary Supplements
N-acetyl cysteine
The beneficial effects of ISDN are reduced following long-term treatment with the drug through a process known as tolerance. Controlled studies have shown that using intravenous and oral N-acetyl cysteine (NAC) reverses or prevents tolerance to nitrates.[1, 2] Another controlled study revealed that intravenous NAC enhanced the beneficial effects of ISDN on heart function.[3]

Therefore, people taking isosorbide dinitrate might benefit from supplemental NAC.

Interactions with Foods and Other Compounds
Food
Taking sustained-release tablets of ISDN with a high-fat meal might increase the absorption of the drug.[4] Individuals who switch from a high-fat diet to a low-fat diet might require a change in the amount of ISDN taken daily. Therefore, people taking ISDN should talk with their healthcare practitioner before starting a low-fat diet.

Alcohol
People taking ISDN might experience lightheadedness on standing, especially after rising from a lying-down or seated position. Drinking alcohol with ISDN may increase the frequency of this side effect.[5] Therefore, individuals taking ISDN should avoid drinking alcohol.

ISOSORBIDE MONONITRATE

Common names: Angeze, Chemydur 60XL, Dynamin, Elantan LA, Elantan, Imdur, Isib, ISMO Retard, ISMO, Isodur, Isosorbide-5-Mononitrate, Isotard, Isotrate, MCR-50, Modisal XL, Monit SR, Monit XL, Monit, Mono-Cedocard Retard-50, Mono-Cedocard, Monoket, Monomax SR, Monosorb XL 60

Combination drugs: Imazin XL Forte, Imazin XL

Isosorbide mononitrate (ISMN) is a member of the nitrate family of drugs used to prevent angina (chest pain). It is available in immediate-release and extended-release products.

Summary of Interactions for Isosorbide Mononitrate
In some cases, an herb or supplement may appear in more than one category, which may seem contradictory. For clarification, read the full article for details about the summarized interactions.

✓ May be Beneficial: Supportive interaction	N-acetyl cysteine
ⓘ Check: Other	Vitamin C
Depletion or interference	None known
Side effect reduction/prevention	None known
Reduced drug absorption/bioavailability	None known
Adverse interaction	None known

Interactions with Dietary Supplements
N-acetyl cysteine (NAC)
In a double-blind trial, sustained-release ISMN plus oral NAC (2,400 mg twice per day) for two days led to significantly longer exercise time than ISMN plus placebo.[1] This outcome suggests that NAC may have increased the efficacy of ISMN. There were no differences in side effects between the two groups.

Vitamin C
Some persons taking **nitroglycerin** (page 191) or isosorbide mononitrate may find that it loses efficacy over time. This is because the body adapts to the drug, a process known as developing tolerance. One study found that taking 2 grams three times daily of vitamin C can decrease this effect when nitroglycerin patches are simultaneously used.[2] Similar benefits have been confirmed in another study.[3] However, it should be noted that it is also possible to avoid tolerance to these drugs by simply changing the dosing schedule. People taking ISMN or nitroglycerin should talk with their pharmacists about avoiding drug tolerance.

Interactions with Foods and Other Compounds
Food
Isosorbide mononitrate should be taken on an empty stomach with a glass of water.[4] Imdur may be taken with or without food[5] and should be swallowed whole, without chewing or crushing.[6]

Alcohol
Isosorbide mononitrate causes low blood pressure. Alcohol may increase this effect, leading to dangerously low blood pressure and other side effects.[7] To prevent problems, people taking isosorbide mononitrate should avoid alcohol.

ISOTRETINOIN

Common names: Accutane, Isotrex, Roaccutane

Isotretinoin is a modified vitamin A molecule used to treat severe acne vulgaris.

Summary of Interactions for Isotretinoin
In some cases, an herb or supplement may appear in more than one category, which may seem contradictory. For clarification, read the full article for details about the summarized interactions.

✓ May be Beneficial: Side effect reduction/prevention	Vitamin E*
🚫 Avoid: Adverse interaction	Vitamin A
Depletion or interference	None known
Supportive interaction	None known
Reduced drug absorption/bioavailability	None known

Interactions with Dietary Supplements
Vitamin A
Although little is known about how isotretinoin interacts with real vitamin A, the two are structurally similar and have similar toxicities. Therefore, people taking isotretinoin should avoid vitamin A supplements at levels higher than typically found in a multivitamin (10,000 IU per day).

Vitamin E
Preliminary research has found that combined administration of isotretinoin and vitamin E (alpha-tocopherol) substantially reduces the initial toxicity of high-dose isotretinoin without reducing drug efficacy.[1] Additional research is needed to further clarify this potentially beneficial interaction.

KALTEN

Contains the following ingredients:
> **Amiloride** (page 11)
> **Atenolol** (page 28)
> Hydrochlorothiazide

KETOCONAZOLE

Common names: Apo-Ketoconazole, Nizoral Shampoo, Nizoral Topical

Ketoconazole is an antifungal agent applied topically to treat fungal and yeast infections of the skin. It is effective in the treatment of ringworm, jock itch, pityriasis, athlete's foot, and dandruff, as well as yeast infections caused by *Candida*. The shampoo is available over the counter in a 1% strength to treat dandruff, and by prescription as a 2% solution to treat pityriasis. The drug is not absorbed through the skin.

Summary of Interactions for Ketoconazole
In some cases, an herb or supplement may appear in more than one category, which may seem contradictory.

For clarification, read the full article for details about the summarized interactions.

Depletion or interference	None known
Side effect reduction/prevention	None known
Supportive interaction	None known
Reduced drug absorption/bioavailability	None known
Adverse interaction	None known

KETOPROFEN

Common names: Apo-Keto, Fenoket, Jomethid XL, Ketil CR, Ketocid, Ketoprofen CR, Ketotard 200XL, Ketovail, Ketozip XL, Larafen CR, Novo-Keto, Nu-Ketoprofen, Orafen, Orudis, Oruvail, Rhodis, Rhovail

Ketoprofen is used to treat rheumatoid arthritis, osteoarthritis, and ankylosing spondylitis. It is in a class of medications known as **nonsteroidal anti-inflammatory drugs** (page 193) (NSAIDs).

Summary of Interactions for Ketoprofen

In some cases, an herb or supplement may appear in more than one category, which may seem contradictory. For clarification, read the full article for details about the summarized interactions.

✓ May be Beneficial: Depletion or interference	**Lithium** (page 157)*
⊘ Avoid: Reduced drug absorption/ bioavailability	Willow*
⊘ Avoid: Adverse interaction	**Lithium** (page 157)* White willow*
Side effect reduction/prevention	None known
Supportive interaction	None known

Interactions with Dietary Supplements
Lithium (page 157)
Lithium is a mineral that may be present in some supplements and is also used in large amounts to treat mood disorders such as manic-depression. Research has shown that **nonsteroidal anti-inflammatory drugs** (page 193) may increase blood levels of lithium,[1] resulting in side effects such as diarrhea, nausea, muscle weakness, and lack of coordination. Though there is no research available to show that ketoprofen increases

lithium blood levels, until more information is available, people taking ketoprofen should talk with their healthcare practitioner before supplementing with lithium.

Interactions with Herbs
White willow bark (Salix alba)
White willow bark contains salicin, which is related to **aspirin** (page 26). Both salicin and aspirin produce anti-inflammatory effects after they have been converted to salicylic acid in the body. The interaction between salicylic acid and ketoprofen is complex. While it may enhance the effectiveness of ketoprofen, salicylic acid also speeds its elimination from the body.[2] Consequently, people taking ketoprofen should avoid herbal products that contain willow bark.

Interactions with Foods and Other Compounds
Food
Ketoprofen may cause stomach upset and should therefore be taken with food.[3]

Calories and fat
Taking a slow-release form of ketoprofen with low-fat, low-calorie food may increase the absorption of the drug, compared with taking it with a high-fat, high-calorie meal.[4] Individuals who eat a diet high in calories and fat may require an adjustment in the daily amount of ketoprofen taken or may experience greater benefit by switching to a low-fat, low-calorie diet. Consult a qualified professional about matching ketoprofen dosage with dietary fat and calorie intake.

KETOROLAC

Common names: Acular, Toradol

Ketorolac is used orally to treat moderately severe acute pain (e.g., migraine headaches), but should not be used for more than five days. It is also used in the eye to treat itching due to seasonal allergies and to prevent inflammation following cataract surgery.

Summary of Interactions for Ketorolac

In some cases, an herb or supplement may appear in more than one category, which may seem contradictory. For clarification, read the full article for details about the summarized interactions.

⊘ Avoid: Reduced drug absorption/ bioavailability	High-fat meal
⊘ Avoid: Adverse interaction	**Lithium** (page 157)* Potassium White willow*
Depletion or interference	None known
Side effect reduction/prevention	None known
Supportive interaction	None known

Interactions with Dietary Supplements
Lithium (page 157)

Lithium is a mineral that may be present in some supplements and is also used in large amounts to treat mood disorders such as manic-depression (bipolar disorder). Most NSAIDs inhibit the excretion of lithium from the body, resulting in higher blood levels of the mineral, though **sulindac** (page 249) may have an opposite effect.[1] Since major changes in lithium blood levels can produce unwanted side effects or interfere with its efficacy, NSAIDs should be used with caution, and only under medical supervision, in people taking lithium supplements.

Potassium

A 50-year-old male developed high blood levels of potassium following eight days of ketorolac treatment.[2] Additional research is needed to determine whether taking ketorolac together with supplemental potassium might enhance this side effect. individuals taking oral ketorolac should probably avoid potassium supplements and salt substitutes until more information is available.

Interactions with Herbs
White willow bark (Salix alba)

White willow bark contains salicin, which is related to **aspirin** (page 26). Both salicin and aspirin produce anti-inflammatory effects after they have been converted to salicylic acid in the body. The administration of salicylates like aspirin to individuals taking oral NSAIDs may result in reduced blood levels of NSAIDs.[3] Though no studies have investigated interactions between white willow bark and NSAIDs, people taking NSAIDs should avoid the herb until more information is available.

Interactions with Foods and Other Compounds
Food

Taking ketorolac with a high-fat breakfast slows the speed of drug absorption by about an hour, but it does not affect overall blood levels of the drug.[4] To lessen stomach upset, ketorolac tablets should be taken with a meal or a snack.

KLIOFEM

Contains the following ingredients:
   Estradiol (page 108)
   Norethisterone

KLIOVANCE

Contains the following ingredients:
   Estradiol (page 108)
   Norethisterone

LABETALOL

Common names: Normodyne, Trandate

Labetalol is used to treat high blood pressure.

Summary of Interactions for Labetalol

In some cases, an herb or supplement may appear in more than one category, which may seem contradictory. For clarification, read the full article for details about the summarized interactions.

✓ May be Beneficial: Supportive interaction	Food
⊘ Avoid: Adverse interaction	High-potassium foods* Pleurisy root* Potassium
Depletion or interference	None known
Side effect reduction/prevention	None known
Reduced drug absorption/bioavailability	None known

Interaction with Dietary Supplements
Potassium

Three kidney transplant patients developed hyperkalemia (high blood potassium levels), a potentially dangerous condition, following intravenous administration of labetalol.[1] Additional research is needed to determine whether taking oral labetalol together with potassium supplements might also lead to elevated blood levels of potassium. However, some other beta-blockers (called "nonselective" beta-blockers) are known to decrease the uptake of potassium from the blood into the cells,[2] leading to hyperkalemia.[3] People taking beta-blockers should therefore avoid taking potassium supplements, or eating large quantities of fruit (e.g., bananas), unless directed to do so by their doctor.

Interactions with Herbs
Pleurisy root
As pleurisy root and other plants in the *Aesclepius* genus contain cardiac glycosides, it is best to avoid use of pleurisy root with heart medications such as beta-blockers.[4]

Interaction with Food and Other Compounds
Food
Taking labetalol with food greatly increases the absorption of the drug.[5] Therefore, labetalol should be taken with a meal.

LACTASE

Common names: Dairy Ease, Dairyaid, LactAid, Lactrase, SureLac, Tilactase

Lactase is a nonprescription enzyme used by people who have an impaired ability to digest lactose (milk sugar) because their bodies make insufficient lactase.

Summary of Interactions for Lactase
In some cases, an herb or supplement may appear in more than one category, which may seem contradictory. For clarification, read the full article for details about the summarized interactions.

ⓘ Check: Other	Calcium
Depletion or interference	None known
Side effect reduction/prevention	None known
Supportive interaction	None known
Reduced drug absorption/bioavailability	None known
Adverse interaction	None known

Interactions with Dietary Supplements
Calcium
Dairy products are rich in calcium. Lactase-deficient people may not consume milk and therefore have fewer

dietary sources of calcium available to them. Lactase products allow lactase-deficient people to digest milk products, increasing their sources and intake of dietary calcium.

LACTIC ACID

Common names: Ammonium Lactate, Lac-Hydrin, Lactinol

Combination drug: Calmurid HC

Lactic acid is an alpha-hydroxy acid applied to the skin to treat scaling and abnormal dryness.

Summary of Interactions for Lactic Acid
In some cases, an herb or supplement may appear in more than one category, which may seem contradictory. For clarification, read the full article for details about the summarized interactions.

Depletion or interference	None known
Side effect reduction/prevention	None known
Supportive interaction	None known
Reduced drug absorption/bioavailability	None known
Adverse interaction	None known

LACTULOSE

Common names: Acilac, Cephulac, Cholac, Chronulac, Duphalac, Enulose Syrup, Generlac, Lactugal, Laxilose, Laxose, Osmolax, PMS-Lactulose, Regulose

Lactulose is used to treat constipation and is a type of drug called a synthetic disaccharide.

Summary of Interactions for Lactulose
In some cases, an herb or supplement may appear in more than one category, which may seem contradictory. For clarification, read the full article for details about the summarized interactions.

Depletion or interference	None known
Side effect reduction/prevention	None known
Supportive interaction	None known
Reduced drug absorption/bioavailability	None known
Adverse interaction	None known

LAMIVUDINE

Common names: 3TC, Epivir, Zeffix

Combination drug: Combivir

Lamivudine is used to treat human immunodeficiency virus (HIV) infection and is in a class of drugs known as antivirals.

Summary of Interactions for Lamivudine

In some cases, an herb or supplement may appear in more than one category, which may seem contradictory. For clarification, read the full article for details about the summarized interactions.

✓ May be Beneficial: Supportive interaction	Sho-saiko-to*
Depletion or interference	None known
Side effect reduction/prevention	None known
Reduced drug absorption/bioavailability	None known
Adverse interaction	None known

Interactions with Herbs
Sho-saiko-to

Test tube studies show that the herbal combination sho-saiko-to enhances the antiviral activity of lamivudine.[1] Sho-saiko-to contains extracts of seven herbs, including *Bupleuri radix, Pinelliae tuber, Scutellariae radix, Zizyphi fructus,* ginseng *(Ginseng radix),* licorice *(Glycyrrhizae radix),* and ginger *(Zingiber rhizoma).* Controlled studies are needed to determine whether taking sho-saiko-to might enhance the beneficial effects of lamivudine.

LANSOPRAZOLE

Common names: Prevacid, Zoton

Lansoprazole is a "proton pump inhibitor" drug that blocks production of stomach acid. Lansoprazole is used to treat diseases in which stomach acid causes damage, including stomach and duodenal ulcers, esophagitis, and Zollinger-Ellison syndrome.

Summary of Interactions for Lansoprazole

In some cases, an herb or supplement may appear in more than one category, which may seem contradictory.

For clarification, read the full article for details about the summarized interactions.

✓ May be Beneficial: Depletion or interference	Beta-carotene* Folic acid Vitamin B$_{12}$* (dietary, not supplemental B$_{12}$)
✓ May be Beneficial: Supportive interaction	Cranberry*
Side effect reduction/prevention	None known
Reduced drug absorption/bioavailability	None known
Adverse interaction	None known

Interactions with Dietary Supplements
Beta-carotene

Omeprazole (page 197), a drug closely related to lansoprazole, taken for seven days led to a near-total loss of stomach acid in healthy people and interfered with the absorption of a single administration of 120 mg of beta-carotene.[1] It is unknown whether repeated administration of beta-carotene would overcome this problem or if absorption of carotenoids from food would be impaired. Persons taking omeprazole and related acid-blocking drugs for long periods may want to have carotenoid blood levels checked, eat plenty of fruits and vegetables, and consider supplementing with carotenoids.

Folic acid

Folic acid is needed by the body to utilize vitamin B$_{12}$. Antacids, including lansoprazole, inhibit folic acid absorption.[2] People taking antacids are advised to supplement with folic acid.

Vitamin B$_{12}$

Omeprazole, a drug closely related to lansoprazole, has interfered with the absorption of vitamin B$_{12}$ from food (though not supplements) in some,[3, 4] but not all, studies.[5, 6] This interaction has not yet been reported with lansoprazole. However, a fall in vitamin B$_{12}$ status may result from decreased stomach acid caused by acid blocking drugs, including lansoprazole.[7]

Interactions with Herbs
Cranberry (Vaccinium macrocarpon)

Omeprazole (page 197) was shown to reduce protein-bound vitamin B$_{12}$ absorption and cranberry juice was shown to increase protein-bound vitamin B$_{12}$ absorption in eight people treated with omeprazole (a drug closely related to lansoprazole).[8] While this effect has not been studied with lansoprazole, people taking lansoprazole may choose to drink cranberry juice or other acidic liquids with vitamin B_{12}-containing foods. Unlike vitamin B_{12} found in food, vitamin B_{12} found in supplements is not bound to peptides (pieces of protein). The absorption of B_{12} supplements therefore does not require acid and is unlikely to be improved by drinking cranberry juice.

Interactions with Foods and Other Compounds
Food
The initial dose of lansoprazole should be taken 30 minutes before a meal.[9] Subsequent doses are equally effective taken with or without food but should be taken at the same time every day.[10] Capsules and granule contents should not be chewed or crushed. However, lansoprazole capsules may be opened, the granule contents sprinkled on one tablespoon of applesauce, then immediately swallowed.

LATANOPROST

Common names: Xalatan

Latanoprost is a prostaglandin analog that is applied to the eye to treat glaucoma. There are currently no reported nutrient or herb interactions involving latanoprost.

Summary of Interactions for Latanoprost
In some cases, an herb or supplement may appear in more than one category, which may seem contradictory. For clarification, read the full article for details about the summarized interactions.

Depletion or interference	None known
Side effect reduction/prevention	None known
Supportive interaction	None known
Reduced drug absorption/bioavailability	None known
Adverse interaction	None known

LEVODOPA

Common names: Dopar, L-dopa, Larodopa

Levodopa is the precursor required by the brain to produce dopamine, a neurotransmitter (chemical messenger in the nervous system). People with Parkinson's disease have depleted levels of dopamine. Levodopa is used to increase dopamine in the brain, which reduces the symptoms of Parkinson's disease. Levodopa is broken down by the body before it reaches the brain. To avoid this, levodopa is used with **carbidopa** (page 49), a drug that protects levodopa from breakdown. Levodopa is available alone or in a combination product.

Summary of Interactions for Levodopa
In some cases, an herb or supplement may appear in more than one category, which may seem contradictory. For clarification, read the full article for details about the summarized interactions.

✓ May be Beneficial: Depletion or interference	Vitamin B_6
Side effect reduction/prevention	None known
Supportive interaction	None known
Reduced drug absorption/bioavailability	None known
Adverse interaction	None known

Interactions with Dietary Supplements
Vitamin B_6
Levodopa is broken down in the body by a process requiring vitamin B_6. Breakdown may deplete available vitamin B_6. **Carbidopa** (page 49) blocks levodopa breakdown and prevents vitamin B_6 depletion. People taking **carbidopa/levodopa** (page 49) (Sinemet), or levodopa plus carbidopa (Lodosyn) have no risk for levodopa-induced vitamin B_6 deficiency; it is not a problem for people to supplement vitamin B_6 while taking Sinemet.

For people taking levodopa alone, small amounts of vitamin B_6 (5–10 mg per day) may prevent levodopa-induced vitamin B_6 deficiency.[1] Amounts of vitamin B_6 slightly higher than those required to replace depleted levels, may reduce the effectiveness of levodopa therapy and should not be taken.[2]

Interactions with Foods and Other Compounds
Food
Food, especially foods high in protein, compete with levodopa for absorption. However, levodopa may be taken with food to avoid stomach upset.[3] It is important to take levodopa at the same time every day, always with or always without food. People with questions about levodopa and food should ask their prescribing doctor or pharmacist. Taking sustained-release Sinemet CR with food may increase blood levels of levodopa.[4] It

is important to take Sinemet CR at the same time every day, always with or always without food. People with questions about Sinemet CR and food should ask their prescribing doctor or pharmacist.

LEVOFLOXACIN

Common names: Levaquin, Tavanic

Levofloxacin is an **antibiotic** (page 19) used to treat bacterial infections of the lungs, sinuses, skin, urinary tract, and kidneys.

Summary of Interactions for Levofloxacin

In some cases, an herb or supplement may appear in more than one category, which may seem contradictory. For clarification, read the full article for details about the summarized interactions.

✓	May be Beneficial: Depletion or interference	Vitamin K*
✓	May be Beneficial: Side effect reduction/prevention	Bifidobacterium longum* Lactobacillus acidophilus* Lactobacillus casei* Saccharomyces boulardii* Saccharomyces cerevisiae* Vitamin K*
✓	May be Beneficial: Supportive interaction	Saccharomyces boulardii*
⊘	Avoid: Reduced drug absorption/ bioavailability	Iron Magnesium
⊘	Avoid: Adverse interaction	**Caffeine** (page 44)*

Interactions with Dietary Supplements

Magnesium

Taking magnesium supplements at the same time as levofloxacin can reduce the intestinal absorption—and thus the effectiveness—of the drug.[1] Consequently, nutritional supplements or **antacids** (page 18) containing magnesium, if used, should be taken two hours before or after taking levofloxacin.

Iron

Taking iron supplements concomitantly with levofloxacin can reduce the absorption—and thus the ef-

fectiveness—of the drug.[2] Therefore, nutritional supplements containing iron, if used, should be taken two hours before or after taking levofloxacin.

Probiotics

A common side effect of antibiotics is diarrhea, which may be caused by the elimination of beneficial bacteria normally found in the colon. Controlled studies have shown that taking probiotic microorganisms—such as *Lactobacillus casei, Lactobacillus acidophilus, Bifidobacterium longum*, or *Saccharomyces boulardii*—helps prevent antibiotic-induced diarrhea.[3]

The diarrhea experienced by some people who take antibiotics also might be due to an overgrowth of the bacterium *Clostridium difficile*, which causes a disease known as pseudomembranous colitis. Controlled studies have shown that supplementation with harmless yeast—such as *Saccharomyces boulardii*[4] or *Saccharomyces cerevisiae* (baker's or brewer's yeast)[5]—helps prevent recurrence of this infection. In one study, taking 500 mg of *Saccharomyces boulardii* twice daily enhanced the effectiveness of the antibiotic vancomycin in preventing recurrent clostridium infection.[6] Therefore, people taking antibiotics who later develop diarrhea might benefit from supplementing with saccharomyces organisms.

Treatment with antibiotics also commonly leads to an overgrowth of yeast *(Candida albicans)* in the vagina (candida vaginitis) and the intestines (sometimes referred to as "dysbiosis"). Controlled studies have shown that *Lactobacillus acidophilus* might prevent candida vaginitis.[7]

Vitamin K

Several cases of excessive bleeding have been reported in people who take antibiotics.[8, 9, 10, 11] This side effect may be the result of reduced vitamin K activity and/or reduced vitamin K production by bacteria in the colon. One study showed that people who had taken broad-spectrum antibiotics had lower liver concentrations of vitamin K_2 (menaquinone), though vitamin K_1 (phylloquinone) levels remained normal.[12] Several antibiotics appear to exert a strong effect on vitamin K activity, while others may not have any effect. Therefore, one should refer to a specific antibiotic for information on whether it interacts with vitamin K. Doctors of natural medicine sometimes recommend vitamin K supplementation to people taking antibiotics. Additional research is needed to determine whether the amount of vitamin K_1 found in some multivitamins is sufficient to prevent antibiotic-induced bleeding. Moreover, most multivitamins do not contain vitamin K.

Levofloxacin

Interactions with Foods and Other Compounds
Caffeine (page 44)

Caffeine may have an intensified effect in people taking levofloxacin. Drugs similar to levofloxacin have been shown to cause caffeine to persist longer in the blood.[13] However, the effects of levofloxacin on caffeine blood levels or symptoms of caffeine ingestion have not been studied.

LINDANE

Common names: Hexit, Kwell Shampoo, PMS-Lindane

Lindane lotion is used topically to treat scabies; lindane shampoo is used to treat head and pubic lice. They are used in situations where treatment with other drugs has failed or cannot be tolerated by the individual.

Summary of Interactions for Lindane

In some cases, an herb or supplement may appear in more than one category, which may seem contradictory. For clarification, read the full article for details about the summarized interactions.

✓ May be Beneficial: Side effect reduction/prevention	Vitamin E*
Depletion or interference	None known
Supportive interaction	None known
Reduced drug absorption/bioavailability	None known
Adverse interaction	None known

Interactions with Dietary Supplements
Vitamin E

Test tube studies reveal that vitamin E protects white blood cells from damage caused by lindane.[1] Lindane is known to promote the formation of tumors,[2] and more research is needed to determine whether vitamin E, when applied at the same time as lindane, can prevent this adverse effect.

Interactions with Foods and Other Compounds
Oils

Applying oils, creams, and ointments at the same time as lindane may enhance the absorption of the drug through the skin.[3] Therefore, to avoid side effects, other drugs and herbal formulas in cream or ointment form should be applied at other times during the day.

LISINOPRIL

Common names: Apo-Lisinopril, Carace, Prinivil, Zestril

Combination drugs: Carace Plus, Prinzide, Zestoretic

Lisinopril is an **angiotensin-converting enzyme (ACE) inhibitor** (page 17), a family of drugs used to treat high blood pressure and some types of heart failure. Lisinopril is also used in some cases to improve survival after a heart attack.

Summary of Interactions for Lisinopril

In some cases, an herb or supplement may appear in more than one category, which may seem contradictory. For clarification, read the full article for details about the summarized interactions.

✓ May be Beneficial: Depletion or interference	Zinc*
⊘ Avoid: Adverse interaction	High-potassium foods* Potassium supplements* Salt substitutes*
Side effect reduction/prevention	None known
Supportive interaction	None known
Reduced drug absorption/bioavailability	None known

Interactions with Dietary Supplements
Potassium

An uncommon yet potentially serious side effect of taking ACE inhibitors is increased blood potassium levels.[1, 2, 3] This problem is more likely to occur in people with advanced kidney disease. Taking potassium supplements,[4] potassium-containing salt substitutes (No Salt, Morton Salt Substitute, and others),[5, 6, 7] or large amounts of high-potassium foods at the same time as ACE inhibitors could cause life-threatening problems.[8] Therefore, people should consult their healthcare practitioner before supplementing additional potassium and should have their blood levels of potassium checked periodically while taking ACE inhibitors.

Zinc

In a study of 34 people with hypertension, six months of **captopril** (page 47) or **enalapril** (page 103) (ACE inhibitors related to lisinopril) treatment led to decreased zinc levels in certain white blood cells,[9] raising concerns about possible ACE inhibitor–induced zinc depletion.

While zinc depletion has not been reported with lisinopril, until more is known, it makes sense for people taking lisinopril long term to consider, as a precaution, taking a zinc supplement or a multimineral tablet containing zinc. (Such multiminerals usually contain no more than 99 mg of potassium, probably not enough to trigger the above-mentioned interaction.) Supplements containing zinc should also contain copper, to protect against a zinc-induced copper deficiency.

Interactions with Foods and Other Compounds
Food
Lisinopril may be taken with or without food.[10]

LITHIUM

Common names: Camcolit, Carbolith, Duralith, Eskalith, Li-Liquid, Liskonum, Litarex, Lithane, Lithionate, Lithobid, Lithonate, Lithotabs, PMS-Lithium, Priadel

The prescription drug lithium is a mineral with antidepressant and antimanic actions. It is used to treat bipolar disorder (manic-depression) and severe depression.

Summary of Interactions for Lithium
In some cases, an herb or supplement may appear in more than one category, which may seem contradictory. For clarification, read the full article for details about the summarized interactions.

✓	May be Beneficial: Depletion or interference	Inositol
✓	May be Beneficial: Side effect reduction/prevention	Essential fatty acids* Inositol
✓	May be Beneficial: Supportive interaction	Folic acid L-tryptophan*
ⓘ	Check: Other	Coffee Psyllium Sodium
	Reduced drug absorption/bioavailability	None known
	Adverse interaction	None known

Interactions with Dietary Supplements
Essential fatty acids
In one report, supplementation with essential fatty acids in the form of safflower oil (3–5 grams per day)

reversed symptoms of lithium toxicity such as tremor and ataxia (an abnormality of gait).[1] Controlled studies are needed to confirm the benefit of a lithium-essential fatty acid combination.

Folic acid
Some studies have found that people taking lithium long term who have high blood levels of folic acid respond better to lithium.[2, 3] Not all studies have confirmed these findings, however.[4]

A double-blind study was conducted combining 200 mcg folic acid per day with lithium therapy.[5] Even though the volunteers in this study were doing well on lithium alone before the study, addition of folic acid further improved their condition, whereas placebo did not. There is no evidence that folic acid reduces side effects of lithium. Based on the available evidence, it is suggested people taking lithium also take at least 200 mcg of folic acid per day.

Inositol
Lithium therapy has been shown to deplete brain stores of inositol.[6] While it has been suggested that inositol supplementation (e.g., 500 mg three times daily) could reduce adverse effects of lithium therapy without reducing the drug's therapeutic effectiveness,[7, 8] the safety and efficacy of this combination has not been proven.

Treatment with lithium can trigger or worsen psoriasis. In a double-blind study, supplementing with inositol (6 grams per day) for ten weeks significantly improved lithium-induced psoriasis, but had no effect on psoriasis in people who were not taking lithium.[9]

L-tryptophan
A small double-blind study found that combining 2–4 grams three times per day of L-tryptophan with lithium significantly improved symptoms in people with bipolar disorder or a mild form of schizophrenia.[10] L-tryptophan is only available from doctors. It should be taken several hours before or after meals.

Sodium
Lithium may cause sodium depletion, especially during initial therapy until consistent blood levels are achieved.[11] A low-sodium (salt-restricted) diet can decrease lithium elimination, leading to increased lithium levels and risk of toxicity in lithium users who reduce their salt intake.[12] Changing to a higher salt intake may cause increased losses of lithium, resulting in the return of mood symptoms.[13, 14] People using lithium therapy should maintain adequate water intake

as well as a normal diet and salt intake. Sodium loss due to diarrhea, illness, extreme sweating, or other causes may alter lithium levels.

Interactions with Herbs
Psyllium (Plantago ovata)
Addition of psyllium husk two times per day to the regimen of a woman treated with lithium was associated with decreased lithium blood levels and lithium levels increased after psyllium was stopped.[15]

Interactions with Foods and Other Compounds
Food
Lithium should be taken with food to avoid stomach upset.[16]

Foods that alkalinize the urine may increase elimination of lithium from the body, potentially decreasing the actions of the drug.[17] Urine-alkalinizing foods include dairy products, nuts, fruits, vegetables (except corn and lentils), and others.

Coffee
Mild hand tremor is a common side effect of lithium therapy. Two cases of women treated with lithium who experienced increased tremor when they stopped drinking coffee have been reported.[18] Lithium levels increased almost 50% in one of the women, who had been drinking 17 cups of coffee per day, requiring a 20% reduction in her lithium dose. In 11 people treated with lithium who drank four to six cups of coffee per day, two weeks without coffee resulted in increased lithium blood levels, anxiety, and depression.[19] Lithium levels, anxiety, and depression ratings returned to base line two weeks after resuming coffee consumption. Until more is known, people taking lithium should avoid abrupt changes in their coffee consumption.

LIVE INFLUENZA VACCINE INTRANASAL

Common names: FluMist

Live influenza vaccine is used to provide active immunization against specific strains of influenza virus. The intranasal formulation contains a weakened influenza virus, which, when sprayed in the nose, stimulates the development of immunity against the disease.

Summary of Interactions for Live influenza Vaccine
In some cases, an herb or supplement may appear in more than one category, which may seem contradictory. For clarification, read the full article for details about the summarized interactions.

⊘ Avoid: Adverse interaction	Willow
Depletion or interference	None known
Side effect reduction/prevention	None known
Supportive interaction	None known
Reduced drug absorption/bioavailability	None known

Interactions with Herbs
White willow bark (Salix alba)
White willow bark contains salicin, a substance similar to **aspirin** (page 26). Aspirin should not be given to children receiving live influenza virus due to the possible link to Reye's syndrome. The same adverse interaction result could theoretically happen if children were to take a willow-containing product following FluMist.

LOCOID C

Contains the following ingredients:
   Chlorquinaldol
   Hydrocortisone

LOMOTIL/LONOX

This is a combination drug containing two ingredients, diphenoxylate and **atropine** (page 30), that is used in the treatment of diarrhea. Diphenoxylate is in a class of drugs known as antidiarrheals.

Summary of Interactions for Lomotil/Lonox
In some cases, an herb or supplement may appear in more than one category, which may seem contradictory. For clarification, read the full article for details about the summarized interactions.

⊘ Avoid: Reduced drug absorption/ bioavailability	Tannin-containing herbs* such as green tea, black tea, uva ursi, black walnut, red raspberry, oak, and witch hazel

Depletion or interference	None known
Side effect reduction/prevention	None known
Supportive interaction	None known
Adverse interaction	None known

Interactions with Herbs

Tannin-containing herbs

Tannins are a group of unrelated chemicals that give plants an astringent taste. Herbs containing high amounts of tannins, such as green tea *(Camellia sinensis)*, black tea, uva ursi *(Arctostaphylos uva-ursi)*, black walnut *(Juglans nigra)*, red raspberry *(Rubus idaeus)*, oak *(Quercus spp.)*, and witch hazel *(Hamamelis virginiana)*, may interfere with the absorption of the drug when taken by mouth.[1]

Interactions with Foods and Other Compounds

Alcohol

Diphenoxylate may enhance the actions of alcohol,[2] resulting in increased drowsiness, dizziness, imbalance, and poor response times. Therefore, people taking diphenoxylate should avoid alcohol, especially when staying alert is necessary.

LOOP DIURETICS

Common names: Apo-Furosemide, Betinex, Bumetanide, Bumex, Burinex, Demadex, Dryptal, Edecrin, Ethacrynic Acid, Froop, Frusol, Furosemide, Lasix, Rusyde, Sodium Edecrin, Torem, Torsemide

Loop diuretics constitute a family of drugs that remove water from the body. They are referred to as potassium-depleting, as they cause the body to lose potassium as well as water. Potassium-depleting diuretics also cause the body to lose magnesium. Loop diuretics are more potent than **thiazide diuretics** (page 258). They are used to lower blood pressure in people with hypertension and to reduce the amount of work the heart has to do, allowing it to pump better in people with congestive heart failure. Loop diuretics are also used to reduce water accumulation caused by other diseases.

The information in this article pertains to loop diuretics in general. The interactions reported here may not apply to all the Also Indexed As terms. Talk to your doctor or pharmacist if you are taking any of these drugs.

Summary of Interactions for Loop Diuretics

In some cases, an herb or supplement may appear in more than one category, which may seem contradictory. For clarification, read the full article for details about the summarized interactions.

✓	May be Beneficial: Depletion or interference	Folic acid* Magnesium Potassium Vitamin B₁
🚫	Avoid: Adverse interaction	Alder Buckthorn* Buchu Buckthorn* Cleavers Dandelion Digitalis Gravel root Horsetail Juniper Licorice Uva ursi
ⓘ	Check: Other	Sodium
	Side effect reduction/prevention	None known
	Supportive interaction	None known
	Reduced drug absorption/bioavailability	None known

Interactions with Dietary Supplements

Folic acid

One study showed that people taking diuretics for more than six months had dramatically lower blood levels of folic acid and higher levels of homocysteine compared with individuals not taking diuretics.[1] Homocysteine, a toxic amino acid by-product, has been associated with atherosclerosis. Until further information is available, people taking diuretics for longer than six months should probably supplement with folic acid.

Magnesium and potassium

Potassium-depleting diuretics, including loop diuretics, cause the body to lose potassium. Loop diuretics may also cause cellular magnesium depletion,[2] although this deficiency may not be reflected by a low blood level of magnesium.[3] Magnesium loss induced by potassium-depleting diuretics can cause additional potassium loss. Until more is known, it has been suggested that people taking potassium-depleting diuretics, including loop diuretics, should supplement both potassium and magnesium.[4]

People taking loop diuretics should be monitored by their doctor, who will prescribe potassium supplements if needed. Such supplementation is particularly critical

Loop Diuretics

before surgery in patients with a history of heart disease. In a preliminary study, people with low blood levels of potassium (in part related to diuretic use) had a higher incidence of serious problems resulting from surgery (including death) compared with those having normal potassium levels.[5] Fruit is high in potassium, and increasing fruit intake is another way of supplementing potassium. Magnesium supplementation is typically 300–400 mg per day.

Vitamin B₁

Vitamin B$_1$

People with congestive heart failure (CHF) treated with the loop diuretic furosemide may be at risk for vitamin B$_1$ deficiency due to: 1) the disease, 2) treatment with furosemide, and/or 3) inadequate dietary vitamin B$_1$ intake.[6] In a study of people with CHF, long-term furosemide therapy was associated with clinically significant vitamin B$_1$ deficiency due to urinary losses.[7] This furosemide-induced vitamin B$_1$ deficiency may worsen heart function in patients with CHF and may be prevented or corrected with vitamin B$_1$ supplementation.[8]

Sodium

Diuretics, including loop diuretics, cause increased loss of sodium in the urine. By removing sodium from the body, diuretics also cause water to leave the body. This reduction of body water is the purpose of taking diuretics. Therefore, there is usually no reason to replace lost sodium, although strict limitation of salt intake in combination with the actions of diuretics can sometimes cause excessive sodium depletion. On the other hand, people who restrict sodium intake and in the process reduce blood pressure may need to have their dose of diuretics lowered.

Interactions with Herbs

Herbs that have a diuretic effect should be avoided when taking diuretic medications, as they may enhance the effect of these drugs and lead to possible cardiovascular side effects. These herbs include dandelion, uva ursi, juniper, buchu, cleavers, horsetail, and gravel root.[9]

Alder buckthorn, buckthorn (Rhamnus catartica, Rhamnus frangula, Frangula alnus)

Use buckthorn or alder buckthorn for more than ten days consecutively may cause a loss of electrolytes (especially the mineral potassium). Medications that also cause potassium loss, such as some diuretics, should be used with caution when taking buckthorn or alder buckthorn.[10]

Digitalis (Digitalis purpurea)

Digitalis refers to a family of plants commonly called foxglove that contain digitalis glycosides, chemicals with actions and toxicities similar to the prescription drug **digoxin** (page 90). Loop diuretics can increase the risk of digitalis-induced heart disturbances.[11] Loop diuretics and digitalis-containing products should only be used under the direct supervision of a doctor trained in their use.

Licorice (Glycyrrhiza glabra)

Licorice may enhance the side effects of potassium-depleting diuretics, including loop diuretics.[12] Loop diuretics and licorice should be used together only under careful medical supervision. Deglycyrrhizinated licorice (DGL) may be used safely with all diuretics.

Interactions with Foods and Other Compounds

Food

Furosemide (Lasix) is most effective taken on an empty stomach, one hour before eating.[13] However, furosemide may be taken with food to prevent gastrointestinal (GI) upset.[14] Torsemide (Demadex) may be taken with or without food.[15]

LOPERAMIDE

Common names: Apo-Loperamide, Arret, Boots Diareze, Diarreze, Diarrhea Relief, Diasorb, Diocalm Ultra, Diocaps, Dom-Loperamide, Imodium, Lodiar, Loperacap, LoperaGen, Norimode, Normaloe, Novo-Loperamide, PMS Loperamide, Rho-Loperamide

Loperamide is a drug used to treat diarrhea. It is available as a prescription and a nonprescription product.

Summary of Interactions for Loperamide

In some cases, an herb or supplement may appear in more than one category, which may seem contradictory. For clarification, read the full article for details about the summarized interactions.

Depletion or interference	None known
Side effect reduction/prevention	None known
Supportive interaction	None known
Reduced drug absorption/bioavailability	None known
Adverse interaction	None known

Interactions with Foods and Other Compounds

Alcohol

Loperamide may cause drowsiness or dizziness.[1] Alcohol may intensify these effects and increase the risk of accidental injury. To prevent problems, people taking loperamide should avoid alcohol.

LOPRESSOR HCT

Contains the following ingredients:
   Hydrochlorothiazide
   Metoprolol (page 176)

LORACARBEF

Common names: Lorabid

Loracarbef is used to treat bacterial infections in people with bronchitis and pneumonia, as well as infections of the middle ear, sinuses, throat, skin, and urinary tract. It belongs to a new class of beta-lactam **antibiotics** (page 19) called carbacephems.

Summary of Interactions for Loracarbef

In some cases, an herb or supplement may appear in more than one category, which may seem contradictory. For clarification, read the full article for details about the summarized interactions.

✓ May be Beneficial: Depletion or interference	Vitamin K*
✓ May be Beneficial: Side effect reduction/prevention	Bifidobacterium longum* Lactobacillus acidophilus* Lactobacillus casei* Saccharomyces boulardii* Saccharomyces cerevisiae* Vitamin K*
✓ May be Beneficial: Supportive interaction	Saccharomyces boulardii*
Reduced drug absorption/bioavailability	None known
Adverse interaction	None known

Interactions with Dietary Supplements

Probiotics

A common side effect of antibiotics is diarrhea, which may be caused by the elimination of beneficial bacteria normally found in the colon. Controlled studies have shown that taking probiotic microorganisms—such as *Lactobacillus casei, Lactobacillus acidophilus, Bifidobacterium longum,* or *Saccharomyces boulardii*—helps prevent antibiotic-induced diarrhea.[1]

The diarrhea experienced by some people who take antibiotics also might be due to an overgrowth of the bacterium *Clostridium difficile,* which causes a disease known as pseudomembranous colitis. Controlled studies have shown that supplementation with harmless yeast—such as *Saccharomyces boulardii*[2] or *Saccharomyces cerevisiae* (baker's or brewer's yeast)[3]—helps prevent recurrence of this infection. In one study, taking 500 mg of *Saccharomyces boulardii* twice daily enhanced the effectiveness of the antibiotic vancomycin in preventing recurrent clostridium infection.[4] Therefore, people taking antibiotics who later develop diarrhea might benefit from supplementing with saccharomyces organisms.

Treatment with antibiotics also commonly leads to an overgrowth of yeast *(Candida albicans)* in the vagina (candida vaginitis) and the intestines (sometimes referred to as "dysbiosis"). Controlled studies have shown that *Lactobacillus acidophilus* might prevent candida vaginitis.[5]

Vitamin K

Several cases of excessive bleeding have been reported in people who take antibiotics.[6, 7, 8, 9] This side effect may be the result of reduced vitamin K activity and/or reduced vitamin K production by bacteria in the colon. One study showed that people who had taken broad-spectrum antibiotics had lower liver concentrations of vitamin K_2 (menaquinone), though vitamin K_1 (phylloquinone) levels remained normal.[10] Several antibiotics appear to exert a strong effect on vitamin K activity, while others may not have any effect. Therefore, one should refer to a specific antibiotic for information on whether it interacts with vitamin K. Doctors of natural medicine sometimes recommend vitamin K supplementation to people taking antibiotics. Additional research is needed to determine whether the amount of vitamin K_1 found in some multivitamins is sufficient to prevent antibiotic-induced bleeding. Moreover, most multivitamins do not contain vitamin K.

LORATADINE

Common names: Boots Hayfever Relief, Claritin, Clarityn Allergy, Clarityn

Combination drug: Claritin-D

Loratadine is a selective antihistamine used to relieve allergic rhinitis (seasonal allergy) symptoms, including sneezing, runny nose, itching, and watery eyes. It is also used to treat people with idiopathic urticaria. Loratadine is available alone and in a combination product.

Summary of Interactions for Loratadine

In some cases, an herb or supplement may appear in more than one category, which may seem contradictory. For clarification, read the full article for details about the summarized interactions.

Depletion or interference	None known
Side effect reduction/prevention	None known
Supportive interaction	None known
Reduced drug absorption/bioavailability	None known
Adverse interaction	None known

Interactions with Foods and Other Compounds
Food
Food slows the absorption of loratadine and also increases the total amount of the drug absorbed.[1] It is recommended that loratadine be taken on an empty stomach.[2]

Alcohol
Selective antihistamines, including loratadine, may cause drowsiness or dizziness, although it is less likely than with nonselective antihistamines.[3] Alcohol can intensify drowsiness and dizziness, increasing the risk of accidental injury. People taking loratadine should use alcohol only with caution.

LORTAB

Contains the following ingredients:
Acetaminophen (page 3)
Hydrocodone (page 137)

LOSARTAN

Common names: Cozaar

Combination drugs: Cozaar-Comp, Hyzaar

Losartan is used alone or in combination with hydrochlorothiazide (Hyzaar) in the treatment of high blood pressure. It is a type of drug called an angiotensin II receptor antagonist.

Summary of Interactions for Losartan

In some cases, an herb or supplement may appear in more than one category, which may seem contradictory. For clarification, read the full article for details about the summarized interactions.

ⓘ Check: Other	Potassium
Depletion or interference	None known
Side effect reduction/prevention	None known
Supportive interaction	None known
Reduced drug absorption/bioavailability	None known
Adverse interaction	None known

Interactions with Dietary Supplements
Potassium
Losartan has caused significant increases in blood potassium levels.[1] Potassium supplements, potassium-containing salt substitutes (No Salt, Morton Salt Substitute, and others), and even high-potassium foods (primarily fruit) should be avoided by those taking losartan, unless directed otherwise by their doctor.

Interactions with Foods and Other Compounds
Food
The intestinal absorption of losartan may be reduced up to 10% if taken with food.[2] Although this is a minor reduction, losartan should be taken an hour before or two hours after food for maximum effectiveness.

LOTREL

Contains the following ingredients:
Amlodipine (page 13)
Benazepril (page 34)

LOTRIDERM

Contains the following ingredients:
Betamethasone (page 73)
Clotrimazole (page 73)

LOTRISONE

Contains the following ingredients:
Clotrimazole
Betamethasone (page 73)

LOVASTATIN

Common names: Apo-Lovastatin, Mevacor

Lovastatin is a member of the HMG-CoA reductase inhibitor family of drugs, which blocks the body's production of cholesterol. Lovastatin is used to lower elevated cholesterol levels. Cholestin, a dietary supplement advertised to help maintain healthy cholesterol, but not to lower high cholesterol, contains several HMG-CoA reductase inhibitor chemicals, including lovastatin.

Summary of Interactions for Lovastatin

In some cases, an herb or supplement may appear in more than one category, which may seem contradictory. For clarification, read the full article for details about the summarized interactions.

✓ May be Beneficial: Depletion or interference	Coenzyme Q10
✓ May be Beneficial: Side effect reduction/prevention	Milk thistle*
⊘ Avoid: Reduced drug absorption/ bioavailability	Fiber (soluble)
⊘ Avoid: Adverse interaction	Red yeast rice
ⓘ Check: Other	Grapefruit or grapefruit juice Niacin Vitamin A Vitamin E
Supportive interaction	None known

Interactions with Dietary Supplements

Coenzyme Q10

It has been clearly documented that HMG Co-A reductase inhibitors, including lovastatin,[1] deplete coenzyme Q_{10} (CoQ_{10}) levels in the blood, an effect that may be responsible for other side effects of the drug, such as abnormal liver function. In a double-blind trial, blood levels of CoQ_{10} were measured in 45 people with high cholesterol treated with lovastatin (20–80 mg per day) or **pravastatin** (page 220) (10–40 mg per day) for 18 weeks.[2] A significant decline in blood levels of CoQ_{10} occurred with both drugs. Supplementation with 90–100 mg per day CoQ_{10} has been shown to prevent reductions in blood levels of CoQ_{10} due to **simvastatin** (page 239).[3, 4] However, some investigators have questioned whether it is worthwhile or necessary for individuals taking HMG-CoA reductase inhibitors to supplement with CoQ_{10}.[5] Until more is known, people taking lovastatin should ask a doctor about supplementation with 30–100 mg CoQ_{10} per day.

Fiber (soluble)

Soluble fiber is found primarily in fruit, beans, and oats, but it is also available separately as pectin, oat bran, and glucomannan. Two sources of soluble fiber—pectin (found in fruit) and oat bran (a component of oatmeal also available by itself)—have been reported to interact with lovastatin.[6] The fiber from these two sources appears to bind the drug in the gastrointestinal tract and reduce absorption of the drug as a consequence. People taking this drug should avoid concentrated intake of soluble fiber, as taking lovastatin with a high soluble-fiber diet leads to reduced drug effectiveness.

Niacin (vitamin B3, nicotinic acid)

Niacin is a vitamin used to lower cholesterol. Large amounts of niacin taken with lovastatin have been reported to cause potentially serious muscle disorders (myopathy or rhabdomyolysis).[7] However, niacin also enhances the cholesterol-lowering effect of lovastatin.[8] Taking as little as 500 mg three times per day of niacin with lovastatin has been shown to have these complementary, supportive actions with almost none of the side effects seen when higher amounts of niacin are taken.[9] Nevertheless, individuals taking lovastatin should consult with their doctor before taking niacin.

Vitamin A

A study of 37 people with high cholesterol treated with diet and HMG-CoA reductase inhibitors found serum vitamin A levels increased over two years of therapy.[10] It remains unclear whether this moderate increase should suggest that people taking lovastatin have a particular need to restrict vitamin A supplementation.

Vitamin E
Oxidative damage to LDL ("bad") cholesterol is widely believed to contribute to heart disease. In a double-blind trial, lovastatin was found to increase oxidative damage to LDL cholesterol and vitamin E was reported to protect against such damage, though not to completely overcome the negative effect of lovastatin.[11] This study suggests that people taking lovastatin might benefit from supplemental vitamin E.

Interactions with Herbs
Milk thistle (Silybum marianum)
One of the possible side effects of lovastatin is liver toxicity. Although there are no clinical studies to substantiate its use with lovastatin, a milk thistle extract standardized to 70–80% silymarin may reduce the potential liver toxicity of lovastatin. The suggested use is 200 mg of the extract three times daily.

Red yeast rice (Monascus purpureas)
A supplement containing red yeast rice (Cholestin) has been shown to effectively lower cholesterol and triglycerides in people with moderately elevated levels of these blood lipids.[12] This extract contains small amounts of naturally occurring HMG-CoA reductase inhibitors such as lovastatin and should not be used if you are currently taking lovastatin or **pravastatin** (page 220).

Interactions with Foods and Other Compounds
Food
Food increases blood levels of lovastatin.[13] Lovastatin should be taken with a meal, at the same time every day.[14] Due to the possibility of reduced lovastatin absorption in the presence of soluble fiber, it makes sense to avoid eating fruit or oatmeal within two hours before or after taking lovastatin.

Grapefruit or grapefruit juice
In a small, single-dose trial with healthy volunteers, blood levels of lovastatin increased to a significantly greater extent when the drug was taken with grapefruit juice than when it was taken with water.[15] The same effect might be seen from eating grapefruit as from drinking its juice. There is one case report of a woman developing severe muscle damage from simvastatin (a drug similar to lovastatin) after she began eating one grapefruit per day.[16] To be on the safe side, people taking lovastatin should not eat grapefruit or drink grapefruit juice.

MAALOX

Contains the following ingredients:
   Aluminum hydroxide (page 10)
   Magnesium hydroxide (page 166)

MAALOX PLUS

Contains the following ingredients:
   Aluminium hydroxide (page 10)
   Dimethicone
   Magnesium hydroxide (page 166)

MAALOX PLUS TABLETS

Contains the following ingredients:
   Aluminium
   Dimethicone
   Magnesium

MACLEAN

Contains the following ingredients:
   Aluminium
   Calcium
   Magnesium

MACROLIDES

Common names: Dirithromycin, Dynabac, Tao, Troleandomycin

Macrolides are a family of **antibiotics** (page 19) used to treat a wide range of bacterial infections. Each drug within the family slows the growth of or kills specific bacteria; therefore, healthcare practitioners prescribe macrolides based on the individual's current needs.

There are interactions that are common to **antibacterial drugs** (page 19) and interactions involving a specific macrolide. For the latter interactions, refer to the highlighted drugs listed below.

- **Azithromycin** (page 31) (Zithromax)
- **Clarithromycin** (page 68) (Biaxin)
- Dirithromycin (Dynabac)
- **Erythromycin** (page 106) oral (EES, EryPed, Ery-Tab, PCE Dispertab, Pediazole)
- Erythromycin topical (A/T/S, Akne-Mycin, Erygel, Erycette, Eryderm, Erygel)
- Troleandomycin (Tao)

Summary of Interactions for Macrolides

In some cases, an herb or supplement may appear in more than one category, which may seem contradictory. For clarification, read the full article for details about the summarized interactions.

✓ May be Beneficial: Depletion or interference	Vitamin K*
✓ May be Beneficial: Side effect reduction/prevention	*Bifidobacterium longum* * *Lactobacillus acidophilus* * *Lactobacillus casei* * *Saccharomyces boulardii* * *Saccharomyces cerevisiae* * Vitamin K
✓ May be Beneficial: Supportive interaction	*Saccharomyces boulardii* *
Reduced drug absorption/bioavailability	None known
Adverse interaction	None known

Interactions common to many, if not all, Macrolides are described in this article. Interactions reported for only one or several drugs in this class may not be listed in this article. Some drugs listed in this article are linked to articles specific to that respective drug; please refer to those individual drug articles. The information in this article may not necessarily apply to drugs in this class for which no separate article exists. If you are taking a Macrolide for which no separate article exists, talk with your doctor or pharmacist.

Interactions with Dietary Supplements
Probiotics
A common side effect of antibiotics is diarrhea, which may be caused by the elimination of beneficial bacteria normally found in the colon. Controlled studies have shown that taking probiotic microorganisms—such as *Lactobacillus casei, Lactobacillus acidophilus, Bifidobacterium longum*, or *Saccharomyces boulardii*—helps prevent antibiotic-induced diarrhea.[1]

The diarrhea experienced by some people who take antibiotics also might be due to an overgrowth of the bacterium *Clostridium difficile*, which causes a disease known as pseudomembranous colitis. Controlled studies have shown that supplementation with harmless yeast—such as *Saccharomyces boulardii*[2] or *Saccharomyces cerevisiae* (baker's or brewer's yeast)[3]—helps prevent recurrence of this infection. In one study, taking 500 mg of *Saccharomyces boulardii* twice daily enhanced the effectiveness of the antibiotic vancomycin in preventing recurrent clostridium infection.[4] Therefore, people taking antibiotics who later develop diarrhea might benefit from supplementing with saccharomyces organisms.

Treatment with antibiotics also commonly leads to an overgrowth of yeast *(Candida albicans)* in the vagina (candida vaginitis) and the intestines (sometimes referred to as "dysbiosis"). Controlled studies have shown that *Lactobacillus acidophilus* might prevent candida vaginitis.[5]

Vitamin K
Several cases of excessive bleeding have been reported in people who take antibiotics.[6, 7, 8, 9] This side effect may be the result of reduced vitamin K activity and/or reduced vitamin K production by bacteria in the colon. One study showed that people who had taken broad-spectrum antibiotics had lower liver concentrations of vitamin K_2 (menaquinone), though vitamin K_1 (phylloquinone) levels remained normal.[10] Several antibiotics appear to exert a strong effect on vitamin K activity, while others may not have any effect. Therefore, one should refer to a specific antibiotic for information on whether it interacts with vitamin K. Doctors of natural medicine sometimes recommend vitamin K supplementation to people taking antibiotics. Additional research is needed to determine whether the amount of vitamin K_1 found in some multivitamins is sufficient to prevent antibiotic-induced bleeding. Moreover, most multivitamins do not contain vitamin K.

MAGNATOL

Contains the following ingredients:
  Alexitol
  Magnesium
  Potassium bicarbonate
  Xanthan gum

MAGNESIUM HYDROXIDE

Common names: Cream of Magnesia, Magnesium Hydroxide Mixture (BP), Milk of Magnesia, MOM

Combination drugs: Advanced Formula Di-Gel Tablets, Calcium Rich Rolaids, Co-Magaldrox, Maalox Plus, Maalox, Mucaine, Mylanta, Tempo Tablets

Magnesium hydroxide is used as an **antacid** (page 18) for short-term relief of stomach upset and as a laxative for short-term treatment of constipation. Magnesium hydroxide is available in nonprescription products alone and in combination with other nonprescription ingredients to relieve stomach upset.

Summary of Interactions for Magnesium Hydroxide

In some cases, an herb or supplement may appear in more than one category, which may seem contradictory. For clarification, read the full article for details about the summarized interactions.

✓	May be Beneficial: Depletion or interference	Folic acid Iron*
ⓘ	Check: Other	Potassium
	Side effect reduction/prevention	None known
	Supportive interaction	None known
	Reduced drug absorption/bioavailability	None known
	Adverse interaction	None known

Interactions with Dietary Supplements
Folic acid

Folic acid is needed by the body to utilize vitamin B_{12}. Antacids, including magnesium hydroxide, inhibit folic acid absorption.[1] People taking antacids are advised to supplement with folic acid.

Iron

Antacids (page 18), including magnesium hydroxide, may reduce the absorption of dietary iron. Iron supplements do not require stomach acid for absorption and one human study found that a magnesium hydroxide/**aluminum hydroxide** (page 10) antacid did not decrease supplemental iron absorption.[2]

Potassium

Individuals taking potassium-depleting **diuretics** (page 94) and those who are otherwise at risk of developing potassium deficiency (such as people with chronic diar-

rhea or vomiting) may experience a fall in serum potassium levels if they take magnesium without taking additional potassium.[3] This could lead to muscle cramps or, in individuals taking **digoxin** (page 90) or digitalis, more serious problems such as cardiac arrhythmias. Individuals who have a history of potassium deficiency and those who are at risk of developing potassium deficiency, as well as people taking digoxin or digitalis, should consult a physician before taking magnesium-containing products.

MAXZIDE

Contains the following ingredients:
   Hydrochlorothiazide
   Triamterene (page 268)

MECLIZINE

Common names: Antivert, Bonamine, Bonikraft, Histamethizine, Medivert, Sea-Legs

Meclizine is used to prevent nausea, vomiting, and dizziness associated with motion sickness, and may be effective in treating vertigo associated with inner ear conditions. It is in a class of drugs known as antihistamines.

Summary of Interactions for Meclizine

In some cases, an herb or supplement may appear in more than one category, which may seem contradictory. For clarification, read the full article for details about the summarized interactions.

Depletion or interference	None known
Side effect reduction/prevention	None known
Supportive interaction	None known
Reduced drug absorption/bioavailability	None known
Adverse interaction	None known

Interactions with Foods and Other Compounds
Alcohol

Drinking alcoholic beverages while taking meclizine can result in added drowsiness.[1] Consequently, people taking meclizine should avoid alcohol, especially when staying alert is necessary.

MEDROXYPROGESTERONE

Common names: Adgyn Medro, Alti-MPA, Cycrin, Depo-Provera, Farlutal, Gen-Medroxy, Novo-Medrone, Provera

Combination drugs: Indivina, Premique, Prempro, Tridestra

Medroxyprogesterone is a semisynthetic compound that differs in structure from the naturally occurring human hormone progesterone. It is added to estrogen replacement therapy to prevent uterine cancer caused by unopposed estrogen. It is also used to treat absence of menstrual bleeding (amenorrhea) and abnormal menstrual bleeding. Medroxyprogesterone is available alone and in a combination product. An injection product is used for contraception.

Summary of Interactions for Medroxyprogesterone

In some cases, an herb or supplement may appear in more than one category, which may seem contradictory. For clarification, read the full article for details about the summarized interactions.

ⓘ Check: Other	Folic acid Magnesium Vitamin A Vitamin D Zinc
Depletion or interference	None known
Side effect reduction/prevention	None known
Supportive interaction	None known
Reduced drug absorption/bioavailability	None known
Adverse interaction	None known

Interactions with Dietary Supplements

Vitamin A and folic acid

In a one-year study of predominantly malnourished women in India and Thailand, medroxyprogesterone used for contraception was associated with increased blood levels of vitamin A and folic acid.[1] The clinical meaning of these changes remains unclear.

Zinc and magnesium

In a group of 37 postmenopausal women treated with conjugated estrogens and medroxyprogesterone for 12 months, urinary zinc and magnesium loss was reduced in those women who began the study with signs of osteoporosis and elevated zinc and magnesium excretion.[2] The clinical significance of this interaction remains unclear.

Vitamin D

In a study of postmenopausal women, treatment with estrogen alone increased vitamin D blood levels, whereas estrogen plus medroxyprogesterone lowered vitamin D back to the level seen without estrogen use.[3] This outcome might suggest that medroxyprogesterone interferes with beneficial effects estrogen may have on vitamin D metabolism and vitamin D supplementation would be called for. However, some research has not found the addition of vitamin D to estrogen/progestin combinations to be helpful.[4] Therefore, while many doctors recommend 400 IU vitamin D to women taking estrogen/progestin combination hormone products, the efficacy of such supplementation has not been proven.

MEMANTINE

Common names: Namenda

Memantine is used to treat moderate to severe Alzheimer dementia. There are currently no reported nutrient or herb interactions involving memantine.

MENTHOL

Menthol is a compound obtained from peppermint oil or other mint oils or made synthetically. Menthol has local anesthetic and counterirritant qualities. It is contained in nonprescription products for short-term relief of minor sore throat and minor mouth or throat irritation. Menthol is also contained in combination products used for relief of muscle aches, sprains, and similar conditions.

There are currently no reported nutrient or herb interactions involving menthol. People using combination products that include menthol are advised to review the other ingredients for possible herb and/or nutrient interactions. Menthol is considered an antidote for many homeopathic remedies and should be avoided by people taking them.

Summary of Interactions for Menthol

In some cases, an herb or supplement may appear in more than one category, which may seem contradictory. For clarification, read the full article for details about the summarized interactions.

✓ May be Beneficial: Depletion or interference	Homeopathics
Side effect reduction/prevention	None known
Supportive interaction	None known
Reduced drug absorption/bioavailability	None known
Adverse interaction	None known

MESALAMINE

Common names: Asacol, Mesalazine, Pentasa, Rowasa, Salofalk

Mesalamine is used to treat mildly to moderately active ulcerative colitis and to prevent recurrence.

Summary of Interactions for Mesalamine

In some cases, an herb or supplement may appear in more than one category, which may seem contradictory. For clarification, read the full article for details about the summarized interactions.

✓ May be Beneficial: Supportive interaction	Psyllium
Depletion or interference	None known
Side effect reduction/prevention	None known
Reduced drug absorption/bioavailability	None known
Adverse interaction	None known

Interactions with Herbs

Psyllium (Plantago ovata)
Taking 20 grams of psyllium seeds together with mesalamine for 12 months was more effective at maintaining remission of ulcerative colitis than taking either the drug or herb alone.[1] People taking mesalamine should consult with their healthcare practitioner to determine whether they should add psyllium seeds to their treatment regimen.

METAXALONE

Common names: Skelaxin

Metaxalone is a muscle relaxant used to treat painful conditions associated with muscle spasm.

Summary of Interactions for Metaxalone

In some cases, an herb or supplement may appear in more than one category, which may seem contradictory.

For clarification, read the full article for details about the summarized interactions.

Depletion or interference	None known
Side effect reduction/prevention	None known
Supportive interaction	None known
Reduced drug absorption/bioavailability	None known
Adverse interaction	None known

Interactions with Foods and Other Compounds

Alcohol
Drinking alcohol while taking metaxalone may enhance the side effects of both compounds, such as drowsiness and dizziness; therefore it should be avoided.[1]

METFORMIN

Common names: Apo-Metformin, Gen-Metformin, Glucamet, Glucophage, Glycon, Novo-Metformin, Nu-Metformin, Rho-Metformin

Metformin is a drug used to lower blood sugar levels in people with non-insulin-dependent (type 2) diabetes.

Summary of Interactions for Metformin

In some cases, an herb or supplement may appear in more than one category, which may seem contradictory. For clarification, read the full article for details about the summarized interactions.

✓ May be Beneficial: Depletion or interference	Folic acid* Vitamin B_{12}
✓ May be Beneficial: Side effect reduction/prevention	Calcium
⃠ Avoid: Reduced drug absorption/ bioavailability	Guar gum*
⃠ Avoid: Adverse interaction	Ginkgo biloba
ⓘ Check: Other	DHEA Magnesium
Supportive interaction	None known

Interactions with Dietary Supplements

Dehydroepiandrosterone (DHEA)
Metformin has been reported to increase blood levels of DHEA-sulfate in at least two studies.[1, 2]

Folic acid and vitamin B_{12}
Metformin therapy has been shown to deplete vitamin B_{12} and sometimes, but not always,[3] folic acid as well.[4]

This depletion occurs through the interruption of a calcium-dependent mechanism. Supplementation with calcium has reversed this effect in a clinical trial.[5] People taking metformin should supplement vitamin B_{12} and folic acid or ask their doctor to monitor folic acid and vitamin B_{12} levels.

Magnesium
In a study of patients with poorly controlled type 2 diabetes, low blood levels of magnesium, and high urine magnesium loss, metformin therapy was associated with reduced urinary magnesium losses but no change in low blood levels of magnesium.[6] Whether this interaction has clinical importance remains unclear.

Guar gum
In a small, controlled study, guar gum plus metformin slowed the rate of metformin absorption.[7] In people with diabetes this interaction could reduce the blood sugar–lowering effectiveness of metformin. Until more is known, metformin should be taken two hours before or two hours after guar gum–containing supplements. It remains unclear whether the small amounts of guar gum found in many processed foods is enough to significantly affect metformin absorption.

Interactions with Herbs
Ginkgo biloba
In a preliminary trial, administration of *Ginkgo biloba* extract (120 mg per day) for three months to patients with type 2 diabetes who were taking oral anti-diabetes medication resulted in a significant worsening of glucose tolerance. Ginkgo did not impair glucose tolerance in individuals whose diabetes was controlled by diet.[8] Individuals taking oral anti-diabetes medication should consult a doctor before taking *Ginkgo biloba*.

Interactions with Foods and Other Compounds
Food
Food interferes with metformin absorption.[9, 10, 11] Taking metformin with food can reduce the absorption of the drug. Therefore, metformin should be taken an hour before or two hours after a meal unless stomach upset occurs.

Alcohol
Lactic acidosis is a rare but serious side effect of metformin. Alcohol increases the production of lactic acid caused by metformin, increasing the risk of lactic acidosis.[12] People taking metformin should avoid alcohol or consult with their doctor before consuming alcohol.

METHOCARBAMOL

Common names: Carbacot, Glyceryl Guaiacolate Carbamate, Robaxin

Methocarbamol is used to treat acute, painful conditions, and is in a class of drugs known as centrally acting skeletal muscle relaxants.

Summary of Interactions for Methocarbamol
In some cases, an herb or supplement may appear in more than one category, which may seem contradictory. For clarification, read the full article for details about the summarized interactions.

Depletion or interference	None known
Side effect reduction/prevention	None known
Supportive interaction	None known
Reduced drug absorption/bioavailability	None known
Adverse interaction	None known

Interactions with Foods and Other Compounds
Alcohol
Drinking alcoholic beverages while taking methocarbamol can result in added drowsiness and dizziness.[1] Consequently, people taking methocarbamol should avoid alcohol, especially when staying alert is necessary.

METHOTREXATE

Common names: Folex, Maxtrex, Rheumatrex

Methotrexate (MTX) is a **chemotherapy** (page 54) drug that interferes with folic acid activation, preventing cell reproduction. Methotrexate is used to treat some forms of cancer; severe, disabling psoriasis; and severe, active rheumatoid arthritis.

Note: Many of the interactions described below, in the text and in the Summary of Interactions, have been reported only for specific chemotherapeutic drugs, and may not apply to other chemotherapeutic drugs. There are many unknowns concerning interactions of nutrients, herbs, and chemotherapy drugs. People receiving chemotherapy who wish to supplement with vitamins, minerals, herbs, or other natural substances should always consult a physician.

Methotrexate

Summary of Interactions for Methotrexate

In some cases, an herb or supplement may appear in more than one category, which may seem contradictory. For clarification, read the full article for details about the summarized interactions.

✓ May be Beneficial: Side effect reduction/prevention	Beta-carotene* (mouth sores) Chamomile* (mouth sores) Eleuthero* (see text) Folic acid (for people with rheumatoid arthritis)* Folic acid* (for people with psoriasis) Ginger* (nausea) Glutamine* Spleen peptide extract* (see text) Vitamin A* Zinc* (taste alterations)
✓ May be Beneficial: Supportive interaction	Antioxidants* Glutamine* Melatonin* Milk thistle* PSK*
⊘ Avoid: Reduced drug absorption/ bioavailability	Folic acid*
⊘ Avoid: Adverse interaction	Folic acid (for people with cancer) PABA*
ⓘ Check: Other	Echinacea* Multivitamin-mineral* Vitamin A* Vitamin C*
Depletion or interference	None known

Interactions with Dietary Supplements

Antioxidants

Chemotherapy can injure cancer cells by creating oxidative damage. As a result, some oncologists recommend that patients avoid supplementing antioxidants if they are undergoing chemotherapy. Limited test tube research occasionally does support the idea that an antioxidant can interfere with oxidative damage to cancer cells.[1] However, most scientific research does not support this supposition.

A modified form of vitamin A has been reported to work synergistically with chemotherapy in test tube research.[2] Vitamin C appears to increase the effectiveness of chemotherapy in animals[3] and with human breast cancer cells in test tube research.[4] In a double-blind study, Japanese researchers found that the combination of vitamin E, vitamin C, and N-acetyl cysteine (NAC)—all antioxidants—protected against chemotherapy-induced heart damage without interfering with the action of the chemotherapy.[5]

A comprehensive review of antioxidants and chemotherapy leaves open the question of whether supplemental antioxidants definitely help people with chemotherapy side effects, but it clearly shows that antioxidants need not be avoided for fear that the actions of chemotherapy are interfered with.[6] Although research remains incomplete, the idea that people taking chemotherapy should avoid antioxidants is not supported by scientific research.

A new formulation of selenium (Seleno-Kappacarrageenan) was found to reduce kidney damage and white blood cell–lowering effects of **cisplatin** (page 64) in one human study. However, the level used in this study (4,000 mcg per day) is potentially toxic and should only be used under the supervision of a doctor.[7]

Glutathione, the main antioxidant found within cells, is frequently depleted in individuals on chemotherapy and/or radiation. Preliminary studies have found that intravenously injected glutathione may decrease some of the adverse effects of chemotherapy and radiation, such as diarrhea.[8]

Folic acid

In cancer treatment, methotrexate works by blocking activation of folic acid. Folic acid-containing supplements may interfere with methotrexate therapy in people with cancer.[9] Methotrexate therapy can lead to folic acid deficiency. People using methotrexate for cancer treatment should ask their prescribing doctor before using any folic acid-containing supplements. There is no concern about folic acid supplementation for people with cancer using **chemotherapy drugs** (page 54) other than methotrexate.

Until recently, it was believed that methotrexate helped people with rheumatoid arthritis also by interfering with folic acid metabolism. However, this is not necessarily so, as some studies have shown that folic acid supplementation in amounts ranging from 5–50 mg per week did not alter the efficacy of methotrexate in the treatment of rheumatoid arthritis.[10, 11, 12] Many doctors now believe that people with rheumatoid arthritis taking methotrexate should supplement large amounts of folic acid. In separate double-blind trials, 5 mg per week of folic acid and 2.5–5 mg per week of folinic acid (an activated form of folic acid) have substantially reduced side effects of methotrexate without interfering with the therapeutic action in rheumatoid patients.[13, 14] Folic or folinic acid was taken at a different time from methotrexate and sometimes only five days per week. Daily (as opposed to weekly) supplementation with folic acid (5 mg per day for 13 days) was found to reduce blood levels of methotrexate;[15] however, the researchers in this study suggest that the reduction in blood methotrexate levels by folic acid does not necessarily mean that the folic acid is interfering with the therapeutic action of the drug. It is possible that the lower blood levels of methotrexate are simply an indication that the drug is being taken up more rapidly by the cells as a result of folic acid supplementation. In most of the studies cited here, folic acid supplementation was begun 24 hours after the administration of methotrexate. Because of the uncertainty regarding this interaction, persons taking methotrexate for rheumatoid arthritis who are considering supplementation with folic acid should first consult with their doctor.

People who are prescribed methotrexate to treat severe psoriasis experience fewer side effects if they also supplement high amounts (5 mg per day) of folic acid.[16] As is the case with methotrexate and rheumatoid arthritis, supplementing folic acid did not interfere with the activity of methotrexate. Such high levels of folic acid should not be taken without clinical supervision.

Glutamine

Though cancer cells use glutamine as a fuel source, studies in humans have not found that glutamine stimulates growth of cancers in people taking chemotherapy.[17, 18] In fact, animal studies show that glutamine may actually decrease tumor growth while increasing susceptibility of cancer cells to radiation and chemotherapy,[19, 20] though such effects have not yet been studied in humans.

Glutamine has successfully reduced chemotherapy-induced mouth sores. In one trial, people were given 4 grams of glutamine in an oral rinse, which was swished around the mouth and then swallowed twice per day.[21] Thirteen of fourteen people in the study had fewer days with mouth sores as a result. These excellent results have been duplicated in some,[22] but not all[23] double-

blind research. In another study, patients receiving high-dose **paclitaxel** (page 205) and melphalan had significantly fewer episodes of oral ulcers and bleeding when they took 6 grams of glutamine four times daily along with the chemotherapy.[24]

One double-blind trial suggested that 6 grams of glutamine taken three times per day can decrease diarrhea caused by chemotherapy.[25] However, other studies using higher amounts or intravenous glutamine have not reported this effect.[26, 27]

Intravenous use of glutamine in people undergoing bone marrow transplants, a procedure sometimes used to allow very high amounts of chemotherapy to be used, has led to reduced hospital stays, leading to a savings of over $21,000 for each patient given glutamine.[28]

Animal studies have demonstrated that administration of methotrexate with intravenous or oral glutamine may enhance the ability of methotrexate to kill tumor cells, while decreasing methotrexate toxicity and improving survival.[29, 30, 31, 32, 33, 34] The effects of oral glutamine supplementation in humans taking methotrexate remains unknown.

Melatonin

High amounts of melatonin have been combined with a variety of chemotherapy drugs to reduce their side effects or improve drug efficacy. One study gave melatonin at night in combination with the drug triptorelin to men with metastatic prostate cancer.[35] All of these men had previously become unresponsive to triptorelin. The combination decreased PSA levels—a marker of prostate cancer progression—in eight of fourteen patients, decreased some side effects of triptorelin, and helped nine of fourteen to live longer than one year. The outcome of this preliminary study suggests that melatonin may improve the efficacy of triptorelin even after the drug has apparently lost effectiveness.

N-acetyl cysteine (NAC)

NAC, an amino acid–like supplement that possesses antioxidant activity, has been used in four human studies to decrease the kidney and bladder toxicity of the chemotherapy drug ifosfamide.[36, 37, 38, 39] These studies used 1–2 grams NAC four times per day. There was no sign that NAC interfered with the efficacy of ifosfamide in any of these studies. Intakes of NAC over 4 grams per day may cause nausea and vomiting.

The newer anti-nausea drugs prescribed for people taking chemotherapy lead to greatly reduced nausea and vomiting for most people. Nonetheless, these drugs often do not totally eliminate all nausea. Natural sub-

Methotrexate

stances used to reduce nausea should not be used instead of prescription anti-nausea drugs. Rather, under the guidance of a doctor, they should be added to those drugs if needed. At least one trial suggests that NAC, at 1,800 mg per day, may reduce nausea and vomiting caused by chemotherapy.[40]

Spleen extract
Patients with inoperable head and neck cancer were treated with a spleen peptide preparation (Polyerga) in a double-blind trial during chemotherapy with cisplatin and 5-FU.[41] The spleen preparation had a significant stabilizing effect on certain white blood cells. People taking it also experienced stabilized body weight and a reduction in the fatigue and inertia that usually accompany this combination of chemotherapy agents.

Beta-carotene and vitamin E
Chemotherapy frequently causes mouth sores. In one trial, people were given approximately 400,000 IU of beta-carotene per day for three weeks and then 125,000 IU per day for an additional four weeks.[42] Those taking beta-carotene still suffered mouth sores, but the mouth sores developed later and tended to be less severe than mouth sores that formed in people receiving the same chemotherapy without beta-carotene.

In a study of chemotherapy-induced mouth sores, six of nine patients who applied vitamin E directly to their mouth sores had complete resolution of the sores compared with one of nine patients who applied placebo.[43] Others have confirmed the potential for vitamin E to help people with chemotherapy-induced mouth sores.[44] Applying vitamin E only once per day was helpful to only some groups of patients in another trial,[45] and not all studies have found vitamin E to be effective.[46] Until more is known, if vitamin E is used in an attempt to reduce chemotherapy-induced mouth sores, it should be applied topically twice per day and should probably be in the tocopherol (versus tocopheryl) form.

Vitamin A
A controlled French trial reported that when postmenopausal late-stage breast cancer patients were given very large amounts of vitamin A (350,000–500,000 IU per day) along with chemotherapy, remission rates were significantly better than when the chemotherapy was not accompanied by vitamin A.[47] Similar results were not found in premenopausal women. The large amounts of vitamin A used in the study are toxic and require clinical supervision.

In a study of children with cancer who were receiving high-dose methotrexate, administration of 180,000 IU of vitamin A on the day before methotrexate treatment reduced the severity of intestinal damage caused by the drug.[48] Because of the complex nature of cancer therapy and the large amount of vitamin A involved, this treatment should be done only with the supervision of a doctor.

Zinc
Irradiation treatment, especially of head and neck cancers, frequently results in changes to normal taste sensation.[49, 50] Zinc supplementation may be protective against taste alterations caused or exacerbated by irradiation. A double-blind trial found that 45 mg of zinc sulfate three times daily reduced the alteration of taste sensation during radiation treatment and led to significantly greater recovery of taste sensation after treatment was concluded.[51]

Multivitamin-mineral
Many chemotherapy drugs can cause diarrhea, lack of appetite, vomiting, and damage to the gastrointestinal tract. Recent anti-nausea prescription medications are often effective. Nonetheless, nutritional deficiencies still occur.[52] It makes sense for people undergoing chemotherapy to take a high-potency multivitamin-mineral to protect against deficiencies.

Taurine
Taurine has been shown to be depleted in people taking chemotherapy.[53] It remains unclear how important this effect is or if people taking chemotherapy should take taurine supplements.

Thymus peptides
Peptides or short proteins derived from the thymus gland, an important immune organ, have been used in conjunction with chemotherapy drugs for people with cancer. One study using thymosin fraction V in combination with chemotherapy, compared with chemotherapy alone, found significantly longer survival times in the thymosin fraction V group.[54] A related substance, thymostimulin, decreased some side effects of chemotherapy and increased survival time compared with chemotherapy alone.[55] A third product, thymic extract TP1, was shown to improve immune function in people treated with chemotherapy compared with effects of chemotherapy alone.[56] Thymic peptides need to be administered by injection. People interested in their combined use with chemotherapy should consult a doctor.

PABA (para-aminobenzoic acid)
PABA can increase methotrexate levels, activity, and side effects.[57] The incidence and severity of this interaction remains unclear.

Interactions with Herbs

Echinacea (Echinacea purpurea, Echinacea angustifolia)
Echinacea is a popular immune-boosting herb that has been investigated for use with chemotherapy. One study investigated the actions of **cyclophosphamide** (page 79), echinacea, and thymus gland extracts to treat advanced cancer patients. Although small and uncontrolled, this trial suggested that the combination modestly extended the life span of some patients with inoperable cancers.[58] Signs of restoration of immune function were seen in these patients.

Eleuthero (Eleutherococcus senticosus)
Russian research has looked at using eleuthero with chemotherapy. One study of patients with melanoma found that chemotherapy was less toxic when eleuthero was given simultaneously. Similarly, women with inoperable breast cancer given eleuthero were reported to tolerate more chemotherapy.[59] Eleuthero treatment was also associated with improved immune function in women with breast cancer treated with chemotherapy and radiation.[60]

Milk thistle (Silybum marianum)
Milk thistle's major flavonoids, known collectively as silymarin, have shown synergistic actions with the chemotherapy drugs **cisplatin** (page 64) and **doxorubicin** (page 100) (Adriamycin) in test tubes.[61] Silymarin also offsets the kidney toxicity of cisplatin in animals.[62] Silymarin has not yet been studied in humans treated with cisplatin. There is some evidence that silymarin may not interfere with some chemotherapy in humans with cancer.[63]

Ginger (Zingiber officinale)
Ginger can be helpful in alleviating nausea and vomiting caused by chemotherapy.[64, 65] Ginger, as tablets, capsules, or liquid herbal extracts, can be taken in 500 mg amounts every two or three hours, for a total of 1 gram per day.

German chamomile (Matricaria recutita)
A liquid preparation of German chamomile has been shown to reduce the incidence of mouth sores in people receiving radiation and systemic chemotherapy treatment in an uncontrolled study. [66]

PSK (Coriolus versicolor)
The mushroom *Coriolus versicolor* contains an immune-stimulating substance called polysaccharide krestin, or PSK. PSK has been shown in several studies to help cancer patients undergoing chemotherapy. One study involved women with estrogen receptor-negative breast cancer. PSK combined with chemotherapy significantly prolonged survival time compared with chemotherapy alone.[67] Another study followed women with breast cancer who were given chemotherapy with or without PSK. The PSK-plus-chemotherapy group had a 25% better chance of survival after ten years compared with those taking chemotherapy without PSK.[68] Another study investigated people who had surgically removed colon cancer. They were given chemotherapy with or without PSK. Those given PSK had a longer disease-free period and longer survival time.[69] Three grams of PSK were taken orally each day in these studies.

Although PSK is rarely available in the United States, hot-water extract products made from *Coriolus versicolor* mushrooms are available. These products may have activity related to that of PSK, but their use with chemotherapy has not been studied.

Interactions with Foods and Other Compounds

Food
Food can interfere with methotrexate absorption, and methotrexate causes stomach upset.[70]

Fruit drinks
Often, people who undergo chemotherapy develop aversions to certain foods, sometimes making it permanently difficult to eat those foods. Exposing people to what researchers have called a "scapegoat stimulus" just before the administration of chemotherapy can direct the food aversion to the "scapegoat" food instead of more important parts of the diet. In one trial, fruit drinks administered just before chemotherapy were most effective in protecting against aversions to other foods.[71]

Alcohol
Alcohol should be avoided during methotrexate therapy, due to concerns of increased risk of liver damage.[72]

METHYLCELLULOSE

Common names: Celevac, Citrucel

Methylcellulose is a semisynthetic, bulk laxative used for short-term treatment of constipation. It is available as a nonprescription drug.

Summary of Interactions for Methylcellulose

In some cases, an herb or supplement may appear in more than one category, which may seem contradictory.

For clarification, read the full article for details about the summarized interactions.

Depletion or interference	None known
Side effect reduction/prevention	None known
Supportive interaction	None known
Reduced drug absorption/bioavailability	None known
Adverse interaction	None known

METHYLDOPA

Common names: Aldomet, Apo-Methyldopa, Novo-Medopa, Nu-Medopa

Combination drugs: Aldoclor, Aldoril

Methyldopa is a drug used to lower blood pressure in people with hypertension (high blood pressure).

Summary of Interactions for Methyldopa

In some cases, an herb or supplement may appear in more than one category, which may seem contradictory. For clarification, read the full article for details about the summarized interactions.

✓ May be Beneficial: Depletion or interference	Vitamin B$_{12}$*
⊘ Avoid: Reduced drug absorption/ bioavailability	Iron
⊘ Avoid: Adverse interaction	Sodium
Side effect reduction/prevention	None known
Supportive interaction	None known

Interactions with Dietary Supplements

Iron

Iron supplements have been found to decrease methyldopa absorption.[1, 2] Taking methyldopa two hours before or after iron-containing products can help avoid this interaction.

Vitamin B$_{12}$

Methyldopa can decrease vitamin B$_{12}$ levels, thus increasing the risk of vitamin B$_{12}$ deficiency.[3]

Sodium

Excess dietary sodium (salt) intake can cause fluid retention and interfere with the blood pressure lowering action of methyldopa.[4] Reducing the use of table salt

and heavily salted foods during methyldopa therapy reduces the likelihood of this interference.

Interactions with Foods and Other Compounds

Food

Food can interfere with methyldopa absorption.[5] Taking methyldopa one hour before or two hours after eating can prevent this interference.

METHYLPHENIDATE

Common names: Metadate ER, Methylin, PMS-Methylphenidate, Riphenidate, Ritalin, Ritalin-SR

Methylphenidate is a stimulant drug with actions similar to amphetamines. It is used as an adjunct to a complete program to treat children with attention deficit-hyperactivity disorder. Methylphenidate is also used to treat people with narcolepsy.

Summary of Interactions for Methylphenidate

In some cases, an herb or supplement may appear in more than one category, which may seem contradictory. For clarification, read the full article for details about the summarized interactions.

⊘ Avoid: Adverse interaction	Alcohol
Depletion or interference	None known
Side effect reduction/prevention	None known
Supportive interaction	None known
Reduced drug absorption/bioavailability	None known

Interactions with Foods and Other Compounds

Food

Some researchers have recommended that methylphenidate be taken 30 to 45 minutes before meals,[1] although it has been reported that methylphenidate was absorbed faster[2] and was equally effective[3] taken with food. Sustained-release methylphenidate (Ritalin-SR) tablets should be swallowed whole, without crushing or chewing.[4]

Alcohol

Methylphenidate may impair physical coordination and cause dizziness or drowsiness.[5] Alcohol may intensify these effects, increasing the risk of accidental injury. To prevent problems, people taking methylphenidate should avoid alcohol.

METHYLTESTOSTERONE

Common names: Android, Testosterone Cypionate, Testred, Virilon

Combination drug: Estratest/Estratest HS

Methyltestosterone is a hormone used in men to treat testosterone deficiency, and in women to treat breast cancer, as well as breast pain and swelling following pregnancy. It is also combined with estrogen (**Estratest** [page 109]) to treat symptoms associated with menopause.

Summary of Interactions for Methyltestosterone

In some cases, an herb or supplement may appear in more than one category, which may seem contradictory. For clarification, read the full article for details about the summarized interactions.

✓ May be Beneficial: Depletion or interference	Beta-carotene* Vitamin A*
⃠ Avoid: Adverse interaction	Zinc
ⓘ Check: Other	Androstenedione (Andro)* Dehydroepiandrosterone (DHEA)*
Side effect reduction/prevention	None known
Supportive interaction	None known
Reduced drug absorption/bioavailability	None known

Interactions with Dietary Supplements

Vitamin A and beta-carotene

A 59-year-old man developed an inability to see well at night following treatment with methyltestosterone.[1] Laboratory tests revealed low blood levels of vitamin A and beta-carotene, which may have resulted from taking the drug. More research is needed to determine if vitamin A and beta-carotene supplementation is required for people taking methyltestosterone.

Zinc

Taking methyltestosterone increased the amount of zinc in the blood and hair of boys with short stature or growth retardation.[2] It is not known whether this increase would occur in other people or whether zinc supplementation by people taking methyltestosterone would result in zinc toxicity. Until more is known, zinc supplementation should be combined with methyltestosterone therapy only under the supervision of a doctor.

Dehydroepiandrosterone (DHEA)

DHEA supplementation has been shown to increase blood levels of testosterone,[3, 4, 5] as does methyltestosterone. No studies have investigated the possible additive effects of taking DHEA and methyltestosterone, but either increased drug effectiveness or more severe side effects are possible. Until more is known, these agents should be combined only under the supervision of a doctor.

Androstenedione (Andro)

Andro supplementation has been shown to increase blood levels of testosterone in women,[6] but not in men.[7] No studies have investigated the possible additive effects of taking andro and methyltestosterone, but either increased drug effectiveness or more severe side effects are possible. Until more is known, these agents should be combined only under the supervision of a doctor.

METOCLOPRAMIDE

Common names: Apo-Metoclop, Gastrobid Continuous, Gastroflux, Gastromax, Maxeran, Nu-Metoclopramide, Ocatmide, Parmid, PMS-Metoclopramide, Primperan, Reglan

Metoclopramide is used to treat heartburn and regurgitation; to prevent vomiting in people receiving drugs to treat cancer; and to prevent nausea, vomiting, heartburn, and fullness after a meal in certain individuals with diabetes.

Summary of Interactions for Metoclopramide

In some cases, an herb or supplement may appear in more than one category, which may seem contradictory. For clarification, read the full article for details about the summarized interactions.

✓ May be Beneficial: Supportive interaction	Willow*
⃠ Avoid: Adverse interaction	N-acetyl cysteine*
Depletion or interference	None known
Side effect reduction/prevention	None known
Reduced drug absorption/bioavailability	None known

Interactions with Dietary Supplements

N-acetyl cysteine

A single case report described a 15-year-old girl who suffered oxygen deprivation in her body tissues after being given high amounts of metoclopramide and N-acetyl-

Metoclopramide

cysteine to treat her for an overdose of **acetaminophen** (page 3).[1] It is unknown whether N-acetyl-cysteine supplementation in the absence of acetaminophen overdose could cause similar effects in people taking metoclopramide. Until controlled research determines the safety of this combination, it should be used only under the supervision of a qualified physician.

Interactions with Herbs
White willow bark (Salix alba)
Salicylic acid is a compound formed in the body from either **aspirin** (page 26) or white willow bark. Taking metoclopramide before aspirin or white willow bark results in higher concentrations of salicylic acid and greater pain relief in people suffering from an acute migraine headache.[2] Controlled studies are necessary to confirm the benefit of this interaction.

Interaction with Foods and Other Compounds
Lactose-containing foods
Individuals who have lactose intolerance (difficulty digesting milk sugar) may experience more severe symptoms while taking metoclopramide.[3] Lactose is the milk sugar present in dairy products.

Caffeine (page 44)
A single case report described a 42-year-old man taking metoclopramide who experienced mental depression after he abruptly quit using caffeine.[4] People who are advised to quit caffeine should probably reduce their coffee or tea consumption gradually if they are taking metoclopramide.

Alcohol
Drinking alcohol while taking metoclopramide may significantly increase the amount and speed of alcohol absorption, resulting in enhanced alcohol effects such as drowsiness.[5] Consequently, people taking metoclopramide should avoid alcohol, especially when staying alert is necessary.

METOPROLOL

Common names: Apo-Metoprolol, Arbralene, Betaloc-SA, Betaloc, Lopresor SR, Lopressor, Mepranix, Novo-Metoprol, Nu-Metop, PMS-Metoprolol, Toprol XL

Combination drugs: Co-Betaloc SA, Co-Betaloc, Lopressor HCT

Metoprolol is a beta-blocker drug used to reduce the symptoms of angina pectoris (chest pain), lower blood pressure in people with hypertension, and treat people after heart attacks. Metoprolol is available alone and in a combination product used to lower blood pressure.

Summary of Interactions for Metoprolol
In some cases, an herb or supplement may appear in more than one category, which may seem contradictory. For clarification, read the full article for details about the summarized interactions.

✓ May be Beneficial: Depletion or interference	High-potassium foods* Pleurisy root* Potassium supplements*
🚫 Avoid: Adverse interaction	Alcohol High-potassium foods* Pleurisy root* Potassium supplements*
Side effect reduction/prevention	None known
Supportive interaction	None known
Reduced drug absorption/bioavailability	None known

Interactions with Dietary Supplements
Potassium
Some **beta-adrenergic blockers** (page 37) (called "nonselective" beta blockers) decrease the uptake of potassium from the blood into the cells,[1] leading to excess potassium in the blood, a potentially dangerous condition known as hyperkalemia.[2] People taking beta-blockers should therefore avoid taking potassium supplements, or eating large quantities of fruit (e.g., bananas), unless directed to do so by their doctor.

Interactions with Herbs
Pleurisy root (Asclepius tuberosa)
As pleurisy root and other plants in the *Aesclepius* genus contain cardiac glycosides, it is best to avoid use of pleurisy root with heart medications such as beta-blockers.[3]

Interactions with Foods and Other Compounds
Food
Food increases the absorption of metoprolol.[4] Metoprolol should be taken at the same time every day[5] always with or always without food.

Alcohol

Metoprolol may cause drowsiness, dizziness, light-headedness, or blurred vision.[6] Alcohol may intensify these effects and increase the risk of accidental injury. To prevent problems, people taking metoprolol should avoid alcohol.

METRONIDAZOLE

Common names: Apo-Metronidazole, Flagyl, MetroCream, MetroGel, MetroLotion, Metronyl, Noritate, Novo-Diazol, Protostat

Combination drug: Helidac

Metronidazole is an **antibiotic** (page 19) used to treat a variety of bacterial and parasitic infections, such as amebiasis, trichomoniasis, and giardiasis. It is also used as a component of multidrug antibiotic combinations to heal stomach and duodenal ulcers caused by *Helicobacter pylori* infections. Metronidazole is available alone and in a combination product.

Summary of Interactions for Metronidazole

In some cases, an herb or supplement may appear in more than one category, which may seem contradictory. For clarification, read the full article for details about the summarized interactions.

✓ May be Beneficial: Side effect reduction/prevention	*Saccharomyces boulardii* (for *Clostridium difficile* only)
✓ May be Beneficial: Supportive interaction	*Saccharomyces boulardii* (for *Clostridium difficile* only)
ⓘ Check: Other	Diosmin Milk thistle
Depletion or interference	None known
Reduced drug absorption/bioavailability	None known
Adverse interaction	None known

Interactions with Dietary Supplements
Diosmin

Diosmin is a flavonoid used to treat hemorrhoids and vein disorders. In a study of healthy male volunteers who took 800 mg of metronidazole, pretreatment with 500 mg of diosmin per day for nine days increased blood levels of metronidazole by 24%.[1] Diosmin appears to increase the availability of metronidazole by inhibiting the enzyme that normally breaks it down. The results of this study suggest that taking diosmin may increase both the effectiveness and toxicity of metronidazole.

Saccharomyces boulardii

The yeast *Saccharomyces boulardii* may help restore microbial balance in the intestines and prevent pseudomembranous colitis (PMC), an intestinal disorder caused by infection with *Clostridium difficile*. Even when *Clostridium difficile* is successfully treated with antibiotics, symptoms recur in about 20% of cases. *Saccharomyces boulardii* has been shown in controlled trials to reduce recurrences when given as an adjunct to antibiotic therapy.[2, 3, 4]

Interactions with Herbs
Milk thistle (Silybum marianum)

Milk thistle has been reported to protect the liver from harm caused by some prescription drugs.[5] While milk thistle has not yet been studied directly for protecting people against the known potentially liver-damaging actions of metronidazole, it is often used for this purpose.

Interactions with Foods and Other Compounds
Food

Metronidazole should be taken with food to avoid stomach upset.

Alcohol

Alcohol may interact with metronidazole, causing facial flushing, headache, light-headedness, nausea, breathlessness, and other symptoms.[6] Vinegar typically contains small amounts of alcohol and should be avoided during metronidazole therapy. People should read all product labels carefully for alcohol content and should avoid alcohol-containing products during metronidazole therapy.

METRONIDAZOLE (VAGINAL)

Common names: MetroGel Vaginal, Nidagel Vaginal Gel, Zidoval Vaginal Gel

Metronidazole (vaginal) is an intravaginal antibiotic used to treat vaginal infections caused primarily by bacteria. **Metronidazole** (page 177) is also available as oral and topical medications.

Summary of Interactions for Metronidazole Vaginal

In some cases, an herb or supplement may appear in more than one category, which may seem contradictory. For clarification, read the full article for details about the summarized interactions.

✓ May be Beneficial: Supportive interaction	Zinc
Depletion or interference	None known
Side effect reduction/prevention	None known
Reduced drug absorption/bioavailability	None known
Adverse interaction	None known

Interactions with Dietary Supplements
Zinc
Four women whose vaginal infections caused by trichomonas (one-celled parasites) were not responding to oral and vaginal metronidazole treatment alone, improved when a zinc sulfate douche was added.[1] Controlled research is needed to determine if zinc enhances the effects of metronidazole in vaginal infections caused by other organisms.

MIDRIN

Contains the following ingredients:
Acetaminophen (page 3)
Dichloralphenazone
Isometheptene

MIFEPRISTONE

Common names: Mifegyne, Mifeprex, RU486

Mifepristone, also known as RU486, is used to induce abortion, and is classified both as a progesterone and a glucocorticosteroid receptor antagonist. It has also been used experimentally to treat Cushing's syndrome (hyperfunctioning adrenal glands), breast cancer, and glaucoma.

Summary of Interactions for Mifepristone

In some cases, an herb or supplement may appear in more than one category, which may seem contradictory. For clarification, read the full article for details about the summarized interactions.

✓ May be Beneficial: Side effect reduction/prevention	Modified shenghua tang
Depletion or interference	None known
Supportive interaction	None known
Reduced drug absorption/bioavailability	None known
Adverse interaction	None known

Interactions with Herbs
Modified shenghua tang
The most common side effect of mifepristone is excess vaginal bleeding. One controlled study showed that drinking modified shenghua tang (a tea made from bupleurum, angelica, ligusticum, peach kernel, baked ginger, and leonurus) greatly reduced the number of days that bleeding occurred following mifepristone therapy.[1]

MINERAL OIL

Common names: Agoral, Kondremul Plain, Liquid Parafin, Milkinol, Neo-Cultol, Petrogalar Plain

Mineral oil is a laxative used to soften stools in people with constipation. Mineral oil is also used as a vehicle to carry other ingredients in some topical skin products.

Summary of Interactions for Mineral Oil

In some cases, an herb or supplement may appear in more than one category, which may seem contradictory. For clarification, read the full article for details about the summarized interactions.

✓ May be Beneficial: Depletion or interference	Beta-carotene Calcium* Phosphorus* Potassium* Vitamin A* Vitamin D* Vitamin E* Vitamin K*
Side effect reduction/prevention	None known
Supportive interaction	None known
Reduced drug absorption/bioavailability	None known
Adverse interaction	None known

Interactions with Dietary Supplements
Vitamins and minerals
Mineral oil has interfered with the absorption of many nutrients, including beta-carotene, calcium, phosphorus,

potassium, and vitamins A, D, K, and E in some,[1] but not all,[2] research. Taking mineral oil on an empty stomach may reduce this interference. It makes sense to take a daily multivitamin-mineral supplement two hours before or after mineral oil. It is important to read labels, because many multivitamins do not contain vitamin K or contain inadequate (less than 100 mcg per day) amounts.

MINOCYCLINE

Common names: Aknemin, Alti-Minocycline, Apo-Minocycline, Blemix, Cyclomin, Gen-Minocycline, Minocin MR, Minocin, Novo-Minocycline

Minocycline is used to treat bacterial infections, and it is in a class of **antibiotics** (page 19) known as tetracyclines. Variations occur between drugs within a class, and therefore minocycline may or may not interact with the same nutrients and herbs as **tetracycline** (page 253).

Summary of Interactions for Minocycline

In some cases, an herb or supplement may appear in more than one category, which may seem contradictory. For clarification, read the full article for details about the summarized interactions.

✓ May be Beneficial: Depletion or interference	Calcium Iron Magnesium Vitamin K* Zinc
✓ May be Beneficial: Side effect reduction/prevention	Bifidobacterium longum* Lactobacillus acidophilus* Lactobacillus casei* Probiotics* Saccharomyces boulardii* Saccharomyces cerevisiae* Vitamin C Vitamin K*
✓ May be Beneficial: Supportive interaction	Nicotinamide* Saccharomyces boulardii*
⊘ Avoid: Reduced drug absorption/ bioavailability	Calcium Iron Magnesium Zinc
⊘ Avoid: Adverse interaction	Vitamin A*

Interactions with Dietary Supplements

Calcium, iron, magnesium, zinc

Taking calcium, iron, magnesium, or zinc at the same time as minocycline can decrease the absorption of both the drug[1, 2] and the mineral. Therefore, calcium, iron, magnesium, or zinc supplements, if used, should be taken an hour before or after the drug.

Vitamin C

Tooth discoloration is a side effect of minocycline observed primarily in young children, but it may occur in adults as well. Vitamin C supplementation may prevent staining in adults taking minocycline.[3]

Nicotinamide (Niacinamide)

Niacinamide taken in combination with minocycline has produced beneficial effects in an individual with cicatricial pemphigoid, an autoimmune blistering disease,[4] as well as in a 46-year-old woman with pemphigus vegetans, another blistering disease.[5] Several other studies have confirmed the efficacy of this combination for bullous (blistering) pemphigoid.[6, 7, 8, 9, 10]

Probiotics

A common side effect of antibiotics is diarrhea, which may be caused by the elimination of beneficial bacteria normally found in the colon. Controlled studies have shown that taking probiotic microorganisms—such as *Lactobacillus casei, Lactobacillus acidophilus, Bifidobacterium longum,* or *Saccharomyces boulardii*—helps prevent antibiotic-induced diarrhea.[11]

The diarrhea experienced by some people who take antibiotics also might be due to an overgrowth of the bacterium *Clostridium difficile*, which causes a disease known as pseudomembranous colitis. Controlled studies have shown that supplementation with harmless yeast—such as *Saccharomyces boulardii*[12] or *Saccharomyces cerevisiae* (baker's or brewer's yeast)[13]—helps prevent recurrence of this infection. In one study, taking 500 mg of *Saccharomyces boulardii* twice daily enhanced the effectiveness of the antibiotic vancomycin in preventing recurrent clostridium infection.[14] Therefore, people taking antibiotics who later develop diarrhea might benefit from supplementing with saccharomyces organisms.

Treatment with antibiotics also commonly leads to an overgrowth of yeast *(Candida albicans)* in the vagina (candida vaginitis) and the intestines (sometimes referred to as "dysbiosis"). Controlled studies have shown that *Lactobacillus acidophilus* might prevent candida vaginitis.[15]

Vitamin A

A 16-year-old girl developed headaches and double vision following treatment for acne with vitamin A and minocycline. These side effects disappeared once the compounds were discontinued.[16] More research is needed to determine whether the symptoms could have been caused by an interaction between vitamin A and the drug.

Vitamin K

Several cases of excessive bleeding have been reported in people who take antibiotics.[17, 18, 19, 20] This side effect may be the result of reduced vitamin K activity and/or reduced vitamin K production by bacteria in the colon. One study showed that people who had taken broad-spectrum antibiotics had lower liver concentrations of vitamin K_2 (menaquinone), though vitamin K_1 (phylloquinone) levels remained normal.[21] Several antibiotics appear to exert a strong effect on vitamin K activity, while others may not have any effect. Therefore, one should refer to a specific antibiotic for information on whether it interacts with vitamin K. Doctors of natural medicine sometimes recommend vitamin K supplementation to people taking antibiotics. Additional research is needed to determine whether the amount of vitamin K_1 found in some multivitamins is sufficient to prevent antibiotic-induced bleeding. Moreover, most multivitamins do not contain vitamin K.

Interactions with Foods and Other Compounds
Food

Food slightly reduces blood levels of minocycline, but the effect is not significant. Unlike other tetracyclines, minocycline may be taken with or without food and is only slightly affected by meals containing dairy.[22]

MIRTAZAPINE

Common names: Remeron, Zispin

Mirtazapine is used to treat people with mental depression, especially those who are also nervous and have trouble sleeping. It is in a class of drugs called tetracyclic antidepressants.

Summary of Interactions for Mirtazapine
In some cases, an herb or supplement may appear in more than one category, which may seem contradictory. For clarification, read the full article for details about the summarized interactions.

ⓘ Check: Other	Melatonin*
Depletion or interference	None known
Side effect reduction/prevention	None known
Supportive interaction	None known
Reduced drug absorption/bioavailability	None known
Adverse interaction	None known

Interactions with Dietary Supplements
Melatonin

Taking mirtazapine results in enhanced secretion of melatonin at night;[1] this may explain part of the mechanism of the effects of mirtazapine. Controlled research is needed to determine whether melatonin supplementation might enhance either the beneficial or the adverse effects of mirtazapine.

Interactions with Foods and Other Compounds
Alcohol

Drinking alcoholic beverages while taking mirtazapine may enhance the effects of the drug, including impairment of thinking, judgment, and performance of difficult tasks; therefore, it should be avoided.[2]

MISOPROSTOL

Common names: Cytotec

Combination drug: Arthrotec

Misoprostol is a type of drug called a prostaglandin E_1 analog that protects the mucosal lining of the stomach and intestines. It is either used alone or in combination with **nonsteroidal anti-inflammatory drugs** (page 193) (NSAIDs) to prevent injury to stomach and intestinal tissue caused by these agents.

Summary of Interactions for Misoprostol
In some cases, an herb or supplement may appear in more than one category, which may seem contradictory. For clarification, read the full article for details about the summarized interactions.

⊘ Avoid: Adverse interaction	Magnesium
Depletion or interference	None known
Side effect reduction/prevention	None known
Supportive interaction	None known
Reduced drug absorption/bioavailability	None known

Interactions with Dietary Supplements

Magnesium

A common side effect of misoprostol is diarrhea, which is aggravated by taking magnesium.[1] Consequently, individuals who experience diarrhea while taking misoprostol should avoid magnesium supplementation.

Interactions with Foods and Other Compounds

Food

Taking misoprostol with food may lower the maximum concentration of the drug in the blood and delay (though not decrease) absorption up to ten hours.[2, 3] However, since ingestion of food with misoprostol may reduce the incidence of diarrhea, it is usually recommended that the drug be taken with a meal.[4]

MIXED AMPHETAMINES

Common names: Adderall, Dexamphetamine, Dexedrine

This drug contains two central nervous system stimulants: amphetamine and dextroamphetamine. It is used to treat narcolepsy and attention deficit disorder (ADD) with hyperactivity.

Summary of Interactions for Mixed Amphetamines

In some cases, an herb or supplement may appear in more than one category, which may seem contradictory. For clarification, read the full article for details about the summarized interactions.

✓	May be Beneficial: Depletion or interference	Veratrum species
✓	May be Beneficial: Side effect reduction/prevention	L-tryptophan* Vitamin B₆
✓	May be Beneficial: Supportive interaction	Magnesium Tyrosine
⊘	Avoid: Reduced drug absorption/ bioavailability	**Lithium** (page 157) Vitamin C
⊘	Avoid: Adverse interaction	Alcohol Magnesium
ⓘ	Check: Other	Ephedra

Interactions with Dietary Supplements

Magnesium

Dextroamphetamine can increase blood levels of magnesium, which causes significant lowering of the calcium to magnesium ratio in the blood. The change in this ratio may in part explain the effectiveness of stimulants like dextroamphetamine in hyperactive boys.[1] Another magnesium-amphetamine interaction involves supplements of **magnesium hydroxide** (page 166), which are known to cause retention of amphetamines in the body.[2] This could theoretically result in increased blood levels of these drugs. Finally, animal studies have suggested that magnesium supplements can increase learning and enhance the behavioral response to stimulants.[3] For these reasons, the use of magnesium along with amphetamines may enhance the effectiveness of these drugs in the treatment of ADD, but controlled studies of this possibility are needed.

Vitamin C

Ingestion of some types of vitamin C results in acidification of the intestinal contents and thus a decreased absorption of amphetamines.[4] Supplements containing vitamin C should be taken an hour before or two hours after taking amphetamines.

Tyrosine

Tyrosine is an amino acid used by the body to produce brain chemicals stimulated by amphetamines. Reduced stimulant effects of amphetamines were observed in individuals who had been made tyrosine deficient.[5] It is possible that a dietary deficiency of tyrosine may reduce the effectiveness of amphetamines. Tyrosine deficiency is not common unless a protein deficiency exists. Adequate tyrosine intake from dietary protein or supplements is necessary in individuals taking amphetamines.

Lithium (page 157)

Lithium is a mineral that may be present in some supplements and is also used in large amounts to treat mood disorders such as bipolar disorder (manic depression). Taking lithium at the same time as amphetamines may inhibit the appetite suppressant and stimulatory effects of the amphetamines.[6] Therefore, people taking amphetamines should take lithium only under the supervision of a doctor.

Vitamin B₆

Occasionally, individuals taking amphetamines develop compulsive behavior and anxiety, even after the drug is discontinued. When this side effect occurred in an eight-year-old boy,[7] supplementation with 200 mg vitamin B₆ each day for one week followed by 100 mg daily, reduced the compulsive behavior and anxiety within three weeks. The symptoms were eliminated after a few months of treatment. Controlled research is needed to determine conclusively the usefulness of vitamin B_6 supplementation for preventing and treating this side effect.

L-tryptophan

In an uncontrolled study of schizophrenic patients, 200 mg per day of L-tryptophan reduced disturbances in thinking, as well as hallucinations caused by dextroamphetamine.[8] Symptoms of psychosis rarely occur in people who take amphetamines and are not schizophrenic. Controlled research is needed to establish the benefits of L-tryptophan and related supplements for people taking amphetamines.

Interactions with Herbs

Ephedra

Ephedra sinica contains a compound called ephedrine. A seven-year-old boy who had 12 mg of ephedrine twice daily added to his dextroamphetamine therapy experienced improvement in hyperactive behavior.[9] He also experienced relief from symptoms, such as headaches and spots before his eyes, that may have been caused by dextroamphetamine. However, concurrent use of amphetamines with other stimulants such as ephedrine or *Ephedra sinica* could cause excessive stimulation of the heart or nervous system. For this reason, such combinations should be used with great caution, and only under the supervision of a doctor.

Veratrum (Veratrum sp.)

Veratrum (Hellebore) is an herb used by doctors of natural medicine to treat high blood pressure;however, amphetamines can inhibit this effect.[10] Therefore, people taking veratrum to treat hypertension should avoid amphetamines.

Interactions with Foods and Other Compounds

Fruit juices

Fruit juices may acidify the intestinal contents, causing reduced absorption of amphetamines.[11] Therefore, juices should be consumed an hour before or two hours after administration of amphetamines.

Alcohol

The combination of alcohol and methamphetamine makes the heart work harder and consume more oxygen, which may produce unwanted effects.[12] Alcohol consumption may also suppress the breakdown of amphetamines, causing elevations in blood levels of the drug.[13] Individuals taking amphetamines should avoid alcoholic beverages, especially if they have known heart problems.

MODUCREN

Contains the following ingredients:
Amiloride (page 11)
Hydrochlorothiazide
Timolol (page 263)

MODURETIC

Contains the following ingredients:
Amiloride (page 11)
Hydrochlorothiazide

MOEXIPRIL

Common names: Perdix, Perdix, Univasc

Moexipril is used to treat high blood pressure, and is in a family of drugs known as **angiotensin-converting enzyme (ACE) inhibitors** (page 17).

Summary of Interactions for Moexipril

In some cases, an herb or supplement may appear in more than one category, which may seem contradictory. For clarification, read the full article for details about the summarized interactions.

✓ May be Beneficial: Depletion or interference	**Lithium** (page 157) (prescription) Potassium
✓ May be Beneficial: Side effect reduction/prevention	Iron
⊘ Avoid: Reduced drug absorption/ bioavailability	Food
⊘ Avoid: Adverse interaction	High-potassium foods* Lithium (supplements) Low-salt diet Potassium supplements* Salt substitutes*
Supportive interaction	None known

Interactions with Dietary Supplements

Potassium

An uncommon yet potentially serious side effect of taking ACE inhibitors is increased blood potassium levels.[1, 2, 3] This problem is more likely to occur in people with advanced kidney disease. Taking potassium supplements,[4] potassium-containing salt substitutes (No Salt, Morton Salt Substitute, and others),[5, 6, 7] or large amounts of high-potassium foods (such as bananas and other fruit) at the same time as taking ACE inhibitors could cause life-threatening problems.[8] Therefore, people should consult their healthcare practitioner before supplementing additional potassium and should have their blood levels of potassium checked periodically while taking ACE inhibitors.

Lithium (page 157)

Lithium is a mineral that may be present in some supplements and is also used in large amounts to treat mood disorders, such as bipolar disorder. Taking lithium at the same time as ACE inhibitors may increase blood levels of the mineral.[9] Controlled studies are needed to determine whether taking moexipril together with the tiny amounts of lithium present in some supplements might produce similar side effects. People taking moexipril should exercise caution when supplementing with lithium until more information is available.

Iron

In a double-blind study of patients who had developed a cough attributed to an ACE inhibitor, supplementation with iron (in the form of 256 mg of ferrous sulfate per day) for four weeks reduced the severity of the cough by a statistically significant 45%, compared with a nonsignificant 8% improvement in the placebo group.[10]

Interactions with Foods and Other Compounds

Food

Taking moexipril with food dramatically reduces the absorption of the drug, especially when taken with a high-fat meal.[11] Therefore, moexipril should be taken an hour before or two hours after a meal.

Low-salt diet

Taking moexipril while on a low-salt diet might cause excessively low blood pressure.[12] Therefore, people taking moexipril should notify their healthcare practitioner before starting a low-salt diet.

MONOZIDE

Contains the following ingredients:
Bisoprolol (page 41)
Hydrochlorothiazide

MONTELUKAST

Common names: Singular

Montelukast is a type of drug known as a leukotriene receptor antagonist (LTRA) used to prevent and treat asthma.

Summary of Interactions for Montelukast

In some cases, an herb or supplement may appear in more than one category, which may seem contradictory. For clarification, read the full article for details about the summarized interactions.

Depletion or interference	None known
Side effect reduction/prevention	None known
Supportive interaction	None known
Reduced drug absorption/bioavailability	None known
Adverse interaction	None known

MOORLAND

Contains the following ingredients:
Aluminium
Bismuth (page 40)
Calcium
Kaolin
Magnesium

MOXIFLOXACIN

Common names: Vigamox Ophthalmic Solution

Moxifloxacin is used to treat bacterial infections in the eye. It belongs to a class of antibiotic drugs called **quinolones** (page 228). There are currently no reported nutrient or herb interactions involving moxifloxacin ophthalmic solution.

Mucaine

MUCAINE

Contains the following ingredients:
Aluminum hydroxide (page 10)
Magnesium hydroxide (page 166)
Oxetacaine

MUPIROCIN

Common names: Bactroban, Bactroban Nasal

Mupirocin is an **antibiotic** (page 19) applied to the skin to treat bacterial skin infections. It is also used to prevent hospital outbreaks of dangerous antibiotic-resistant *Staph aureus* infections.

Summary of Interactions for Mupirocin

In some cases, an herb or supplement may appear in more than one category, which may seem contradictory. For clarification, read the full article for details about the summarized interactions.

Depletion or interference	None known
Side effect reduction/prevention	None known
Supportive interaction	None known
Reduced drug absorption/bioavailability	None known
Adverse interaction	None known

MYCOLOG II

Contains the following ingedients:
Nystatin (page 195)
Triamcinolone

MYLANTA

Contains the following ingredients:
Aluminum hydroxide (page 10)
Magnesium hydroxide (page 166)

NABUMETONE

Common names: Relafen, Relifex

Nabumetone is a member of the **nonsteroidal anti-inflammatory drug** (page 193) (NSAIDs) family.

NSAIDs reduce inflammation (swelling), pain, and temperature. Nabumetone is used to treat osteoarthritis and rheumatoid arthritis.

Summary of Interactions for Nabumetone

In some cases, an herb or supplement may appear in more than one category, which may seem contradictory. For clarification, read the full article for details about the summarized interactions.

✓ May be Beneficial: Depletion or interference	Iron
✓ May be Beneficial: Side effect reduction/prevention	Copper* Licorice
✓ May be Beneficial: Supportive interaction	Copper*
🚫 Avoid: Adverse interaction	**Lithium** (page 157)* Sodium* White willow*
ⓘ Check: Other	Potassium
Reduced drug absorption/bioavailability	None known

Interactions with Dietary Supplements

Copper

Supplementation may enhance the anti-inflammatory effects of NSAIDs while reducing their ulcerogenic effects. One study found that when various anti-inflammatory drugs were chelated with copper, the anti-inflammatory activity was increased.[1] Animal models of inflammation have found that the copper chelate of **aspirin** (page 26) was active at one-eighth the effective amount of aspirin. These copper complexes are less toxic than the parent compounds, as well.

Iron

NSAIDs cause gastrointestinal (GI) irritation, bleeding, and iron loss.[2] Iron supplements can cause GI irritation.[3] However, iron supplementation is sometimes needed in people taking NSAIDs if those drugs have caused enough blood loss to lead to iron deficiency. If both iron and nabumetone are prescribed, they should be taken with food to reduce GI irritation and bleeding risk.

Lithium (page 157)

Lithium is a mineral that may be present in some supplements and is also used in large amounts to treat mood disorders such as manic-depression (bipolar disorder). Most NSAIDs inhibit the excretion of lithium from the body, resulting in higher blood levels of the mineral, though **sulindac** (page 249) may have an opposite effect.[4] Since major changes in lithium blood levels can produce unwanted side effects or interfere with its efficacy, NSAIDs should be used with caution, and only under medical supervision, in people taking lithium supplements.

Potassium

NSAIDs have caused kidney dysfunction and increased blood potassium levels, especially in older people.[5] People taking NSAIDs, including nabumetone, should not supplement potassium without consulting with their doctor.

Sodium

Nabumetone may cause sodium and water retention.[6] It is healthful to reduce dietary salt intake by eliminating table salt and heavily salted foods.

Interactions with Herbs
Licorice (Glycyrrhiza glabra)

The flavonoids found in the extract of licorice known as DGL (deglycyrrhizinated licorice) are helpful for avoiding the irritating actions NSAIDs have on the stomach and intestines. One study found that 350 mg of chewable DGL taken together with each dose of **aspirin** (page 26) reduced gastrointestinal bleeding caused by the aspirin.[7] DGL has been shown in controlled human research to be as effective as drug therapy (**cimetidine** [page 61]) in healing stomach ulcers.[8]

White willow bark (Salix alba)

White willow bark contains salicin, which is related to **aspirin** (page 26). Both salicin and aspirin produce anti-inflammatory effects after they have been converted to salicylic acid in the body. The administration of salicylates like aspirin to individuals taking oral NSAIDs may result in reduced blood levels of NSAIDs.[9] Though no studies have investigated interactions between white willow bark and NSAIDs, people taking NSAIDs should avoid the herb until more information is available.

Interactions with Foods and Other Compounds
Food

Nabumetone should be taken with food to prevent gastrointestinal upset.[10]

Alcohol

Nabumetone may cause drowsiness, dizziness, or blurred vision.[11] Alcohol may intensify these effects and increase the risk of accidental injury. Use of alcohol during nabumetone therapy increases the risk of stom-

ach irritation and bleeding. People taking nabumetone should avoid alcohol.

NADOLOL

Common names: Alti-Nadolol, Apo-Nadol, Corgard, Novo-Nadolol

Combination drug: Corgaretic

Nadolol is used to treat both angina pectoris (chest pain) and high blood pressure, and it is in a class of drugs known as beta-adrenergic blockers. Since nadolol is related to **propranolol** (page 224), it may have similar interactions with dietary supplements and herbs.

Summary of Interactions for Nadolol

In some cases, an herb or supplement may appear in more than one category, which may seem contradictory. For clarification, read the full article for details about the summarized interactions.

✓ May be Beneficial: Depletion or interference	Pleurisy root*
⊘ Avoid: Reduced drug absorption/ bioavailability	Calcium* Willow*
⊘ Avoid: Adverse interaction	High-potassium foods* Potassium*
Side effect reduction/prevention	None known
Supportive interaction	None known

Interactions with Dietary Supplements
Calcium

Calcium supplements, if taken at the same time as some beta-blocker drugs, may reduce blood levels of the drug.[1] However, whether calcium affects nadolol in this manner is unknown. Until more information is available, people on nadolol should take calcium supplements an hour before or two hours after the drug.

Potassium

People taking nadolol may experience significant increases in blood levels of potassium,[2] though it is unknown whether supplementation with potassium might enhance this effect. People taking beta-blockers should therefore avoid taking potassium supplements, or eating large quantities of high-potassium foods, such as fruit (e.g., bananas), unless directed to do so by their doctor.

Interactions with Herbs

Pleurisy root

As pleurisy root and other plants in the *Aesclepius* genus contain cardiac glycosides, it is best to avoid use of pleurisy root with heart medications such as beta-blockers.[3]

White willow bark (Salix alba)

The active compound in white willow bark, salicin, is converted to salicylic acid in the body. Taking salicylates with other beta-adrenergic blocking drugs has resulted in decreased absorption of the drugs.[4] Therefore, until more is known about the interaction between willow and nadolol, they should not be taken at the same time.

Interactions with Foods and Other Compounds

Potassium

People taking nadolol may experience significant increases in blood levels of potassium,[5] though it is unknown whether supplementation with potassium might enhance this effect. People taking beta-blockers should therefore avoid taking potassium supplements, or eating large quantities of high-potassium foods, such as fruit (e.g., bananas), unless directed to do so by their doctor.

NAPROXEN/ NAPROXEN SODIUM

Common names: Aleve, Anaprox, Apo-Napro-Na, Apo-Naproxyn, Arthrosin, Arthroxen, Napralen, Napron X, Naprosyn, Naxen, Novo-Naprox Sodium, Novo-Naprox, Nu-Naprox, Nycopren, Rhodiaprox, Synflex, Timpron

Naproxen/naproxen sodium are members of the **non-steroidal anti-inflammatory drug** (page 193) (NSAIDs) family. NSAIDs reduce inflammation (swelling), pain, and temperature. Naproxen is used to treat mild to moderate pain, osteoarthritis, rheumatoid arthritis, ankylosing spondylitis, primary dysmenorrhea, tendinitis, bursitis, and other conditions. Naproxen and naproxen sodium are available in prescription strength; naproxen sodium is also available in nonprescription strength.

Summary of Interactions for Naproxen

In some cases, an herb or supplement may appear in more than one category, which may seem contradictory. For clarification, read the full article for details about the summarized interactions.

✓	May be Beneficial: Depletion or interference	Iron
✓	May be Beneficial: Side effect reduction/prevention	Copper* Licorice
✓	May be Beneficial: Supportive interaction	Copper*
🚫	Avoid: Adverse interaction	**Lithium** (page 157)* Sodium* White willow*
ⓘ	Check: Other	Potassium
Reduced drug absorption/bioavailability		None known

Interactions with Dietary Supplements

Copper

Supplementation with copper may enhance the anti-inflammatory effects of NSAIDs while reducing their ulcerogenic effects. One study found that when various anti-inflammatory drugs were chelated with copper, the anti-inflammatory activity was increased.[1] Animal models of inflammation have found that the copper chelate of **aspirin** (page 26) was active at one-eighth the effective dose of aspirin. These copper complexes are less toxic than the parent compounds, as well.

Lithium (page 157)

Lithium is a mineral that may be present in some supplements and is also used in large amounts to treat mood disorders such as manic-depression (bipolar disorder). Most NSAIDs inhibit the excretion of lithium from the body, resulting in higher blood levels of the mineral, though **sulindac** (page 249) may have an opposite effect.[2] Since major changes in lithium blood levels can produce unwanted side effects or interfere with its efficacy, NSAIDs should be used with caution, and only under medical supervision, in people taking lithium supplements.

Iron

NSAIDs cause gastrointestinal (GI) irritation, bleeding, and iron loss.[3] Iron supplements can cause GI irritation.[4] However, iron supplementation is sometimes needed in people taking NSAIDs if those drugs have caused enough blood loss to lead to iron deficiency. If both iron and naproxen are prescribed, they should be taken with food to reduce GI irritation and bleeding risk.

Potassium

Naproxen has caused kidney problems and increased blood potassium levels, especially in older people.[5, 6]

People taking naproxen should not supplement potassium without consulting with their doctor.

Sodium

Naproxen may cause sodium and water retention.[7] It is healthful to reduce dietary salt intake by decreasing the use of table salt and avoiding heavily salted foods.

Interactions with Herbs

Licorice (Glycyrrhiza glabra)

The flavonoids found in the extract of licorice known as DGL (deglycyrrhizinated licorice) are helpful for avoiding the irritating actions NSAIDs have on the stomach and intestines. One study found that 350 mg of chewable DGL taken together with each dose of **aspirin** (page 26) reduced gastrointestinal bleeding caused by the aspirin.[8] DGL has been shown in controlled human research to be as effective as drug therapy (**cimetidine** [page 61]) in healing stomach ulcers.[9]

White willow bark (Salix alba)

White willow bark contains salicin, which is related to **aspirin** (page 26). Both salicin and aspirin produce anti-inflammatory effects after they have been converted to salicylic acid in the body. The administration of salicylates like aspirin to individuals taking oral NSAIDs may result in reduced blood levels of NSAIDs.[10] Though no studies have investigated interactions between white willow bark and NSAIDs, people taking NSAIDs should avoid the herb until more information is available.

Interactions with Foods and Other Compounds

Food

Naproxen should be taken with food to prevent gastrointestinal upset.[11]

Alcohol

Naproxen may cause drowsiness, dizziness, or blurred vision.[12] Alcohol may intensify these effects and increase the risk of accidental injury. Use of alcohol during naproxen therapy increases the risk of stomach irritation and bleeding. People taking naproxen should avoid alcohol.

NEFAZODONE

Common names: Dutonin, Serzone

Nefazodone is a drug used to treat people with depression.

Summary of Interactions for Nefazodone

In some cases, an herb or supplement may appear in more than one category, which may seem contradictory. For clarification, read the full article for details about the summarized interactions.

🚫 Avoid: Adverse interaction	St. John's wort*
ⓘ Check: Other	Digitalis
Depletion or interference	None known
Side effect reduction/prevention	None known
Supportive interaction	None known
Reduced drug absorption/bioavailability	None known

Interactions with Herbs

Digitalis (Digitalis lanata, Digitalis purpurea)

Digitalis refers to a family of plants commonly called foxglove that contain digitalis glycosides, chemicals with actions and toxicities similar to the prescription drug **digoxin** (page 90).

Nefazodone increased serum digoxin levels in a three-way crossover study of 18 healthy men.[1] No interactions between nefazodone and digitalis have been reported. Until more is known, nefazodone and digitalis-containing products should be used only under the direct supervision of a doctor trained in their use.

St. John's wort (Hypericum perforatum)

Although there have been no interactions reported in the medical literature, it is best to avoid using nefazodone with St. John's wort unless you are under the supervision of a qualified healthcare professional.

Interactions with Foods and Other Compounds

Food

Nefazodone may be taken with or without food.[2]

Alcohol

People taking nefazodone are advised to avoid alcohol.[3]

NEOMYCIN

Common names: Mycifradin, Myciguent, NeoTab, Nivemycin

Combination drugs: Adcortyl with Graneodin, Betnovate-N, Dermovate-NN, Gregoderm, Synalar N, Tri-Adcortyl, Trimovate

Neomycin is an **antibacterial** (page 19) drug that is poorly absorbed when taken by mouth. It is combined with enteric coated **erythromycin** (page 106) to suppress gastrointestinal (GI) bacteria before surgery to avoid infection. Neomycin is used to treat hepatic coma in cases of liver failure and is included in some antibiotic products used to treat infections of the eyes, ears, or skin.

Summary of Interactions for Neomycin

In some cases, an herb or supplement may appear in more than one category, which may seem contradictory. For clarification, read the full article for details about the summarized interactions.

✓ May be Beneficial: Depletion or interference	Beta-carotene Calcium Carbohydrates Fats Folic acid Iron Magnesium Potassium Sodium Vitamin A Vitamin B$_{12}$ Vitamin B$_6$ Vitamin D Vitamin K Vitamin K*
✓ May be Beneficial: Side effect reduction/prevention	*Bifidobacterium longum* *Lactobacillus acidophilus* *Lactobacillus casei* *Saccharomyces boulardii* *Saccharomyces cerevisiae* Vitamin K*
✓ May be Beneficial: Supportive interaction	*Saccharomyces boulardii**
Reduced drug absorption/bioavailability	None known
Adverse interaction	None known

Interactions with Dietary Supplements
Probiotics

A common side effect of antibiotics is diarrhea, which may be caused by the elimination of beneficial bacteria normally found in the colon. Controlled studies have shown that taking probiotic microorganisms—such as *Lactobacillus casei, Lactobacillus acidophilus, Bifidobacterium longum,* or *Saccharomyces boulardii*—helps prevent antibiotic-induced diarrhea.[1]

The diarrhea experienced by some people who take antibiotics also might be due to an overgrowth of the bacterium *Clostridium difficile,* which causes a disease known as pseudomembranous colitis. Controlled studies have shown that supplementation with harmless yeast—such as *Saccharomyces boulardii*[2] or *Saccharomyces cerevisiae* (baker's or brewer's yeast)[3]—helps prevent recurrence of this infection. In one study, taking 500 mg of *Saccharomyces boulardii* twice daily enhanced the effectiveness of the antibiotic vancomycin in preventing recurrent clostridium infection.[4] Therefore, people taking antibiotics who later develop diarrhea might benefit from supplementing with saccharomyces organisms.

Treatment with antibiotics also commonly leads to an overgrowth of yeast *(Candida albicans)* in the vagina (candida vaginitis) and the intestines (sometimes referred to as "dysbiosis"). Controlled studies have shown that *Lactobacillus acidophilus* might prevent candida vaginitis.[5]

Vitamins and minerals

Neomycin can decrease absorption or increase elimination of many nutrients, including calcium, carbohydrates, beta-carotene, fats, folic acid, iron, magnesium, potassium, sodium, and vitamin A, vitamin B$_{12}$, vitamin D, and vitamin K.[6, 7] Surgery preparation with oral neomycin is unlikely to lead to deficiencies. It makes sense for people taking neomycin for more than a few days to also take a multivitamin-mineral supplement.

Vitamin B$_6$

Neomycin may inactivate vitamin B$_6$.[8] Surgery preparation with oral neomycin is unlikely to lead to vitamin B$_6$ deficiency. People taking oral neomycin for more than a few days should ask their doctor about vitamin B$_6$ supplementation to prevent deficiency.

Vitamin K

Several cases of excessive bleeding have been reported in people who take antibiotics.[9, 10, 11, 12] This side effect may be the result of reduced vitamin K activity and/or reduced vitamin K production by bacteria in the colon. One study showed that people who had taken broad-spectrum antibiotics had lower liver concentrations of vitamin K$_2$ (menaquinone), though vitamin K$_1$ (phylloquinone) levels remained normal.[13] Several antibiotics appear to exert a strong effect on vitamin K activity, while others may not have any effect. Therefore, one should refer to a specific antibiotic for information on whether it interacts with vitamin K. Doctors of natural medicine sometimes recommend vitamin K supplementation to people taking antibiotics. Additional research is needed to determine whether the amount of vitamin K_1 found in some multivitamins is sufficient to prevent antibiotic-induced bleeding. Moreover, most multivitamins do not contain vitamin K.

NICOTINE ALTERNATIVES

Common names: Habitrol, Nicoderm, Nicorette Microtab Tablets, Nicorette, Nicorette Gum, Nicorette Patches, Nicorette Spray, Nicotinell TTS Patches, Nicotinell, Nicotinell Gum, Nicotinell Lozenges, Nicotrol, Nicotrol Inhaler, Nicotrol NS, NiQuitin CQ Patches, Prostep

Nicotine is available in various forms as an aid to quitting smoking. Nicotine skin patches are available in nonprescription and prescription strengths. Nicotine gum is available without prescription. Nicotine nasal spray and oral inhaler are available by prescription.

Summary of Interactions for Nicotine Alternatives

In some cases, an herb or supplement may appear in more than one category, which may seem contradictory. For clarification, read the full article for details about the summarized interactions.

⊘ Avoid: Reduced drug absorption/ bioavailability	Acidic foods and beverages
ⓘ Check: Other	Lobelia
Depletion or interference	None known
Side effect reduction/prevention	None known
Supportive interaction	None known
Adverse interaction	None known

Interactions with Herbs
Lobelia (Lobelia inflata)
Lobelia is the plant from which the drug lobeline was isolated. Lobeline produces effects similar to nicotine.[1] Combined use of nicotine and lobeline may increase the risk of nicotine side effects. No interactions have been reported with nicotine and lobelia, and in fact research has suggested lobeline may be useful as an aid to stopping smoking.[2]

Interactions with Foods and Other Compounds
Food
Absorption of nicotine from nicotine gum requires mildly alkaline saliva.[3] Acidic foods and beverages (cof-fee, colas, fruit, fruit juices, and others) may reduce nicotine absorption. This potential interaction may be avoided by chewing nicotine gum one hour before or after consuming acidic food and beverages.

NIFEDIPINE

Common names: Adalat LA, Adalat Retard, Adalat, Adipine MR, Angiopine LA, Angiopine MR, Angiopine, Apo-Nifed, Calanif, Cardilate MR, Coracten SR, Coracten XL, Coracten, Coroday MR, Fortipine LA 40, Gen-Nifedipine, Hypolar Retard 20, Nifedipress MR, Nifedotard 20 MR, Nifelease, Nifopress Retard, Nimodrel MR, Nivaten Retard, Novo-Nifedin, Nu-Nifedipine-PA, Nu-Nifed, PMS-Nifedipine, Procardia, Slofedipine XL, Tensipine MR, Unipine XL

Combination drugs: Beta-Adalat, Tenif

Nifedipine is a calcium-channel blocker used to treat angina pectoris and high blood pressure.

Summary of Interactions for Nifedipine

In some cases, an herb or supplement may appear in more than one category, which may seem contradictory. For clarification, read the full article for details about the summarized interactions.

⊘ Avoid: Adverse interaction	Pleurisy root* Tobacco*
ⓘ Check: Other	Grapefruit juice
Depletion or interference	None known
Side effect reduction/prevention	None known
Supportive interaction	None known
Reduced drug absorption/bioavailability	None known

Interactions with Herbs
Pleurisy root
As pleurisy root and other plants in the *Aesclepius* genus contain cardiac glycosides, it is best to avoid use of pleurisy root with heart medications such as calcium-channel blockers.[1]

Interactions with Foods and Other Compounds
Grapefruit juice
Ingestion of grapefruit juice has been shown to increase the absorption of **felodipine** (page 113) (a drug similar in structure and action to that of nifedipine) and to increase the adverse effects of the medication in patients with hypertension. People taking nifedipine

Nifedipine

or similar drugs should not consume grapefruit juice or grapefruit, unless they have discussed it with their physician.[2]

Food

Nifedipine may be taken with or without food.[3] Nifedipine products should be swallowed whole, without crushing or chewing.[4]

Tobacco

In a double-blind study of ten cigarette smokers with angina treated with nifedipine for one week, angina episodes were significantly reduced during the non-smoking phase compared to the smoking phase.[5] People with angina taking nifedipine should not smoke tobacco.

NITROFURANTOIN

Common names: Apo-Nitrofurantoin, Furadantin, Macrobid, Macrodantin, Novo-Furantoin

Nitrofurantoin is an **antibiotic** (page 19) used to treat urinary tract bacterial infections.

Summary of Interactions for Nitrofurantoin

In some cases, an herb or supplement may appear in more than one category, which may seem contradictory. For clarification, read the full article for details about the summarized interactions.

✓ May be Beneficial: Depletion or interference	Vitamin K*
✓ May be Beneficial: Side effect reduction/prevention	Bifidobacterium longum* Lactobacillus acidophilus* Lactobacillus casei* Saccharomyces boulardii* Saccharomyces cerevisiae* Vitamin K*
✓ May be Beneficial: Supportive interaction	Saccharomyces boulardii*
⊘ Avoid: Reduced drug absorption/ bioavailability	Magnesium*
Adverse interaction	None known

Interactions with Dietary Supplements

Magnesium

In six healthy men, nitrofurantoin absorption was reduced by also taking magnesium trisilicate.[1] Another magnesium compound, magnesium oxide (commonly found in supplements) was shown to bind with nitrofurantoin in a test tube.[2]

In a study of 11 people, the rate of nitrofurantoin absorption was delayed despite the fact that the amount of nitrofurantoin ultimately absorbed remained the same when the drug was administered in a colloidal magnesium aluminum silicate suspension.[3] It remains unclear whether this interaction is clinically important or if typical magnesium supplements would have the same effect.

Probiotics

A common side effect of antibiotics is diarrhea, which may be caused by the elimination of beneficial bacteria normally found in the colon. Controlled studies have shown that taking probiotic microorganisms—such as *Lactobacillus casei*, *Lactobacillus acidophilus*, *Bifidobacterium longum*, or *Saccharomyces boulardii*—helps prevent antibiotic-induced diarrhea.[4]

The diarrhea experienced by some people who take antibiotics also might be due to an overgrowth of the bacterium *Clostridium difficile*, which causes a disease known as pseudomembranous colitis. Controlled studies have shown that supplementation with harmless yeast—such as *Saccharomyces boulardii*[5] or *Saccharomyces cerevisiae* (baker's or brewer's yeast)[6]—helps prevent recurrence of this infection. In one study, taking 500 mg of *Saccharomyces boulardii* twice daily enhanced the effectiveness of the antibiotic vancomycin in preventing recurrent clostridium infection.[7] Therefore, people taking antibiotics who later develop diarrhea might benefit from supplementing with saccharomyces organisms.

Treatment with antibiotics also commonly leads to an overgrowth of yeast (*Candida albicans*) in the vagina (candida vaginitis) and the intestines (sometimes referred to as "dysbiosis"). Controlled studies have shown that *Lactobacillus acidophilus* might prevent candida vaginitis.[8]

Vitamin K

Several cases of excessive bleeding have been reported in people who take antibiotics.[9, 10, 11, 12] This side effect may be the result of reduced vitamin K activity and/or reduced vitamin K production by bacteria in the colon. One study showed that people who had taken broad-spectrum antibiotics had lower liver concentrations of vitamin K_2 (menaquinone), though vitamin K_1 (phylloquinone) levels remained normal.[13] Several antibiotics appear to exert a strong effect on vitamin K activity, while others may not have any effect. Therefore, one should refer to a specific antibiotic for information on whether it interacts with vitamin K. Doctors of natural medicine sometimes recommend vitamin K supplementation to people taking antibiotics. Additional research is needed to determine whether the amount of vitamin K_1 found in some multivitamins is sufficient to prevent antibiotic-induced bleeding. Moreover, most multivitamins do not contain vitamin K.

Interactions with Foods and Other Compounds
Food
Taking nitrofurantoin with food improves absorption[14] and reduces gastrointestinal (GI) upset.[15]

NITROGLYCERIN

Common names: Coro-Nitro Pump Spray, Deponit, Glyceryl Trinitrate, Glytrin Spray, GTN 300 mcg, Minitran, Nitrek, Nitro-Bid, Nitro-Dur, Nitro-Time, Nitrodisc, Nitrogard, Nitroglyn, Nitrolingual Pumpspray, Nitrolingual, Nitrol, Nitromin, Nitrong SR, Nitrostat, Percutol, Suscard, Sustac, Transderm-Nitro, Transiderm-Nitro, Tridil, Trini-patch

Nitroglycerin dilates blood vessels by relaxing the smooth muscles surrounding them, increasing blood flow. Nitroglycerin is used to treat or prevent chest pain in people with angina pectoris and to treat instances of congestive heart failure.

Summary of Interactions for Nitroglycerin
In some cases, an herb or supplement may appear in more than one category, which may seem contradictory. For clarification, read the full article for details about the summarized interactions.

✓ May be Beneficial: Supportive interaction	N-acetyl cysteine* Vitamin C
⃠ Avoid: Adverse interaction	N-acetyl cysteine*
Depletion or interference	None known
Side effect reduction/prevention	None known
Reduced drug absorption/bioavailability	None known

Interactions with Dietary Supplements
N-acetyl cysteine (NAC)
Continuous nitroglycerin use leads to development of nitroglycerin tolerance and loss of effectiveness. Intravenous (iv) N-acetyl cysteine (NAC), during short-term studies of people receiving continuous nitroglycerin, was reported to reverse nitroglycerin tolerance.[1, 2] In a double-blind study of patients with unstable angina, transdermal nitroglycerin plus oral NAC (600 mg three times per day) was associated with fewer failures of medical treatment than placebo, NAC, or nitroglycerin alone. However, when combined with nitroglycerin use, NAC has led to intolerable headaches.[3, 4] In two double-blind, randomized trials of angina patients treated with transdermal nitroglycerin, oral NAC 200 mg or 400 mg three times per day failed to prevent nitroglycerin tolerance.[5, 6]

Vitamin C
Vitamin C may help maintain the blood vessel dilation response to nitroglycerin. A double-blind study found that individuals taking 2 grams of vitamin C three times per day did not tend to develop nitroglycerin tolerance over time compared to those taking placebo.[7] In another controlled clinical trial, similar protection was achieved with 500 mg three times daily.[8]

People using long-acting nitroglycerin can avoid tolerance with a ten- to twelve-hour nitroglycerin-free period every day. People taking long-acting nitroglycerin should ask their prescribing doctor or pharmacist about preventing nitroglycerin tolerance.

Interactions with Foods and Other Compounds
Alcohol
Alcohol, when consumed during nitroglycerin therapy, may cause low blood pressure and circulatory collapse in extreme cases.[9] People using nitroglycerin should avoid alcohol.

NITROUS OXIDE

Nitrous oxide is an anesthetic gas. It is used during dental work and with patients who are not candidates for more commonly used **anesthetics** (page 129) during surgery.

Summary of Interactions for Nitrous Oxide
In some cases, an herb or supplement may appear in more than one category, which may seem contradictory.

For clarification, read the full article for details about the summarized interactions.

✓ May be Beneficial: Depletion or interference	Folic acid Vitamin B$_{12}$
✓ May be Beneficial: Side effect reduction/prevention	Catechin* Ginger* Milk thistle*
Supportive interaction	None known
Reduced drug absorption/bioavailability	None known
Adverse interaction	None known

Interactions with Dietary Supplements

Folic acid and vitamin B$_{12}$

Nitrous oxide interferes with activity of vitamin B$_{12}$, which further interferes with the activity of folic acid, causing adverse actions.[1, 2] Administration of folic acid or folinic acid (activated folic acid) has reversed nitrous oxide-induced bone marrow changes.[3, 4] People with vitamin B$_{12}$ deficiency may be especially susceptible.[5] People who will undergo nitrous oxide anesthesia for several hours may benefit from vitamin B$_{12}$ and folic acid supplementation.[6] Some doctors recommend 100 mcg of vitamin B$_{12}$ and 1,000 mcg folic acid, starting one week before through one week after prolonged exposure to nitrous oxide. People with normal vitamin B$_{12}$ levels who undergo short-duration nitrous oxide anesthesia (less than two hours) do not require supplementation.

Catechin

Some general anesthetic drugs have infrequently caused liver damage. One animal study showed that taking catechin (a bioflavonoid) prior to halothane exposure reduced the amount of liver damage caused by the drug.[7] Additional research is needed to determine whether this protective effect occurs in humans and with other general anesthetics.

Interactions with Herbs

Ginger (Zingiber officinale)

General anesthetics commonly cause nausea upon waking. In a double-blind study, taking 1 gram of ginger one hour before surgery was as effective at reducing nausea and vomiting as the anti-nausea drug **metoclopramide** (page 175).[8] Individuals taking ginger in order to avoid side effects should disclose this to their doctor prior to surgery, since the herb might affect blood clotting.

Milk thistle (Silybum marianum)

Some general anesthetic drugs have infrequently caused liver damage. One animal study showed that taking silybine, an active compound found in milk thistle, prior to halothane exposure reduced the amount of liver damage caused by the drug.[9] Though controlled research in humans is necessary, some doctors of natural medicine currently suggest taking milk thistle standardized to contain 140 mg of silymarin three times a day, beginning a week before surgery and continuing for at least one week after surgery.

NIZATIDINE

Common names: Apo-Nizatidine, Axid, Axid AR, Zinga

Nizatidine is a member of the H-2 blocker (histamine blocker) family of drugs that prevents the release of acid into the stomach. Nizatidine is used to treat stomach and duodenal ulcers and reflux of stomach acid into the esophagus. Nizatidine is available as the prescription drug and as a nonprescription product for relief of heartburn, acid indigestion, and sour stomach.

Summary of Interactions for Nizatidine

In some cases, an herb or supplement may appear in more than one category, which may seem contradictory. For clarification, read the full article for details about the summarized interactions.

✓ May be Beneficial: Depletion or interference	Folic acid Iron* Vitamin B$_{12}$
⊘ Avoid: Adverse interaction	Tobacco
ⓘ Check: Other	Copper Folic acid Magnesium
Side effect reduction/prevention	None known
Supportive interaction	None known
Reduced drug absorption/bioavailability	None known

Interactions with Dietary Supplements

Folic acid

Folic acid is needed by the body to utilize vitamin B$_{12}$. Antacids, including nizatidine, inhibit folic acid absorption.[1] People taking antacids are advised to supplement with folic acid.

Iron

Stomach acid may increase absorption of iron from food. H-2 blocker drugs reduce stomach acid and are associated with decreased dietary iron absorption.[2] The iron found in supplements is available to the body without the need for stomach acid. People with ulcers may be iron deficient due to blood loss. If iron deficiency is present, iron supplementation may be beneficial. Iron levels in the blood can be checked with lab tests.

Magnesium-containing antacids

In healthy people, a **magnesium hydroxide** (page 166)/**aluminum hydroxide** (page 10) antacid, taken with nizatidine, decreased nizatidine absorption by 12%.[3] People can avoid this interaction by taking nizatidine two hours before or after any aluminum/magnesium-containing antacids. Some magnesium supplements such as magnesium hydroxide are also antacids.

Vitamin B$_{12}$

Stomach acid is needed for vitamin B$_{12}$ in food to be absorbed by the body. H-2 blocker drugs reduce stomach acid and may therefore inhibit absorption of the vitamin B$_{12}$ naturally present in food. However, the vitamin B$_{12}$ found in supplements does not depend on stomach acid for absorption.[4] Lab tests can determine vitamin B$_{12}$ levels in people.

Other vitamins and minerals

There is some evidence that other vitamins and minerals, such as folic acid[5] and copper,[6] require the presence of stomach acid for optimal absorption. Long-term use of H-2 blockers may therefore promote a deficiency of these nutrients. Individuals requiring long-term use of H-2 blockers may therefore benefit from a multiple vitamin/mineral supplement.

Interactions with Foods and Other Compounds

Food

To prevent heartburn after meals, nizatidine is best taken 30 minutes before meals.[7] For other conditions, nizatidine works best taken with an early evening meal.[8]

Tobacco

In a randomized, double-blind, one-year study of 513 patients with recently healed duodenal ulcers, smokers were found to have a significantly higher recurrence rate than nonsmokers during maintenance therapy with nizatidine.[9]

NONSTEROIDAL ANTI-INFLAMMATORY DRUGS

Common names: Dalfon, Diflunisal, Dolobid, Fenoprofen, Meclofenamate, Meclomen, Mefenamic Acid, Meloxicam, Mobic, Nonsteroidal Anti-Inflammatory Analgesics, NSAIDs, Ponstel, Tolectin, Tolmetin

Nonsteroidal anti-inflammatory drugs (NSAIDs) are a family of medications used to treat rheumatoid arthritis, osteoarthritis, mild-to-moderate pain, menstrual cramps, bursitis, gout, and migraine headaches, as well as other conditions. Ophthalmic formulations of certain NSAIDs are used during or after eye surgery. NSAIDs are divided into two categories, based on their action within the body: COX-1 and COX-2 inhibitors.

Interactions involving oral NSAIDs in general are described on this page. For interactions involving specific NSAIDs, refer to the highlighted drugs listed below.

COX-1 Inhibitors

- **Diclofenac** (page 87) (Voltaren, Cataflam)
- Diclofenac and **misoprostol** (page 180) (Arthrotec)
- Diflunisal (Dolobid)
- **Etodolac** (page 111) (Lodine)
- Fenoprofen (Dalfon)
- **Flurbiprofen** (page 121) (Ansaid)
- **Ibuprofen** (page 139) (Motrin and others)
- **Indomethacin** (page 141) (Indocin)
- **Ketoprofen** (page 150) (Orudis, Oruvail)
- **Ketorolac** (page 150) (Toradol)
- Meclofenamate (Meclomen)
- Mefenamic acid (Ponstel)
- Meloxicam (Mobic)
- **Nabumetone** (page 184) (Relafen)
- **Naproxen** (page 186) (Anaprox, Naprosyn)
- **Oxaprozin** (page 203) (Daypro)
- **Piroxicam** (page 219) (Feldene)
- **Salsalate** (page 235) (Disalcid, Salflex)
- **Sulindac** (page 249) (Clinoril)
- Tolmetin (Tolectin)

COX-2 Inhibitors

- **Celecoxib** (page 51) (Celebrex)
- Valdecoxib (Bextra)

Nonsteroidal Anti-Inflammatory Drugs

Summary of Interactions for NSAIDs

In some cases, an herb or supplement may appear in more than one category, which may seem contradictory. For clarification, read the full article for details about the summarized interactions.

⊘ Avoid: Adverse interaction	**Lithium** (page 157) White willow
Depletion or interference	None known
Side effect reduction/prevention	None known
Supportive interaction	None known
Reduced drug absorption/bioavailability	None known

Interactions common to many, if not all, NSAIDs are described in this article. Interactions reported for only one or several drugs in this class may not be listed in this article. Some drugs listed in this article are linked to articles specific to that respective drug; please refer to those individual drug articles. The information in this article may not necessarily apply to drugs in this class for which no separate article exists. If you are taking an NSAID for which no separate article exists, talk with your doctor or pharmacist.

Interactions with Dietary Supplements

Lithium *(page 157)*

Lithium is a mineral that may be present in some supplements and is also used in large amounts to treat mood disorders such as manic-depression (bipolar disorder). Most NSAIDs inhibit the excretion of lithium from the body, resulting in higher blood levels of the mineral, though **sulindac** (page 249) may have an opposite effect.[1] Since major changes in lithium blood levels can produce unwanted side effects or interfere with its efficacy, NSAIDs should be used with caution, and only under medical supervision, in people taking lithium supplements.

Interactions with Herbs

White willow bark (Salix alba)

White willow bark contains salicin, which is related to **aspirin** (page 26). Both salicin and aspirin produce anti-inflammatory effects after they have been converted to salicylic acid in the body. The administration of salicylates like aspirin to individuals taking oral NSAIDs may result in reduced blood levels of NSAIDs.[2] Though no studies have investigated interactions between white willow bark and NSAIDs, people taking NSAIDs should avoid the herb until more information is available.

NULACIN

Contains the following ingredients:
Calcium
Magnesium
Peppermint oil

NUVELLE

Contains the following ingredients:
Estradiol (page 108)
Levonorgestrel

NUVELLE TS

Contains the following ingredients:
Estradiol (page 108)
Levonorgestrel

NYQUIL

Contains the following ingredients:
Acetaminophen (page 3)
Alcohol
Dextromethorphan (page 87)
Doxylamine (page 102)
Pseudoephedrine

NYQUIL HOT THERAPY POWDER

Contains the following ingredients:
Acetaminophen (page 3)
Dextromethorphan (page 87)
Doxylamine (page 102)
Pseudoephedrine

NYSTAFORM-HC

Contains the following ingredients:
Chlorhexidine (page 58)
Hydrocortisone
Nystatin (page 195)

NYSTATIN ORAL

Common names: Mycostatin (oral), Nilstat (oral), Nystamont, Nystex, Nystop

Oral nystatin is an antifungal drug used to treat yeast infections of the mouth (thrush), primarily in people with weakened immune systems. Doctors of natural medicine occasionally prescribe nystatin to treat yeast overgrowth in the intestines.

Summary of Interactions for Nystatin Oral

In some cases, an herb or supplement may appear in more than one category, which may seem contradictory. For clarification, read the full article for details about the summarized interactions.

Depletion or interference	None known
Side effect reduction/prevention	None known
Supportive interaction	None known
Reduced drug absorption/bioavailability	None known
Adverse interaction	None known

NYSTATIN TOPICAL

Common names: Mycostatin (topical), Nilstat (topical), Nystex Ointment, Pedi Dri Topical Powder

Combination drugs: Dermovate-NN, Gregoderm, Mycolog II, Nystaform-HC, Terra-Cortril Nystatin, Timodine, Tri-Adcortyl, Trimovate

Nystatin is used topically, either alone or in combination with triamcinolone (Mycolog II), to treat yeast infections of the skin. It is classified as an antifungal drug.

Summary of Interactions for Nystatin Topical

In some cases, an herb or supplement may appear in more than one category, which may seem contradictory. For clarification, read the full article for details about the summarized interactions.

Depletion or interference	None known
Side effect reduction/prevention	None known
Supportive interaction	None known
Reduced drug absorption/bioavailability	None known
Adverse interaction	None known

OFLOXACIN

Common names: Apo-Oflox, Exocin, Floxin, Ocuflox, Tarivid

Ofloxacin is a "fluoroquinolone" **antibiotic** (page 19) used to treat bacterial infections. Ofloxacin is available in special preparations to treat eye infections and ear infections.

Summary of Interactions for Ofloxacin

In some cases, an herb or supplement may appear in more than one category, which may seem contradictory. For clarification, read the full article for details about the summarized interactions.

✓ May be Beneficial: Side effect reduction/prevention	Bifidobacterium longum* Lactobacillus acidophilus* Lactobacillus casei* Saccharomyces boulardii* Saccharomyces cerevisiae*
✓ May be Beneficial: Supportive interaction	Saccharomyces boulardii*
⃠ Avoid: Reduced drug absorption/bioavailability	Calcium Iron Magnesium Zinc
ⓘ Check: Other	Vitamin K
Depletion or interference	None known
Adverse interaction	None known

Interactions with Dietary Supplements
Minerals
Minerals including calcium, iron, magnesium, and zinc can bind to fluoroquinolones, including ofloxacin, greatly reducing drug absorption.[1] Ofloxacin should be taken four hours before or two hours after consuming **antacids** (page 18) (Maalox, Mylanta, Tumms, Rolaids and others) that may contain these minerals and mineral-containing supplements.[2]

Probiotics
A common side effect of antibiotics is diarrhea, which may be caused by the elimination of beneficial bacteria normally found in the colon. Controlled studies have shown that taking probiotic microorganisms—such as

Lactobacillus casei, Lactobacillus acidophilus, Bifidobacterium longum, or *Saccharomyces boulardii*—helps prevent antibiotic-induced diarrhea.[3]

The diarrhea experienced by some people who take antibiotics also might be due to an overgrowth of the bacterium *Clostridium difficile,* which causes a disease known as pseudomembranous colitis. Controlled studies have shown that supplementation with harmless yeast—such as *Saccharomyces boulardii*[4] or *Saccharomyces cerevisiae* (baker's or brewer's yeast)[5]—helps prevent recurrence of this infection. In one study, taking 500 mg of *Saccharomyces boulardii* twice daily enhanced the effectiveness of the antibiotic vancomycin in preventing recurrent clostridium infection.[6] Therefore, people taking antibiotics who later develop diarrhea might benefit from supplementing with saccharomyces organisms.

Treatment with antibiotics also commonly leads to an overgrowth of yeast *(Candida albicans)* in the vagina (candida vaginitis) and the intestines (sometimes referred to as "dysbiosis"). Controlled studies have shown that *Lactobacillus acidophilus* might prevent candida vaginitis.[7]

Vitamin K

Unlike with most other antibiotics, preliminary research suggests that people taking ofloxacin do not need to supplement vitamin K to protect against possible drug-induced depletion.[8]

Interactions with Foods and Other Compounds
Food

Ofloxacin may be taken with or without food; food slows the absorption but not the total amount of ofloxacin absorbed from.[9, 10] Milk does not alter ofloxacin absorption.[11]

OLANZAPINE

Common names: Zyprexa

Olanzapine is used to treat the symptoms associated with psychotic disorders, especially schizophrenia.

Summary of Interactions for Olanzapine

In some cases, an herb or supplement may appear in more than one category, which may seem contradictory. For clarification, read the full article for details about the summarized interactions.

✓ May be Beneficial: Supportive interaction	Glycine
🚫 Avoid: Adverse interaction	Alcohol Smoking
Depletion or interference	None known
Side effect reduction/prevention	None known
Reduced drug absorption/bioavailability	None known

Interactions with Dietary Supplements
Glycine

In a small double-blind study, people with schizophrenia being treated with olanzapine experienced an improvement in their symptoms when glycine was added to their treatment regimen.[1] The initial amount of glycine used was 4 grams per day; this was increased gradually over a period of 10 to 17 days to a maximum of 0.8 grams per 2.2 pounds of body weight per day.

Interactions with Foods and Other Compounds
Smoking

Cigarette smoking increases the elimination of risperidone from the body.[2] This interaction becomes a problem when an individual who has been taking olanzapine voluntarily starts or quits smoking. People who start smoking while taking risperidone may experience increased disease symptoms, while those who stop smoking while taking the drug may experience increased side effects. Individuals who change their smoking habits while on risperidone should notify their doctor.

Alcohol

Ingestion of alcohol may decrease blood levels of olanzapine by stimulating the liver to break down the drug.[3] Consequently, individuals who begin using alcohol while taking olanzapine may experience increased disease symptoms due to the reduced effectiveness of the drug. In addition, people who take antipsychotic agents such as olanzapine should avoid alcohol because it may intensify the effects of the drug on the nervous system and may cause low blood pressure.[4]

OLOPATADINE

Common names: Patanol

Olopatadine is used short-term to prevent itching due to allergic inflammation of the eye (conjunctivitis). At the time of this writing, no evidence of nutrient or herb interactions involving olopatadine was found in the medical literature.

Summary of Interactions for Olopatadine

In some cases, an herb or supplement may appear in more than one category, which may seem contradictory. For clarification, read the full article for details about the summarized interactions.

Depletion or interference	None known
Side effect reduction/prevention	None known
Supportive interaction	None known
Reduced drug absorption/bioavailability	None known
Adverse interaction	None known

OMALIZUMAB

Common names: Xolair

Omalizumab is used to treat moderate to severe asthma caused by perennial air-borne allergens in people with symptoms not controlled by **inhaled corticosteroids** (page 143). There are currently no reported nutrient or herb interactions involving omalizumab.

OMEPRAZOLE

Common names: Losec, Prilosec

Omeprazole is a member of the proton pump inhibitor family of drugs, which blocks production of stomach acid. Omeprazole is used to treat diseases in which stomach acid causes damage, including gastric and duodenal ulcers, gastroesophageal reflux disease, erosive esophagitis, and Zollinger-Ellison syndrome.

Summary of Interactions for Omeprazole

In some cases, an herb or supplement may appear in more than one category, which may seem contradictory. For clarification, read the full article for details about the summarized interactions.

✓	May be Beneficial: Depletion or interference	Folic acid Vitamin B_{12}*
✓	May be Beneficial: Side effect reduction/prevention	Cranberry*

⊘	Avoid: Reduced drug absorption/ bioavailability	St. John's wort
	Supportive interaction	None known
	Adverse interaction	None known

Interactions with Dietary Supplements

Folic acid

Folic acid is needed by the body to utilize vitamin B_{12}. Antacids, including omeprazole, inhibit folic acid absorption.[1] People taking antacids are advised to supplement with folic acid.

Vitamin B_{12}

Omeprazole interferes with the absorption of vitamin B_{12} from food (though not from supplements) in some[2, 3, 4, 5] but not all[6, 7] studies. A true deficiency state, resulting in vitamin B_{12}-deficiency anemia, has only been reported in one case.[8] The fall in vitamin B_{12} status may result from the decrease in stomach acid required for vitamin B_{12} absorption from food caused by the drug.[9] This problem may possibly be averted by drinking acidic juices when eating foods containing vitamin B_{12}.[10]

However, all people taking omeprazole need to either supplement with vitamin B_{12} or have their vitamin B_{12} status checked on a yearly basis. Even relatively small amounts of vitamin B_{12} such as 10–50 mcg per day, are likely to protect against drug induced vitamin depletion.

Interactions with Herbs

St. John's wort

In a study of healthy human volunteers, supplementing with St. John's wort greatly decreased omeprazole blood levels by accelerating the metabolism of the drug.[11] Use of St. John's wort may, therefore, interfere with the actions of omeprazole.

Cranberry (Vaccinium marocarpon)

People taking omeprazole may increase absorption of dietary vitamin B_{12} by drinking cranberry juice or other acidic liquids with vitamin B_{12}-containing foods.[12]

ONE TOUCH TEST STRIP

One Touch Strips are used by people who have diabetes to monitor blood sugar levels.

One Touch Test Strip

Summary of Interactions for One Touch Test Strip

In some cases, an herb or supplement may appear in more than one category, which may seem contradictory. For clarification, read the full article for details about the summarized interactions.

Depletion or interference	None known
Side effect reduction/prevention	None known
Supportive interaction	None known
Reduced drug absorption/bioavailability	None known
Adverse interaction	None known

OPAS

Contains the following ingredients:
Calcium
Magnesium
Sodium bicarbonate (page 240)

ORAL CONTRACEPTIVES

Common names: Alesse-28, Alesse, BiNovum, Brevicon, Brevinor, Cilest, Cyclen, Demulen, Desogen, Desogestrel, Ethynodiol, Eugynon, Femodene, Genora, Jenest, Levlen, Levonorgestrel, Lo/Ovral, Loestrin, Logynon, Marvelon, Mercilon, Mestranol, Microgynon, Micronor, Min-Ovral, Minestrin, Minulet, Modicon, Necon 1/35, Necon, Nelova, Nordette, Norethindrone, Norethin, Norgestrol, Norimin, Norinyl-I, Norinyl, Ortho Tri-Cyclen, Ortho-Cept, Ortho-Cyclen, Ortho-Novum, Ortho, Ovcon, Ovral, Ovranette, Ovran, Ovrette, Ovysmen, Select, Synphase, Synphasic, Tri-Cyclen, Tri-Minulet, Tri-Norinyl, Triadene, Trinordiol, TriNovum, Triphasil, Triquilar

Oral contraceptives, or birth control pills, are primarily used to prevent pregnancy and to treat menstrual irregularities and endometriosis. Oral contraceptives are available as an estrogen and progestin combination or as a progestin-only product. The estrogens used in oral contraceptives are different from those used in hormone-replacement therapy. Consequently, interactions involving estrogens used in birth control pills may or may not be similar to those used in hormone replacement.

Interactions that are common to oral contraceptives are described below. For interactions involving drugs used in hormone-replacement therapy, refer to the article on **estrogen** (page 109).

Mestranol and Norethindrone
- Genora 1/50
- Nelova 1/50
- Norethin 1/50
- Ortho-Novum 1/50

Ethinyl estradiol and Norethindrone
- Brevicon
- Estrostep
- Genora 1/35
- GenCept 1/35
- Jenest-28
- Loestrin 1.5/30
- Loestrin1/20
- Modicon
- Necon 1/25
- Necon 10/11
- Necon 0.5/30
- Necon 1/50
- Nelova 1/35
- Nelova 10/11
- Norinyl 1/35
- Norlestin 1/50
- Ortho Novum 1/35
- Ortho Novum 10/11
- Ortho Novum 7/7/7
- Ovcon-35
- Ovcon-50
- Tri-Norinyl

Ethinyl estradiol and Ethynodiol
- Demulen 1/35
- Demulen 1/50
- Nelulen 1/25
- Nelulen 1/50
- Zovia

Ethinyl estradiol and Norgestrel
- Lo/Ovral
- Ovral

Ethinyl estradiol and Levonorgestrel
- Alesse
- Levlen
- Levlite
- Levora 0.15/30
- Nordette
- Preven Emergency Contraceptive Kit
- Tri-Levlen
- Triphasil
- Trivora

Ethinyl estradiol and Desogestrel
- Desogen
- Ortho-TriCyclen

Levonorgestrel
- Plan B
- Norethindrone
- Micronor
- Nor-QD
- Norgestrel
- Ovrette

Summary of Interactions for Oral Contraceptives

In some cases, an herb or supplement may appear in more than one category, which may seem contradictory. For clarification, read the full article for details about the summarized interactions.

✓ May be Beneficial: Depletion or interference	Folic acid Magnesium* Vitamin B₁* Vitamin B₁₂* Vitamin B₂* Vitamin B₃* Vitamin B₆ Vitamin C* Zinc*
✓ May be Beneficial: Side effect reduction/prevention	Folic acid Vitamin B₆
✓ May be Beneficial: Supportive interaction	Folic acid*
⊘ Avoid: Adverse interaction	St. John's wort* Tobacco
ⓘ Check: Other	Calcium Copper Iron Manganese Vitamin A
Reduced drug absorption/bioavailability	None known

Interactions common to many, if not all, Oral Contraceptives are described in this article. Interactions reported for only one or several drugs in this class may not be listed in this article. Some drugs listed in this article are linked to articles specific to that respective drug; please refer to those individual drug articles. The information in this article may not necessarily apply to drugs in this class for which no separate article exists. If you are taking an Oral Contraceptive for which no separate article exists, talk with your doctor or pharmacist.

Interactions with Dietary Supplements
Folic acid

Oral contraceptive (OC) use can cause folic acid depletion.[1] In a double-blind trial of OC users with cervical dysplasia, supplementation with very large amounts (10 mg per day) of folic acid improved cervical health.[2] Women with cervical dysplasia diagnosed while they are taking OCs should consult a doctor. Mega-folate

supplementation should not be attempted without a doctor's supervision, nor is there any reason to believe that folic acid supplementation would help people with cervical cancer.

Iron

Menstrual blood loss is typically reduced with use of OCs. This can lead to increased iron stores and, presumably, a decreased need for iron in premenopausal women.[3] Premenopausal women taking OCs should have their iron levels monitored and talk with their prescribing doctor before using iron-containing supplements.

Magnesium

Women using OCs were found to have significantly lower serum magnesium levels in a controlled study.[4] In a preliminary study, blood levels of magnesium decreased in women taking an OC containing ethinyl estradiol and levonorgestrel.[5] Although the importance of this interaction remains somewhat unclear, supplementation with 250–350 mg of magnesium per day is a safe and reasonable supplemental level for most adults.

Vitamin B₆

Oral contraceptives have been associated with vitamin B₆ depletion and clinical depression. In a small, double-blind study of women with depression taking OCs, vitamin B₆ (20 mg twice per day) improved depression.[6] Half of the women in the study showed laboratory evidence of vitamin B₆ deficiency.

Other nutrients

A review of literature suggests that women who use OCs may experience decreased vitamin B₁, B₂, B₃, B₁₂, C, and zinc levels.[7, 8, 9] OC use has been associated with increased absorption of calcium and copper and with increased blood levels of copper and vitamin A.[10, 11, 12] OCs may interfere with manganese absorption.[13] The clinical importance of these actions remains unclear.

Interactions with Herbs
St. John's wort

Eight cases reported to the Medical Products Agency of Sweden suggest that St. John's wort may interact with oral contraceptives and cause intramenstrual bleeding and/or changes in menstrual bleeding.[14] One reviewer has suggested that St. John's wort may reduce serum levels of estradiol.[15] It should be noted, however, that only three of the eight Swedish women returned to normal menstrual cycles after stopping St. John's wort. Women taking oral contraceptives for birth control should consult with their doctor before taking St. John's wort.

Interactions with Foods and Other Compounds

Tobacco (Nicotiana species)

Women who smoke and use OCs have a five-times greater risk of dying from a heart attack than OC users who do not smoke.[16] Women over the age of 35 who smoke and use OCs have a greatly increased risk of death related to circulatory disease.[17] Avoiding or quitting smoking is good for health.

ORAL CORTICOSTEROIDS

Common names: Aristocort Oral, Cortef Oral, Decadron Oral, Delta-Cortef Oral, Deltasone Oral, Dexamethasone Oral, Hydrocortisone Oral, Medrol Oral, Methylprednisolone Oral, Orasone Oral, Pediapred Oral, Prednisolone Oral, Prednisone Oral, Prelone Oral, Triamcinolone Oral

Corticosteroids are a family of compounds that include the adrenal steroid hormone cortisol (hydrocortisone) and related synthetic drugs, such as prednisone. Both the natural and synthetic compounds are powerful anti-inflammatory agents. Oral corticosteroids are used to treat autoimmune and inflammatory diseases, including asthma, bursitis, Crohn's disease, tendinitis, ulcerative colitis, rheumatoid arthritis, and lupus, and skin conditions, such as eczema and psoriasis. They are also used to reduce inflammation associated with severe allergic reactions and to prevent organ rejection following transplant surgery.

The information in this article pertains to oral corticosteroids in general. The interactions reported here may not apply to all the Also Indexed As terms. Talk to your doctor or pharmacist if you are taking any of these drugs.

Summary of Interactions for Oral Corticosteroids

In some cases, an herb or supplement may appear in more than one category, which may seem contradictory. For clarification, read the full article for details about the summarized interactions.

✓ May be Beneficial: Depletion or interference	Calcium Chromium Magnesium Melatonin Potassium Selenium Vitamin B$_6$ Vitamin D
✓ May be Beneficial: Side effect reduction/prevention	Chromium Vitamin A
✓ May be Beneficial: Supportive interaction	N-acetyl cysteine (NAC)*

🚫 Avoid: Reduced drug absorption/ bioavailability	Magnesium
🚫 Avoid: Adverse interaction	Alcohol Sodium
ℹ Check: Other	Alder buckthorn* Buckthorn* Diuretic herbs* Grapefruit juice Laxative herbs* Licorice Protein Vitamin A* Vitamin C* Vitamin K* Zinc*

Interactions with Dietary Supplements

Magnesium

Corticosteroids may increase the body's loss of magnesium.[1] Some doctors recommend that people taking corticosteroids for more than two weeks supplement with 300–400 mg of magnesium per day. Magnesium has also been reported to interfere with the absorption of dexamethasone.[2]

N-acetyl cysteine (NAC)

One preliminary study found that in people with fibrosing alveolitis (a rare lung disease), supplementation with 600 mg N-acetyl cysteine three times per day increased the effectiveness of prednisone therapy.[3]

Potassium

Oral corticosteroids increase the urinary loss of potassium.[4] This may not cause a significant problem for most people. Individuals who wish to increase potassium intake should eat more fruits, vegetables, and juices rather than taking over-the-counter potassium supplements, which do not contain significant amounts of potassium.

Vitamin A

In some people, treatment with corticosteroids can impair wound healing. In one study, topical or internal vitamin A improved wound healing in eight of ten patients on corticosteroid therapy.[5] In theory, vitamin A might also reverse some of the beneficial effects of corticosteroids, but this idea has not been investigated and no reports exist of such an interaction in people taking both vitamin A and corticosteroids. People using oral corticosteroids should consult with a doctor to determine whether improved wound healing might outweigh the theoretical risk associated with concomitant vitamin A use.

Although blood levels of vitamin A appear to increase during dexamethasone therapy[6]—most likely due to mobilization of the vitamin from its stores in the liver—evidence from animal studies has also indicated that corticosteroids can *deplete* vitamin A from tissues.[7]

Vitamin B6
Corticosteroids may increase the loss of vitamin B6.[8] One double-blind study of people with asthma failed to show any added benefit from taking 300 mg per day of vitamin B6 along with **inhaled steroids** (page 143).[9] Therefore, while small amounts of vitamin B6 may be needed to prevent deficiency, large amounts may not provide added benefit. Some doctors recommend that people taking corticosteroids for longer than two weeks supplement with at least 2 mg of vitamin B6 per day.

Calcium and vitamin D
Oral corticosteroids reduce absorption of calcium[10] and interfere with the activation and metabolism of the vitamin,[11, 12, 13, 14] increasing the risk of bone loss. Doctors can measure levels of activated vitamin D (called 1,25 dihydroxycholecalciferol) to determine whether a deficiency exists; if so, activated vitamin D is only available by prescription. A study of rheumatoid arthritis patients treated with low amounts of prednisone found that those who received 1,000 mg of calcium per day plus 500 IU of vitamin D per day for two years experienced no bone loss during that time period.[15] An analysis of properly conducted trials concluded that supplementation with vitamin D and calcium was more effective than placebo or calcium alone in protecting against corticosteroid-induced osteoporosis.[16] Most doctors recommend 1,000 mg of calcium and 400–800 IU vitamin D per day for the prevention of osteoporosis.

Chromium
Preliminary data suggest that corticosteroid treatment increases chromium loss and that supplementation with chromium (600 mcg per day in the form of chromium picolinate) can prevent corticosteroid-induced diabetes.[17] Double-blind trials are needed to confirm these observations.

Melatonin
A controlled trial found that a single dose of the synthetic corticosteroid dexamethasone suppressed production of melatonin in nine of 11 healthy volunteers.[18] Further research is needed to determine if long-term use of corticosteroids interferes in a meaningful way with melatonin production, and whether supplemental melatonin would be advisable for people taking corticosteroids.

Sodium
Oral corticosteroids cause both sodium and water retention.[19] People taking corticosteroids should talk with their doctor about whether they should restrict salt intake.

Other nutrients
Oral corticosteroids have been found to increase urinary loss of vitamin K, vitamin C, selenium, and zinc.[20, 21] The importance of these losses is unknown.

Interactions with Herbs
Buckthorn, alder buckthorn (Rhamnus catartica, Rhamnus frangula, Frangula alnus)
Use of buckthorn or alder buckthorn for more than ten days consecutively may cause a loss of electrolytes (especially the mineral potassium). Because corticosteroids also cause potassium loss, buckthorn or alder buckthorn should be used with caution if corticosteroids are being taken.[22]

Licorice (Glycyrrhiza glabra)
Licorice extract was shown to decrease the elimination of prednisone in test tube studies.[23] If this action happens in people, it might prolong prednisone activity and possibly increase prednisone-related side effects. A small, controlled study found that intravenous (iv) glycyrrhizin (an active constituent in licorice) given with iv prednisolone prolonged prednisolone action in healthy men.[24] Whether this effect would occur with oral corticosteroids and licorice supplements is unknown.

An animal study has shown that glycyrrhizin prevents the immune-suppressing actions of cortisone—the natural corticosteroid hormone produced by the body.[25] More research is necessary to determine if this action is significant in humans taking oral corticosteroids. Until more is known, people should not take licorice with corticosteroids without first consulting a doctor.

Diuretic herbs
Use of corticosteroids may be associated with loss of certain minerals, called electrolytes. Herbs with a diuretic action (i.e., they promote fluid loss from the body through an increase in urine production) may accelerate the electrolyte loss caused by corticosteroids.[26] Such herbs include asparagus root, butcher's broom, cleavers, corn silk, juniper, mate, and parsley. This interaction is theoretical and has not been reported in the medical literature.

Laxative herbs

Like diuretic herbs, herbs with a laxative action could theoretically increase electrolyte loss associated with corticosteroid use.[27] Such herbs include aloe, buckthorn, cascara sagrada, rhubarb, and senna. This interaction is theoretical and has not been reported in the medical literature.

Interactions with Foods and Other Compounds
Food

Corticosteroids can cause stomach upset and should be taken with food.[28]

Protein

Oral corticosteroids can cause loss of body protein. For this reason, medical doctors sometimes recommend a high-protein diet for people taking these drugs.[29] However, people with diseases that cause kidney damage should not consume too much protein, as this could worsen their condition. A high-protein diet should be used only after consulting a doctor.

Alcohol

Corticosteroids can irritate the stomach, and alcohol can enhance this adverse reaction.[30]

Grapefruit juice

Taking methylprednisolone with grapefruit juice has been shown to delay the absorption and increase the blood concentration of the drug.[31] The mechanism by which grapefruit juice increases the concentration of methylpredniolone in the blood is not known, but it is suspected that it may interfere with enzymes in the liver responsible for clearing the drug from the body. In certain people, grapefruit juice may, therefore, enhance the effects of methylprednisolone. The combination should be avoided unless approved by the prescribing doctor.

ORLISTAT

Common names: Xenical

Orlistat is used for obesity management, including weight loss and weight maintenance, in association with a low-calorie diet.

Summary of Interactions for Orlistat

In some cases, an herb or supplement may appear in more than one category, which may seem contradictory.

For clarification, read the full article for details about the summarized interactions.

✓	May be Beneficial: Depletion or interference	Beta-carotene Vitamin A Vitamin D Vitamin E
✓	May be Beneficial: Side effect reduction/prevention	Psyllium
✓	May be Beneficial: Supportive interaction	Food
	Reduced drug absorption/bioavailability	None known
	Adverse interaction	None known

Interactions with Dietary Supplements
Beta-carotene

One well-controlled study showed that taking orlistat greatly reduces the absorption of beta-carotene.[1] Therefore, individuals taking orlistat for long periods of time should probably supplement with beta-carotene.

Vitamin E

Taking orlistat dramatically reduces the absorption of vitamin E,[2] which might result in deficiency symptoms. Therefore, people taking orlistat for long periods of time should supplement with vitamin E.

Vitamin A and vitamin D

In one well-controlled study, taking orlistat for six months resulted in reduced blood levels of vitamins A and D, though levels for most individuals remained within the normal range. However, a few people developed levels low enough to require supplementation.[3] Other studies have shown that taking orlistat had no affect on blood vitamin A levels.[4, 5] Although additional research is needed, the current evidence suggests that individuals taking orlistat for more than six months should supplement with vitamins A and D.

Interactions with Herbs
Psyllium

In a group of obese women taking orlistat three times per day, ingestion of 6 grams of psyllium with each dose of orlistat significantly reduced the gastrointestinal side effects of the drug.[6]

Interactions with Foods and Other Compounds
Food

Orlistat blocks enzymes responsible for the breakdown and absorption of fat. Therefore, orlistat should be taken during, or up to one hour after, each main meal that contains fat.[7]

OXAPROZIN

Common names: Daypro

Oxaprozin is a member of the **nonsteroidal anti-inflammatory drug** (page 193) (NSAIDs) family. NSAIDs reduce inflammation (swelling), pain, and temperature. Oxaprozin is used to treat osteoarthritis and rheumatoid arthritis.

Summary of Interactions for Oxaprozin

In some cases, an herb or supplement may appear in more than one category, which may seem contradictory. For clarification, read the full article for details about the summarized interactions.

✓	May be Beneficial: Depletion or interference	Iron
✓	May be Beneficial: Side effect reduction/prevention	Copper* Licorice
✓	May be Beneficial: Supportive interaction	Copper*
🚫	Avoid: Adverse interaction	**Lithium** (page 157)* Sodium* White willow*
ⓘ	Check: Other	Potassium
	Reduced drug absorption/bioavailability	None known

Interactions with Dietary Supplements

Copper

Supplementation may enhance the anti-inflammatory effects of NSAIDs while reducing their ulcerogenic effects. One study found that when various anti-inflammatory drugs were chelated with copper, the anti-inflammatory activity was increased.[1] Animal models of inflammation have found that the copper chelate of **aspirin** (page 26) was active at one-eighth the effective dose of aspirin. These copper complexes are less toxic than the parent compounds, as well.

Iron

NSAIDs cause gastrointestinal (GI) irritation, bleeding, and iron loss.[2] Iron supplements can cause GI irritation.[3] However, iron supplementation is sometimes needed in people taking NSAIDs if those drugs have caused

enough blood loss to lead to iron deficiency. If both iron and oxaprozin are prescribed, they should be taken with food to reduce GI irritation and bleeding risk.

Lithium (page 157)

Lithium is a mineral that may be present in some supplements and is also used in large amounts to treat mood disorders such as manic-depression (bipolar disorder). Most NSAIDs inhibit the excretion of lithium from the body, resulting in higher blood levels of the mineral, though **sulindac** (page 249) may have an opposite effect.[4] Since major changes in lithium blood levels can produce unwanted side effects or interfere with its efficacy, NSAIDs should be used with caution, and only under medical supervision, in people taking lithium supplements.

Potassium

NSAIDs have caused kidney dysfunction and increased blood potassium levels, especially in older people.[5] People taking NSAIDs, including oxaprozin, should not supplement potassium without consulting with their doctor.

Sodium

Oxaprozin may cause sodium and water retention.[6] It is healthful to reduce dietary salt intake by eliminating table salt and heavily salted foods.

Interactions with Herbs

Licorice (Glycyrrhiza glabra)

The flavonoids found in the extract of licorice known as DGL (deglycyrrhizinated licorice) are helpful for avoiding the irritating actions NSAIDs have on the stomach and intestines. One study found that 350 mg of chewable DGL taken together with each dose of aspirin reduced gastrointestinal bleeding caused by the aspirin.[7] DGL has been shown in controlled human research to be as effective as drug therapy (**cimetidine** [page 61]) in healing stomach ulcers.[8]

White willow bark (Salix alba)

White willow bark contains salicin, which is related to **aspirin** (page 26). Both salicin and aspirin produce anti-inflammatory effects after they have been converted to salicylic acid in the body. The administration of salicylates like aspirin to individuals taking oral NSAIDs may result in reduced blood levels of NSAIDs.[9] Though no studies have investigated interactions between white willow bark and NSAIDs, people taking NSAIDs should avoid the herb until more information is available.

Interactions with Foods and Other Compounds
Food
Oxaprozin should be taken with food to prevent gastrointestinal upset.[10]

Alcohol
Oxaprozin may cause drowsiness, dizziness, or blurred vision.[11] Alcohol may intensify these effects and increase the risk of accidental injury. Use of alcohol during oxaprozin therapy increases the risk of stomach irritation and bleeding. People taking oxaprozin should avoid alcohol.

OXAZEPAM

Common names: Apo-Oxazepam, Serax

Oxazepam is used to treat symptoms of anxiety, such as worry, restlessness, and insomnia; symptoms that occur during alcohol withdrawal; and agitation and irritability in elderly individuals. Oxazepam is in a class of drugs known as **benzodiazepines** (page 36).

Summary of Interactions for Oxazepam
In some cases, an herb or supplement may appear in more than one category, which may seem contradictory. For clarification, read the full article for details about the summarized interactions.

✓ May be Beneficial: Supportive interaction	Vinpocetine*
⊘ Avoid: Adverse interaction	Alcohol Smoking
Depletion or interference	None known
Side effect reduction/prevention	None known
Reduced drug absorption/bioavailability	None known

Interactions with Dietary Supplements
Vinpocetine
In a preliminary trial, an extract of periwinkle called vinpocetine was shown to produce minor improvements in short-term memory among people taking flunitrazepam, a benzodiazepine.[1] Further study is needed to determine if vinpocetine would be a helpful adjunct to use of benzodiazepines, or oxazepam specifically.

Interactions with Foods and Other Compounds
Food
Controlled studies have shown that eating diets low in calories, protein, and carbohydrates can reduce the elimination of oxazepam from the body and increase the amount of time it remains in the blood.[2, 3] On the other hand, research indicates that certain foods, such as Brussels sprouts and cabbage, might reduce blood levels of oxazepam and increase the removal of the drug.[4] Further research is needed to determine whether certain foods and diets can result in significant changes in the effectiveness or safety of oxazepam.

Alcohol
Drinking alcoholic beverages with oxazepam can increase side effects of the drug, such as drowsiness, fatigue, and light-headedness.[5] Therefore, alcohol should be avoided by people taking oxazepam, especially when staying alert is necessary.

Smoking
Cigarette smoking can significantly increase the elimination of oxazepam from the body.[6] Problems might occur if people either start or stop smoking while taking oxazepam. Individuals who stop smoking may experience increased side effects, while those who start smoking may notice that the drug is less effective.

OXYBUTYNIN

Common names: Albert Oxybutynin, Apo-Oxybutynin, Contimin, Cystrin, Ditropan, Gen-Oxybutynin, Novo-Oxybutynin, Nu-Oxybutyn, Oxybutyn

Oxybutynin is used to treat symptoms of an overactive bladder, including urinary urgency and frequency, and is in a class of drugs called anticholinergic antispasmodics.

Summary of Interactions for Oxybutynin
In some cases, an herb or supplement may appear in more than one category, which may seem contradictory. For clarification, read the full article for details about the summarized interactions.

Depletion or interference	None known
Side effect reduction/prevention	None known
Supportive interaction	None known
Reduced drug absorption/bioavailability	None known
Adverse interaction	None known

Interactions with Foods and Other Compounds
Alcohol
Drinking alcoholic beverages while taking oxybutynin may enhance the drowsiness caused by the drug.[1] Con-

sequently, people taking oxybutynin should avoid alcohol, especially when staying alert is necessary.

OXYCODONE

Common names: M-Oxy, OxyContin, OxyFast, OxyIR, Percolone, Roxicodone, Supeudol

Combination drugs: Endocet, Percocet, Percodan, Roxicet, Roxiprin

Oxycodone is a narcotic analgesic used to relieve moderate to severe pain. Oxycodone is available in combination products.

Summary of Interactions for Oxycodone

In some cases, an herb or supplement may appear in more than one category, which may seem contradictory. For clarification, read the full article for details about the summarized interactions.

Depletion or interference	None known
Side effect reduction/prevention	None known
Supportive interaction	None known
Reduced drug absorption/bioavailability	None known
Adverse interaction	None known

Interactions with Foods and Other Compounds

Food

Oxycodone may cause gastrointestinal (GI) upset. Oxycodone-containing products may be taken with food to reduce or prevent GI upset.[1] A common side effect of narcotic analgesics is constipation.[2] Increasing dietary fiber (especially vegetables and whole-grain foods) and water intake can ease constipation.

Alcohol

Oxycodone may cause drowsiness, dizziness, or blurred vision. Alcohol may intensify these effects and increase the risk of accidental injury.[3] To prevent problems, people taking oxycodone should avoid alcohol.

PACLITAXEL

Common names: Paxene, Taxol

Paclitaxel is a natural (though quite toxic) substance derived from the yew tree by taking a naturally present substance from the tree and chemically altering it to form the drug. The resultant drug is administered intravenously. It is used as a **chemotherapy** (page 54) drug to treat people with a wide variety of cancers.

Note: Many of the interactions described below, in the text and in the Summary of Interactions, have been reported only for specific chemotherapeutic drugs, and may not apply to other chemotherapeutic drugs. There are many unknowns concerning interactions of nutrients, herbs, and chemotherapy drugs. People receiving chemotherapy who wish to supplement with vitamins, minerals, herbs, or other natural substances should always consult a physician.

Summary of Interactions for Paclitaxel

In some cases, an herb or supplement may appear in more than one category, which may seem contradictory. For clarification, read the full article for details about the summarized interactions.

✓	May be Beneficial: Depletion or interference	Multiple nutrients (malabsorption)* Taurine*
✓	May be Beneficial: Side effect reduction/prevention	Beta-carotene* (mouth sores) Chamomile* (mouth sores) Eleuthero* (see text) Ginger* (nausea) Glutamine Glutamine* (mouth sores) Melatonin N-acetyl cysteine* (NAC) Spleen peptide extract* (see text) Thymus peptides* (see text) Vitamin E*, topical (mouth sores)
✓	May be Beneficial: Supportive interaction	Antioxidants* Melatonin Milk thistle* PSK*
ⓘ	Check: Other	Echinacea* Multivitamin-mineral* Vitamin A*
ⓘ	Check: Other	Vitamin C*
	Reduced drug absorption/bioavailability	None known
	Adverse interaction	None known

Interactions with Dietary Supplements

Antioxidants

Chemotherapy can injure cancer cells by creating oxidative damage. As a result, some oncologists recommend that patients avoid supplementing antioxidants if they are undergoing chemotherapy. Limited test tube research occasionally does support the idea that an antioxidant can interfere with oxidative damage to cancer cells.[1] However, most scientific research does not support this supposition.

A modified form of vitamin A has been reported to work synergistically with chemotherapy in test tube research.[2] Vitamin C appears to increase the effectiveness of chemotherapy in animals[3] and with human breast cancer cells in test tube research.[4] In a double-blind study, Japanese researchers found that the combination of vitamin E, vitamin C, and N-acetyl cysteine (NAC)—all antioxidants—protected against chemotherapy-induced heart damage without interfering with the action of the chemotherapy.[5]

A comprehensive review of antioxidants and chemotherapy leaves open the question of whether supplemental antioxidants definitely help people with chemotherapy side effects, but the article strongly suggests that antioxidants need not be avoided for fear that the actions of chemotherapy would be interfered with.[6]

A new formulation of selenium (Seleno-Kappacarrageenan) was found to reduce kidney damage and white blood cell–lowering effects of **cisplatin** (page 64) in one human study. However, the level used in this study (4,000 mcg per day) is potentially toxic and should only be used under the supervision of a doctor.[7]

Glutathione, the main antioxidant found within cells, is frequently depleted in individuals on chemotherapy and/or radiation. Preliminary studies have found that intravenously injected glutathione may decrease some of the adverse effects of chemotherapy and radiation, such as diarrhea.[8]

Glutamine

Though cancer cells use glutamine as a fuel source, studies in humans have not found that glutamine stimulates growth of cancers in people taking chemotherapy.[9, 10] In fact, animal studies show that glutamine may actually decrease tumor growth while increasing susceptibility of cancer cells to radiation and chemotherapy,[11, 12] though such effects have not yet been studied in humans.

Glutamine has successfully reduced chemotherapy-induced mouth sores. In one trial, people were given 4 grams of glutamine in an oral rinse, which was swished around the mouth and then swallowed twice per day.[13] Thirteen of fourteen people in the study had fewer days with mouth sores as a result. These excellent results have been duplicated in some,[14] but not all[15] double-blind research. In another study, patients receiving high-dose paclitaxel and melphalan had significantly fewer episodes of oral ulcers and bleeding when they took 6 grams of glutamine four times daily along with the chemotherapy.[16] In another preliminary trial, supplementation with 10 grams of glutamine three times per day, beginning 24 hours after administration of high-dose paclitaxel, reduced the severity of drug-induced nerve damage (peripheral neuropathy).[17]

One double-blind trial suggested that 6 grams of glutamine taken three times per day can decrease diarrhea caused by chemotherapy.[18] However, other studies using higher amounts or intravenous glutamine have not reported this effect.[19, 20]

Intravenous use of glutamine in people undergoing bone marrow transplants, a procedure sometimes used to allow very high amounts of chemotherapy to be used, has led to reduced hospital stays, leading to a savings of over $21,000 for each patient given glutamine.[21]

Paclitaxel commonly causes muscle and joint pain. Five cases of people experiencing these symptoms who responded to the amino acid glutamine have been reported.[22] All five were given 10 grams glutamine by mouth three times per day beginning 24 hours after the paclitaxel treatment. Although the report does not state how many days glutamine supplements were taken, it may have been for ten days or less—the typical time it takes for these symptoms to subside following paclitaxel administration. Whereas all five had experienced moderate to severe symptoms from the drug when taken previously without glutamine, none of the five experienced these symptoms when glutamine was added. In another study, patients receiving high-dose paclitaxel and melphalan had significantly fewer episodes of oral ulcers and bleeding when they took 6 g of glutamine four times daily along with the chemotherapy.[23]

Glutamate, an amino acid structurally related to glutamine, had previously been reported to reduce paclitaxel-induced nerve damage in animals.[24]

Melatonin

Melatonin supplementation (20 mg per day) has decreased toxicity and improved effectiveness of chemotherapy with paclitaxel.[25]

N-acetyl cysteine (NAC)

NAC, an amino acid–like supplement that possesses antioxidant activity, has been used in four human studies to decrease the kidney and bladder toxicity of the chemotherapy drug ifosfamide.[26, 27, 28, 29] These studies used 1–2 grams NAC four times per day. There was no sign that NAC interfered with the efficacy of ifosfamide in any of these studies. Intakes of NAC over 4 grams per day may cause nausea and vomiting.

The newer anti-nausea drugs prescribed for people taking chemotherapy lead to greatly reduced nausea and vomiting for most people. Nonetheless, these drugs often do not totally eliminate all nausea. Natural substances used to reduce nausea should not be used instead of prescription anti-nausea drugs. Rather, under the guidance of a doctor, they should be added to those drugs if needed. At least one trial suggests that NAC, at 1,800 mg per day may reduce nausea and vomiting caused by chemotherapy.[30]

Spleen extract

Patients with inoperable head and neck cancer were treated with a spleen peptide preparation (Polyerga) in a double-blind trial during chemotherapy with cisplatin and 5-FU.[31] The spleen preparation had a significant stabilizing effect on certain white blood cells. People taking it also experienced stabilized body weight and a reduction in the fatigue and inertia that usually accompany this combination of chemotherapy agents.

Beta-carotene and vitamin E

Chemotherapy frequently causes mouth sores. In one trial, people were given approximately 400,000 IU of beta-carotene per day for three weeks and then 125,000 IU per day for an additional four weeks.[32] Those taking beta-carotene still suffered mouth sores, but the mouth sores developed later and tended to be less severe than mouth sores that formed in people receiving the same chemotherapy without beta-carotene.

In a study of chemotherapy-induced mouth sores, six of nine patients who applied vitamin E directly to their mouth sores had complete resolution of the sores compared with one of nine patients who applied placebo.[33] Others have confirmed the potential for vitamin E to help people with chemotherapy-induced mouth sores.[34] Applying vitamin E only once per day was helpful to only some groups of patients in another trial,[35] and not all studies have found vitamin E to be effective.[36] Until more is known, if vitamin E is used in an attempt to reduce chemotherapy-induced mouth sores, it should be applied topically twice per day and should probably be in the tocopherol (versus tocopheryl) form.

Vitamin A

A controlled French trial reported that when postmenopausal late-stage breast cancer patients were given very large amounts of vitamin A (350,000–500,000 IU per day) along with chemotherapy, remission rates were significantly better than when the chemotherapy was not accompanied by vitamin A.[37] Similar results were not found in premenopausal women. The large amounts of vitamin A used in the study are toxic and require clinical supervision.

Multivitamin-mineral

Many chemotherapy drugs can cause diarrhea, lack of appetite, vomiting, and damage to the gastrointestinal tract. Recent anti-nausea prescription medications are often effective. Nonetheless, nutritional deficiencies still occur.[38] It makes sense for people undergoing chemotherapy to take a high-potency multivitamin-mineral to protect against deficiencies.

Taurine

Taurine has been shown to be depleted in people taking chemotherapy.[39] It remains unclear how important this effect is or if people taking chemotherapy should take taurine supplements.

Thymus peptides

Peptides or short proteins derived from the thymus gland, an important immune organ, have been used in conjunction with chemotherapy drugs for people with cancer. One study using thymosin fraction V in combination with chemotherapy, compared with chemotherapy alone, found significantly longer survival times in the thymosin fraction V group.[40] A related substance, thymostimulin, decreased some side effects of chemotherapy and increased survival time compared with chemotherapy alone.[41] A third product, thymic extract TP1, was shown to improve immune function in people treated with chemotherapy compared with effects of chemotherapy alone.[42] Thymic peptides need to be administered by injection. People interested in their combined use with chemotherapy should consult a doctor.

Interactions with Herbs

Echinacea (Echinacea purpurea, Echinacea angustifolia)

Echinacea is a popular immune-boosting herb that has been investigated for use with chemotherapy. One study investigated the actions of **cyclophosphamide** (page 79), echinacea, and thymus gland extracts to treat advanced cancer patients. Although small and uncontrolled, this trial suggested that the combination modestly extended the life span of some patients with inoperable cancers.[43] Signs of restoration of immune function were seen in these patients.

Eleuthero (Eleutherococcus senticosus)

Russian research has looked at using eleuthero with chemotherapy. One study of patients with melanoma found that chemotherapy was less toxic when eleuthero was given simultaneously. Similarly, women with inoperable breast cancer given eleuthero were reported to tolerate more chemotherapy.[44] Eleuthero treatment was also associated with improved immune function in women with breast cancer treated with chemotherapy and radiation.[45]

Milk thistle (Silybum marianum)

Milk thistle's major flavonoids, known collectively as silymarin, have shown synergistic actions with the chemotherapy drugs **cisplatin** (page 64) and **doxorubicin** (page 100) (Adriamycin) in test tubes.[46] Silymarin also offsets the kidney toxicity of cisplatin in animals.[47] Silymarin has not yet been studied in humans treated with cisplatin. Research with a limited number of chemotherapy drugs suggest that silymarin does not interfere with their anticancer effect. However, additional research is needed.[48]

Ginger (Zingiber officinale)

Ginger can be helpful in alleviating nausea and vomiting caused by chemotherapy.[49, 50] Tablets or capsules containing powdered ginger can be taken in 500 mg amounts every two or three hours, as needed.

German chamomile (Matricaria recutita)

A liquid preparation of German chamomile has been shown to reduce the incidence of mouth sores in people receiving radiation and systemic chemotherapy treatment in an uncontrolled study. [51]

PSK (Coriolus versicolor)

The mushroom *Coriolus versicolor* contains an immune-stimulating substance called polysaccharide krestin, or PSK. PSK has been shown in several studies to help cancer patients undergoing chemotherapy. One study involved women with estrogen receptor-negative breast cancer. PSK combined with chemotherapy significantly prolonged survival time compared with chemotherapy alone.[52] Another study followed women with breast cancer who were given chemotherapy with or without PSK. The PSK-plus-chemotherapy group had a 25% better chance of survival after ten years compared with

those taking chemotherapy without PSK.[53] Another study investigated people who had surgically removed colon cancer. They were given chemotherapy with or without PSK. Those given PSK had a longer disease-free period and longer survival time.[54] Three grams of PSK were taken orally each day in these studies.

Although PSK is rarely available in the United States, hot-water extract products made from *Coriolus versicolor* mushrooms are available. These products may have activity related to that of PSK, but their use with chemotherapy has not been studied.

Interactions with Foods and Other Compounds
Fruit drinks

Often, people who undergo chemotherapy develop aversions to certain foods, sometimes making it permanently difficult to eat those foods. Exposing people to what researchers have called a "scapegoat stimulus" just before the administration of chemotherapy can direct the food aversion to the "scapegoat" food instead of more important parts of the diet. In one trial, fruit drinks administered just before chemotherapy were most effective in protecting against aversions to other foods.[55]

PAROXETINE

Common names: Paxil, Seroxat

Paroxetine is a member of the selective serotonin reuptake inhibitor (SSRI) family of drugs used to treat people with depression.

Summary of Interactions for Paroxetine

In some cases, an herb or supplement may appear in more than one category, which may seem contradictory. For clarification, read the full article for details about the summarized interactions.

✓	May be Beneficial: Depletion or interference	Sodium
✓	May be Beneficial: Side effect reduction/prevention	*Ginkgo biloba**
⊘	Avoid: Adverse interaction	5-Hydroxytryptophan (5-HTP)* L-tryptophan* St. John's wort*
	Supportive interaction	None known
	Reduced drug absorption/bioavailability	None known

Interactions with Dietary Supplements
5-Hydroxytryptophan (5-HTP) and L-trytophan
Paroxetine increases serotonin activity in the brain. 5-HTP and L-tryptophan are converted to serotonin in the brain, and taking either of these compounds with paroxetine may increase paroxetine-induced side effects. Dietary supplements of L-tryptophan (available only by prescriptions from special compounding pharmacists) taken with paroxetine caused headache, sweating, dizziness, agitation, restlessness, nausea, vomiting, and other symptoms.[1] Some doctors have used small amounts of L-tryptophan in combination with SSRIs, to increase the effectiveness of the latter. However, because of the potential for side effects, 5-HTP and L-tryptophan should never be taken in combination with paroxetine or other SSRIs, unless the combination is being closely monitored by a doctor. Foods rich in L-tryptophan do not appear to interact with paroxtine or other SSRIs.

On the other hand, the combination of 45 mg DL-tryptophan (a synthetic variation of L-tryptophan) per pound of body weight (a relatively high dose) with zimelidine, a drug with a similar action to paroxetine, did not cause these side effects in another trial.[2]

Sodium
SSRI drugs, including paroxetine, have been reported to cause sodium depletion.[3, 4, 5] The risk for SSRI-induced sodium depletion appears to be increased during the first few weeks of treatment in women, the elderly, and patients also using **diuretics** (page 94). Doctors prescribing SSRI drugs, including paroxetine, should monitor their patients for signs of sodium depletion.

Interactions with Herbs
Ginkgo biloba
In three men and two women treated with **fluoxetine** (page 120) or **sertraline** (page 237) (SSRI drugs closely related to paroxetine) for depression who experienced sexual dysfunction, addition of Ginkgo biloba extract (GBE) in the amount of 240 mg per day effectively reversed the sexual dysfunction.[6] This makes sense because ginkgo has been reported to help men with some forms of erectile dysfunction.[7]

St. John's wort (Hypericum perforatum)
One report described a case of serotonin syndrome in a patient who took St. John's wort and **trazodone** (page 267), a weak SSRI drug.[8] The patient reportedly experienced mental confusion, muscle twitching, sweating, flushing, and ataxia. In another case, a patient experienced grogginess, lethargy, nausea, weakness, and fatigue after taking one dose of paroxetine after ten days of St. John's wort use.[9]

Interactions with Foods and Other Compounds
Food
Paroxetine may be taken with or without food.[10]

Alcohol
SSRI drugs, including paroxetine, may cause dizziness or drowsiness.[11] Alcohol may intensify these effects and increase the risk of accidental injury. Alcohol should be avoided during paroxetine therapy.

PENICILLAMINE

Common names: Cuprimine, Depen, Distamine, Pendramine

Penicillamine is a chelating agent (binds metals and carries them out of the body). Penicillamine is used to treat people with Wilson's disease, cystinuria, and severe rheumatoid arthritis.

Summary of Interactions for Penicillamine
In some cases, an herb or supplement may appear in more than one category, which may seem contradictory. For clarification, read the full article for details about the summarized interactions.

✓ May be Beneficial: Depletion or interference	Sodium* Vitamin B6
✓ May be Beneficial: Supportive interaction	Bromelain
⊘ Avoid: Reduced drug absorption/ bioavailability	Guar gum* Iron Zinc
ⓘ Check: Other	Copper
Side effect reduction/prevention	None known
Adverse interaction	None known

Interactions with Dietary Supplements
Copper
One of the main uses of penicillamine is to reduce toxic copper deposits in people with Wilson's disease. People taking a copper supplement can make Wilson's disease worse and may negate the benefits of drugs used to remove copper from the body.

Iron
Penicillamine binds iron. When taken with iron, penicillamine absorption and activity are reduced.[1] Four

cases of penicillamine-induced kidney damage were reported when concomitant iron therapy was stopped, which presumably led to the increased penicillamine absorption and toxicity.[2]

Vitamin B6

Penicillamine may increase vitamin B_6 excretion, reduce activity, and increase the risk for vitamin B_6 deficiency.[3] It makes sense for people taking penicillamine to supplement with small (5–20 mg per day) amounts of vitamin B_6. Some researchers have suggested that as much as 50 mg per day of vitamin B_6 may be necessary.[4]

Zinc

People taking penicillamine should discuss with their doctor whether it would be appropriate to take a zinc supplement (at a separate time of day from the penicillamine).[5] However, people taking penicillamine should not supplement with zinc, unless they are being supervised by a doctor.

Bromelain

One report found bromelain improved the action of antibiotic drugs, including penicillin and erythromycin, in treating a variety of infections. In that trial, 22 out of 23 people who had previously not responded to the antibiotics did so after adding bromelain four times per day.[6] Doctors will sometimes prescribe enough bromelain to equal 2,400 gelatin dissolving units (listed as GDU on labels) per day. This amount would equal approximately 3,600 MCU (milk clotting units), another common measure of bromelain activity.

Guar gum

In a double-blind study with ten healthy people, guar gum reduced penicillin absorption.[7] Until more is known, to avoid this interaction, people taking penicillin should take it two hours before or after any guar gum-containing supplements. It remains unclear whether the smaller amounts of guar gum found in many processed foods would have a significant effect.

Sodium

Penicillamine therapy has been associated with sodium depletion.[8] The frequency of this association remains unclear.

Interactions with Foods and Other Compounds

Food

Food decreases penicillamine absorption.[9] Penicillamine should be taken one hour before or two hours after any food to avoid this interaction.

PENICILLIN V

Common names: Apo-Pen VK, Aspin, Ledercillin VK, Nadopen-V, Novo-Pen-VK, Nu-Pen-VK, Pen-Vee K, Phenoxymethyl Penicillin, Ten-kicin, V-Cillin-K, Veetids

Penicillin V is an **antibiotic** (page 19) used to treat bacterial infections.

Summary of Interactions for Penicillin V

In some cases, an herb or supplement may appear in more than one category, which may seem contradictory. For clarification, read the full article for details about the summarized interactions.

✓	May be Beneficial: Depletion or interference	Vitamin K*
✓	May be Beneficial: Side effect reduction/prevention	*Bifidobacterium longum** *Lactobacillus acidophilus** *Lactobacillus casei** *Saccharomyces boulardii** *Saccharomyces cerevisiae** Vitamin K*
✓	May be Beneficial: Supportive interaction	Bromelain* *Saccharomyces boulardii**
🚫	Avoid: Reduced drug absorption/ bioavailability	Guar Gum*
	Adverse interaction	None known

Interactions with Dietary Supplements

Bromelain

One report found bromelain improved the action of antibiotic drugs, including penicillin and **erythromycin** (page 106), in treating a variety of infections. In that trial, 22 out of 23 people who had previously not responded to the antibiotics did so after adding bromelain four times per day.[1] Doctors will sometimes prescribe enough bromelain to equal 2,400 gelatin dissolving units (listed as GDU on labels) per day. This amount would equal approximately 3,600 MCU (milk clotting units), another common measure of bromelain activity.

Guar gum

In a double-blind study with ten healthy people, guar gum reduced penicillin absorption.[2] Until more is known, to avoid this interaction, people taking penicillin should take it two hours before or after any guar gum–containing supplements. It remains unclear whether the smaller amounts of guar gum found in many processed foods would have a significant effect.

Probiotics
A common side effect of antibiotics is diarrhea, which may be caused by the elimination of beneficial bacteria normally found in the colon. Controlled studies have shown that taking probiotic microorganisms—such as *Lactobacillus casei*, *Lactobacillus acidophilus*, *Bifidobacterium longum*, or *Saccharomyces boulardii*—helps prevent antibiotic-induced diarrhea.[3]

The diarrhea experienced by some people who take antibiotics also might be due to an overgrowth of the bacterium *Clostridium difficile*, which causes a disease known as pseudomembranous colitis. Controlled studies have shown that supplementation with harmless yeast—such as *Saccharomyces boulardii*[4] or *Saccharomyces cerevisiae* (baker's or brewer's yeast)[5]—helps prevent recurrence of this infection. In one study, taking 500 mg of *Saccharomyces boulardii* twice daily enhanced the effectiveness of the antibiotic vancomycin in preventing recurrent clostridium infection.[6] Therefore, people taking antibiotics who later develop diarrhea might benefit from supplementing with saccharomyces organisms.

Treatment with antibiotics also commonly leads to an overgrowth of yeast *(Candida albicans)* in the vagina (candida vaginitis) and the intestines (sometimes referred to as "dysbiosis"). Controlled studies have shown that *Lactobacillus acidophilus* might prevent candida vaginitis.[7]

Vitamin K
Several cases of excessive bleeding have been reported in people who take antibiotics.[8, 9, 10, 11] This side effect may be the result of reduced vitamin K activity and/or reduced vitamin K production by bacteria in the colon. One study showed that people who had taken broad-spectrum antibiotics had lower liver concentrations of vitamin K_2 (menaquinone), though vitamin K_1 (phylloquinone) levels remained normal.[12] Several antibiotics appear to exert a strong effect on vitamin K activity, while others may not have any effect. Therefore, one should refer to a specific antibiotic for information on whether it interacts with vitamin K. Doctors of natural medicine sometimes recommend vitamin K supplementation to people taking antibiotics. Additional research is needed to determine whether the amount of

vitamin K_1 found in some multivitamins is sufficient to prevent antibiotic-induced bleeding. Moreover, most multivitamins do not contain vitamin K.

Interactions with Foods and Other Compounds
Food
Penicillin V should be taken at least one hour before or two hours after eating.[13, 14]

PENICILLINS

Common names: Bacampicillin, Bactocil, Bicillin C-R, Bicillin L-A, Carbenicillin, Clavulanate, Cloxacillin, Cloxapen, Geocillin, Mezlin, Mezlocillin, Nafcillin, Oxacillin, Penicillin G, Pfizerpen, Piperacillin, Pipracil, Spectrobid, Sulbactam, Tazobactam, Ticarcillin, Ticar, Unipen

Penicillins are a family of **antibiotics** (page 19) used to treat a wide variety of bacterial infections occurring in the body. Each drug within the family kills specific bacteria; therefore, healthcare practitioners prescribe penicillins based on the individual's current needs.

There are interactions that are common to **antibacterial drugs** (page 19) in general and interactions involving a specific penicillin drug. For the latter interactions, refer to the highlighted drugs listed below.

- **Amoxicillin** (page 13) (Amoxil, Trimox)
- Amoxicillin and Clavulanate (Augmentin)
- **Ampicillin** (page 15) (Principen, Totacillin)
- Ampicillin and Sulbactam (Unisyn)
- Bacampicillin (Spectrobid)
- Carbenicillin (Geocillin)
- Cloxacillin (Cloxapen)
- **Dicloxacillin** (page 88) (Dynapen, Dycill)
- Mezlocillin (Mezlin)
- Nafcillin (Unipen)
- Oxacillin (Bactocill)
- Penicillin G (Bicillin C-R, Bicillin L-A, Pfizerpen)
- **Penicillin V** (page 210) (Beepen-VK, Veetids)
- Piperacillin (Pipracil)
- Piperacillin and Tazobactam (Zosyn)
- Ticarcillin (Ticar)
- Ticarcillin and Clavulanate (Timentin)

Summary of Interactions for Penicillins
In some cases, an herb or supplement may appear in more than one category, which may seem contradictory. For clarification, read the full article for details about the summarized interactions.

Penicillins

✓ May be Beneficial: Depletion or interference	Vitamin K*
✓ May be Beneficial: Side effect reduction/prevention	Bifidobacterium longum* Lactobacillus acidophilus* Lactobacillus casei* Saccharomyces boulardii* Saccharomyces cerevisiae* Vitamin K
✓ May be Beneficial: Supportive interaction	Saccharomyces boulardii*
Reduced drug absorption/bioavailability	None known
Adverse interaction	None known

Interactions common to many, if not all, Penicillins are described in this article. Interactions reported for only one or several drugs in this class may not be listed in this article. Some drugs listed in this article are linked to articles specific to that respective drug; please refer to those individual drug articles. The information in this article may not necessarily apply to drugs in this class for which no separate article exists. If you are taking a Penicillin for which no separate article exists, talk with your doctor or pharmacist.

Interactions with Dietary Supplements

Probiotics

A common side effect of antibiotics is diarrhea, which may be caused by the elimination of beneficial bacteria normally found in the colon. Controlled studies have shown that taking probiotic microorganisms—such as *Lactobacillus casei, Lactobacillus acidophilus, Bifidobacterium longum,* or *Saccharomyces boulardii*—helps prevent antibiotic-induced diarrhea.[1]

The diarrhea experienced by some people who take antibiotics also might be due to an overgrowth of the bacterium *Clostridium difficile*, which causes a disease known as pseudomembranous colitis. Controlled studies have shown that supplementation with harmless yeast—such as *Saccharomyces boulardii*[2] or *Saccharomyces cerevisiae* (baker's or brewer's yeast)[3]—helps prevent recurrence of this infection. In one study, taking 500 mg of *Saccharomyces boulardii* twice daily enhanced the effectiveness of the antibiotic vancomycin in preventing recurrent clostridium infection.[4] Therefore, people taking antibiotics who later develop diarrhea might benefit from supplementing with saccharomyces organisms.

Treatment with antibiotics also commonly leads to an overgrowth of yeast (*Candida albicans*) in the vagina (candida vaginitis) and the intestines (sometimes referred to as "dysbiosis"). Controlled studies have shown that *Lactobacillus acidophilus* might prevent candida vaginitis.[5]

Vitamin K

Several cases of excessive bleeding have been reported in people who take antibiotics.[6, 7, 8, 9] This side effect may be the result of reduced vitamin K activity and/or reduced vitamin K production by bacteria in the colon. One study showed that people who had taken broad-spectrum antibiotics had lower liver concentrations of vitamin K_2 (menaquinone), though vitamin K_1 (phylloquinone) levels remained normal.[10] Several antibiotics appear to exert a strong effect on vitamin K activity, while others may not have any effect. Therefore, one should refer to a specific antibiotic for information on whether it interacts with vitamin K. Doctors of natural medicine sometimes recommend vitamin K supplementation to people taking antibiotics. Additional research is needed to determine whether the amount of vitamin K_1 found in some multivitamins is sufficient to prevent antibiotic-induced bleeding. Moreover, most multivitamins do not contain vitamin K.

PENTOXIFYLLINE

Common names: Albert Pentoxifylline, Apo-Pentoxifylline, Nu-Pentoxifylline-SR, Oxpentifylline, Pentoxil, Trental

Pentoxifylline decreases blood thickness and improves red blood cell flexibility. Pentoxifylline is used to improve symptoms of intermittent claudication and in the treatment of other circulatory disorders.

Summary of Interactions for Pentoxifylline

In some cases, an herb or supplement may appear in more than one category, which may seem contradictory. For clarification, read the full article for details about the summarized interactions.

✓ May be Beneficial: Supportive interaction	Vitamin E
Depletion or interference	None known
Side effect reduction/prevention	None known
Reduced drug absorption/bioavailability	None known
Adverse interaction	None known

Interactions with Dietary Supplements

Vitamin E

The combination of vitamin E and pentoxifylline has been used successfully to reduce damage to normal tissues caused by radiation therapy.[1]

Interactions with Foods and Other Compounds

Food

Pentoxifylline should be taken with meals.[2]

PERCOCET

Contains the following ingredients:
Acetaminophen (page 3)
Oxycodone (page 205)

PERCODAN

Contains the following ingredients:
Aspirin (page 26)
Oxycodone (page 205)

PERPHENAZINE

Common names: Trilafon

Combination drug: Triavil, Etrafon

Perphenazine is used to treat symptoms associated with psychiatric disorders, as well as severe nausea and vomiting in adults. It is in a class of drugs known as phenothiazine neuroleptics.

Summary of Interactions for Perphenazine

In some cases, an herb or supplement may appear in more than one category, which may seem contradictory. For clarification, read the full article for details about the summarized interactions.

✓ May be Beneficial: Side effect reduction/prevention	Coenzyme Q₁₀*
⊘ Avoid: Adverse interaction	Bacopa **Lithium** (page 157)*
ⓘ Check: Other	Vitamin C*
Depletion or interference	None known
Supportive interaction	None known
Reduced drug absorption/bioavailability	None known

Interactions with Dietary Supplements

Lithium *(page 157)*

Lithium is a mineral that may be present in some supplements and is also used in large amounts to treat mood disorders such as bipolar disorder (manic depression). Taking lithium medication at the same time as phenothiazine drugs might increase the risk of nerve damage resulting in delirium and seizures.[1, 2] Controlled research is needed to determine whether combining perphenazine and with the comparatively small amounts of lithium found in non-prescription supplements might cause similar side effects. Until more information is available, people taking perphenazine should exercise caution when supplementing with products that contain lithium.

Coenzyme Q₁₀

Phenothiazine drugs similar to perphenazine can cause changes in heart activity in some people, which might be prevented by supplementing with coenzyme Q₁₀.[3, 4] Therefore, some health practitioners may recommend coenzyme Q₁₀ supplementation to people taking perphenazine.

Vitamin C

Taking phenothiazine drugs can stop menstruation in some women. Two women taking phenothiazines similar to perphenazine began menstruating following supplementation with 6 grams of vitamin C each day.[5] Controlled studies are needed to determine whether vitamin C supplementation might benefit women specifically taking perphenazine who are experiencing menstrual changes. Some health practitioners recommend vitamin C supplementation to women who stop menstruating while taking perphenazine. Vitamin C might also enhance the effectiveness of neuroleptic drugs such as perphenazine in the treatment of schizophrenia. One uncontrolled study showed that 10 of 13 individuals experienced a reduction in disorganized thoughts, hallucinations, and suspicious thoughts when 8 grams of vitamin C was added to their daily drug therapy.[6] Controlled studies are needed to show whether people taking perphenazine for schizophrenia might benefit from vitamin C supplementation.

Interactions with Herbs

Bacopa

An animal study found that the effects of chlorpromazine, a drug similar to (perphenazine, prochlorperazine, thioridazine), were enhanced when a bacopa extract was given along with it.[7] Until more is known, people taking medications from this family of drugs (called phenothiazines) should not take bacopa.

Interactions with Foods and Other Compounds
Alcohol

Taking perphenazine and alcohol together may enhance the side effects of alcohol, such as drowsiness and dizziness, and might increase the risk of suicide.[8] Consequently, people who are taking perphenazine should avoid alcohol.

PHENAZOPYRIDINE

Common names: Azo Standard Tablet, Azo-100, Phenazo, Pyridiate, Pyridium, Urodine, Urogesic

Phenazopyridine is an analgesic used to treat minor pain, burning, and urinary urgency and frequency resulting from urinary tract infections.

Summary of Interactions for Phenazopyridine

In some cases, an herb or supplement may appear in more than one category, which may seem contradictory. For clarification, read the full article for details about the summarized interactions.

Depletion or interference	None known
Side effect reduction/prevention	None known
Supportive interaction	None known
Reduced drug absorption/bioavailability	None known
Adverse interaction	None known

Interactions with Foods and Other Compounds
Food

Phenazopyridine should be taken with food to prevent stomach and intestinal upset.[1]

PHENELZINE

Common names: Nardil

Phenelzine is a member of a group of drugs called monoamine oxidase (MAO) inhibitors (also called MAOIs). Phenelzine is sometimes used to treat people with depression who do not respond to other antidepressant drug therapy.

Summary of Interactions for Phenelzine

In some cases, an herb or supplement may appear in more than one category, which may seem contradictory.

For clarification, read the full article for details about the summarized interactions.

✓	May be Beneficial: Depletion or interference	Vitamin B$_6$
🚫	Avoid: Adverse interaction	Aspartame* Ephedra* Ginseng (species not specified)* Scotch broom St. John's wort* Tyramine-containing foods
	Side effect reduction/prevention	None known
	Supportive interaction	None known
	Reduced drug absorption/bioavailability	None known

Interactions with Dietary Supplements
Vitamin B$_6$

Phenelzine has a chemical structure similar to other drugs (**isoniazid** [page 146] and **hydralazine** [page 136]) that can cause vitamin B$_6$ deficiency. One case of phenelzine-induced vitamin B$_6$ deficiency has been reported.[1] Little is known about this interaction. People taking phenelzine should ask their doctor about monitoring vitamin B$_6$ levels and considering supplementation.

Interactions with Herbs
Ephedra

Ephedra contains the chemical **ephedrine** (page 104), which may interact with phenelzine, causing potentially dangerous changes to blood pressure.[2] People should read product labels for ephedra/ephedrine content. Ephedra and ephedrine-containing products should be avoided during phenelzine therapy. People with questions about phenelzine and ephedra/ephedrine should ask their doctor or pharmacist.

Ginseng (species not specified)

In a case report of a woman treated with phenelzine, addition of a ginseng-containing tea was associated with insomnia, headache, and tremor.[3] Other contents of the tea were not reported. In a case report of a woman treated with phenelzine for depression, addition of ginseng (not further identified) was associated with hypomania (a mild form of mania), which the patient had not previously experienced.[4] Until more is known, people should combine ginseng and phenelzine with caution after consulting a knowledgeable doctor.

St. John's wort (Hypericum perforatum)
Although St. John's wort contains chemicals that bind MAO in test tubes, it is believed that the action of St. John's wort is not due to MAOI activity.[5] However, because St. John's wort may have serotonin reuptake inhibiting action (similar to the action of drugs such as Prozac, it is best to avoid concomitant use of St. John's wort with MAOI drugs.

Scotch broom (Cytisus scoparius)
Scotch broom contains high levels of tyramine. Combining phenelzine and Scotch broom may cause MAOI-type reactions (diarrhea, flushing, sweating, pounding chest, dangerous changes in blood pressure, and other symptoms).[6] It is important for people taking phenelzine to avoid Scotch broom. People with questions about phenelzine and Scotch broom should ask their doctor.

Interactions with Foods and Other Compounds
Tyramine-containing foods
Phenelzine can alter metabolism of a chemical called tyramine that is present in certain foods, leading to diarrhea, flushing, sweating, pounding chest, dangerous changes in blood pressure, and other symptoms.[7] It is important for people taking phenelzine to avoid tyramine-containing foods. People with questions about phenelzine and tyramine-containing foods should ask their doctor or pharmacist.

Aspartame
Two cases were reported involving men treated with phenelzine who experienced restlessness, agitation, tremor, and insomnia after drinking large quantities of cola beverages containing aspartame.[8] Until more is known, people taking phenelzine should use aspartame-containing foods with caution.

PHENERGAN WITH CODEINE

Contains the following ingredients:
Codeine (page 75)
Promethazine (page 223)

PHENERGAN VC

Contains the following ingredients:
Phenylephrine
Promethazine (page 223)

PHENERGAN VC WITH CODEINE

Contains the following ingredients:
Codeine (page 75)
Phenylephrine
Promethazine (page 223)

PHENOBARBITAL

Common names: Phenobarbitone

Phenobarbital is occasionally used as a sedative before surgery, as a hypnotic (sleeping pill) to treat insomnia, and as an **anticonvulsant** (page 21) to prevent and treat seizure disorders. Phenobarbital is classified as a **barbiturate** (page 34).

Summary of Interactions for Phenobarbital
In some cases, an herb or supplement may appear in more than one category, which may seem contradictory. For clarification, read the full article for details about the summarized interactions.

✓ May be Beneficial: Depletion or interference	Biotin Calcium Folic acid L-carnitine Vitamin A* Vitamin B$_{12}$* Vitamin B$_6$* Vitamin D Vitamin K*
✓ May be Beneficial: Side effect reduction/prevention	Folic acid* L-carnitine* Vitamin B$_{12}$* Vitamin D* Vitamin K*
✓ May be Beneficial: Supportive interaction	Folic acid*
⊘ Avoid: Reduced drug absorption/bioavailability	Vitamin B$_6$
⊘ Avoid: Adverse interaction	Alcohol Folic acid*

Interaction with Dietary Supplements
Biotin
One controlled study showed that long-term use of phenobarbital increases the breakdown of biotin.[1] A

test tube study also showed that primidone, a drug that is converted to phenobarbital by the body, prevents the absorption of biotin.[2] Further research is needed to determine whether people taking phenobarbital might be at risk for biotin deficiency.

Calcium

Individuals on long-term multiple anticonvulsant therapy may develop below-normal blood levels of calcium, which may be related to drug-induced vitamin D deficiency.[3] Two infants born to women taking high doses of phenytoin and phenobarbital while pregnant developed jitteriness and tetany (a syndrome characterized by muscle twitches), cramps, and spasms that can be caused by calcium deficiency during the first two weeks of life.[4] Controlled research is needed to determine whether pregnant women who are taking anticonvulsant medications should supplement with additional amounts of calcium and vitamin D.

L-carnitine

One controlled study showed that taking phenobarbital resulted in reduced blood levels of L-carnitine.[5] Further research is needed to determine whether people taking phenobarbital might benefit from supplemental L-carnitine. Based on the currently available information, some healthcare practitioners may recommend monitoring L-carnitine blood levels or supplementing with L-carnitine.

Folic acid

Long-term treatment with phenobarbital results in dramatic reductions in folic acid blood levels, though the clinical significance of this effect is unclear.[6] Nevertheless, some healthcare practitioners might recommend supplemental folic acid to individuals taking phenobarbital.

One preliminary study showed that pregnant women who use anticonvulsant drugs without folic acid supplementation have an increased risk of having a child with birth defects, such as heart defects, cleft lip and palate, neural tube defects, and skeletal abnormalities. However, supplementation with folic acid greatly reduces the risk.[7] Consequently, some healthcare practitioners recommend that women taking multiple anticonvulsant drugs supplement with 5 mg of folic acid daily, for three months prior to conception and during the first trimester, to prevent folic acid deficiency-induced birth defects.[8] Other practitioners suggest that 1 mg or less of folic acid each day is sufficient to prevent deficiency during pregnancy.[9]

One well-controlled study showed that adding folic acid to multiple anticonvulsant therapy resulted in reduced seizure frequency.[10] In addition, three infants with seizures who were unresponsive to medication experienced immediate relief following supplementation with the active form of folic acid.[11]

Despite the apparent beneficial effects, some studies have indicated that as little as 0.8 mg of folic acid taken daily can increase the frequency and/or severity of seizures.[12, 13, 14, 15] However, a recent controlled study showed that both healthy and epileptic women taking less than 1 mg of folic acid per day had no increased risk for seizures.[16] Until more is known about the risks and benefits of folic acid, individuals taking multiple anticonvulsant drugs should consult with their healthcare practitioner before supplementing with folic acid. In addition, pregnant women or women who might become pregnant while taking anticonvulsant drugs should discuss folic acid supplementation with their practitioner.

Vitamin A

Anticonvulsant drugs can occasionally cause birth defects when taken by pregnant women, and their toxicity might be related to low blood levels of vitamin A. One controlled study showed that taking multiple anticonvulsant drugs results in dramatic changes in the way the body utilizes vitamin A.[17] Further controlled research is needed to determine whether supplemental vitamin A might prevent birth defects in children born to women on multiple anticonvulsant therapy. Other research suggests that ingestion of large amounts of vitamin A may promote the development of birth defects, although the studies are conflicting.

Vitamin B_6

One controlled study revealed that supplementing with 200 mg of vitamin B_6 daily for four weeks resulted in a 45% reduction in phenobarbital blood levels.[18] Therefore, people taking phenobarbital should probably avoid supplementing with large amounts of vitamin B_6.

One controlled study revealed that taking anticonvulsant drugs dramatically reduces blood levels of vitamin B_6.[19] A nutritional deficiency of vitamin B_6 can lead to an increase in homocysteine blood levels, which has been associated with atherosclerosis. Vitamin B_6 deficiency is also associated with symptoms such as dizziness, fatigue, mental depression, and seizures. People taking multiple anticonvulsant drugs should discuss with their doctor whether supplementing with vitamin B_6 is advisable.

Vitamin B₁₂

Anemia is an uncommon side effect experienced by people taking anticonvulsant drugs. Though the cause may be folic acid deficiency in many cases, a deficiency of vitamin B_{12} may also be a factor in some instances. Deficiencies of folic acid and vitamin B_{12} can lead to nerve and mental problems. One study revealed that individuals on long-term anticonvulsant therapy, despite having no laboratory signs of anemia, had dramatically lower levels of vitamin B_{12} in their cerebrospinal fluid (the fluid that bathes the brain) when compared with people who were not taking seizure medications. Improvement in mental status and nerve function was observed in a majority of symptomatic individuals after taking 30 mcg of vitamin B_{12} daily for a few days.[20] Another study found that long-term anticonvulsant therapy had no effect on blood levels of vitamin B_{12}.[21] Despite these contradictory findings, people taking anticonvulsant drugs for several months or years might prevent nerve and mental problems by supplementing with vitamin B_{12}.

Vitamin D

Though research results vary, long-term use of anticonvulsant drugs appears to interfere with vitamin D activity, which might lead to softening of bones (osteomalacia). One study showed that blood levels of vitamin D in males taking anticonvulsants were lower than those found in men who were not taking seizure medication.[22] In a controlled study, bone strength improved in children taking anticonvulsant drugs who were supplemented with the activated form of vitamin D and 500 mg per day of calcium for nine months.[23] Some research suggests that differences in exposure to sunlight—which normally increases blood levels of vitamin D—might explain why some studies have failed to find a beneficial effect of vitamin D supplementation. In one controlled study, blood vitamin D levels in children taking anticonvulsants were dramatically lower in winter months than in summer months.[24] Another study of 450 people in Florida taking anticonvulsants found that few had drug-induced bone disease.[25] Consequently, people taking anticonvulsant drugs who do not receive adequate sunlight should supplement with 400 IU of vitamin D each day to help prevent osteomalacia.

Vitamin E

Two studies showed that individuals taking phenytoin and phenobarbital had lower blood vitamin E levels than those who received no treatment for seizures.[26, 27] Though the consequences of lower blood levels of vitamin E are unknown, people taking multiple anticonvulsant drugs should probably supplement with 100 to 200 IU of vitamin E daily to prevent a deficiency.

Vitamin K

Some studies have shown that babies born to women taking anticonvulsant drugs have low blood levels of vitamin K, which might cause bleeding in the infant.[28] Though some researchers recommend vitamin K supplementation prior to delivery,[29, 30] not all agree that supplementation for women taking anticonvulsant drugs is necessary.[31] Until more information is available, pregnant women or women who might become pregnant while taking anticonvulsant drugs should discuss vitamin K supplementation with their healthcare practitioner.

Interaction with Food and Other Compounds

Alcohol

Drinking alcoholic beverages while taking phenobarbital enhances side effects such as drowsiness, confusion, and dizziness.[32] Consequently, people taking barbiturates should avoid drinking alcohol, especially when they must stay alert.

PHENTERMINE

Common names: Adipex-P, Duromine, Fastin, Ionamin, Obenix, Obephen, Obermine, Obestin, Phentamine, Phentride, T-Diet, Zantril

Phentermine is a nonamphetamine drug used as a short-term adjunct to calorie restriction for weight loss. Phentermine is available in two forms, phentermine hydrochloride (Fastin and others) and phentermine resin (Ionamin and others).

Summary of Interactions for Phentermine

In some cases, an herb or supplement may appear in more than one category, which may seem contradictory. For clarification, read the full article for details about the summarized interactions.

Depletion or interference	None known
Side effect reduction/prevention	None known
Supportive interaction	None known
Reduced drug absorption/bioavailability	None known
Adverse interaction	None known

Interactions with Foods and Other Compounds
Food

Phentermine should be taken on an empty stomach.[1]

Alcohol

Phentermine may cause dizziness or blurred vision.[2] Alcohol may intensify these effects, increasing the risk for accidental injury. People taking phentermine should avoid alcohol.

PHENYLPROPANOLAMINE

Common names: Acutrim, Dex-A-Diet, Dexatrim, Phenldrine, Phenoxine, PPA, Propagest, Rhindecon, Unitrol

Combination drugs: Ami-Tex LA, Appedrine, Contac 12 Hour, DayQuil Allergy Relief, Dex-A-Diet Plus Vitamin C, Diadex Grapefruit Diet Plan, Dimetapp, Entex LA, Robitussin CF, Tavist-D, Triaminic-12

Phenylpropanolamine is a drug used to relieve nasal congestion due to colds, hay fever, upper respiratory allergies, and sinusitis. It is available in nonprescription products alone and in combination with other nonprescription drugs, to treat symptoms of allergy, colds, and upper respiratory infections. Phenylpropanolamine is also used as an adjunct to calorie restriction in short-term weight loss. It is available in nonprescription products alone and in combination with other ingredients for weight loss.

The Food and Drug Administration (FDA) has taken steps to remove phenylpropanolamine from all drug products and has issued a public health advisory concerning phenylpropanolamine hydrochloride. This drug is an ingredient used in many over-the-counter (OTC) and prescription cough and cold medications as a decongestant and in OTC weight loss products. PPA has been found to increase the risk of hemorrhagic stroke (bleeding into the brain or into tissue surrounding the brain) in women. Men may also be at risk. Although the risk of hemorrhagic stroke is very low, the FDA recommends that consumers not use any products that contain PPA.

Summary of Interactions for Phenylpropanolamine

In some cases, an herb or supplement may appear in more than one category, which may seem contradictory. For clarification, read the full article for details about the summarized interactions.

⊘ Avoid: Adverse interaction	**Caffeine** (page 44) Ephedra*
Depletion or interference	None known
Side effect reduction/prevention	None known
Supportive interaction	None known
Reduced drug absorption/bioavailability	None known

Interactions with Herbs
Ephedra

Ephedra is the plant from which the drug **ephedrine** (page 104) was originally isolated. Phenylpropanolamine and ephedrine have similar effects and side effects.[1] Until 2004, ephedra, also called ma huang, was used in many herbal products including supplements promoted for weight loss.

While interactions between phenylpropanolamine and ephedra have not been reported, it seems likely that such interactions could occur. To prevent potential problems, people taking phenylpropanolamine-containing products should avoid using ephedra/ephedrine-containing products.

Interactions with Foods and Other Compounds
Caffeine (page 44)

Phenylpropanolamine can increase blood pressure,[2] a danger especially in people with high blood pressure.[3] In a double-blind study of six healthy people, administration of caffeine and phenylpropanolamine produced an additive increase in blood pressure.[4] Additionally, in a study of 16 healthy people, phenylpropanolamine plus caffeine resulted in higher serum caffeine levels than when caffeine was given alone.[5]

Caffeine is found in coffee, tea, soft drinks, chocolate, guaraná (*Paullinia cupana*), nonprescription drugs, and supplement products containing caffeine or guaraná. People taking phenylpropanolamine-containing products can minimize the interaction with caffeine by limiting or avoiding caffeine.

PHRENILIN

Contains the following ingredients:
    Acetaminophen (page 3)
    Butalbital (page 44)

PIROXICAM

Common names: Alti-Piroxicam, Apo-Piroxicam, Feldene, Fexicam, Flamatrol, Gen-Piroxicam, Kentene, Larapam, Novo-Pirocam, Nu-Pirox, Pirozip

Piroxicam is used to treat rheumatoid arthritis and osteoarthritis. It is in a class of medications known as **nonsteroidal anti-inflammatory drugs** (page 193) (NSAIDs).

Summary of Interactions for Piroxicam

In some cases, an herb or supplement may appear in more than one category, which may seem contradictory. For clarification, read the full article for details about the summarized interactions.

⊘ Avoid: Adverse interaction	Lithium* Potassium*
ⓘ Check: Other	Folic acid* Willow*
Depletion or interference	None known
Side effect reduction/prevention	None known
Supportive interaction	None known
Reduced drug absorption/bioavailability	None known

Interactions with Dietary Supplements

Potassium

An 85-year-old man developed higher than normal blood levels of potassium following several months of treatment with piroxicam.[1] Until more is known, people taking piroxicam for long periods should have their blood checked regularly for high potassium levels and may need to avoid high potassium intake with the guidance of a health practitioner.

Folic acid

Piroxicam may prevent inflammation by blocking the activity of enzymes that depend on folic acid.[2] However, other studies show that people taking NSAIDs such as **aspirin** (page 26) have lower than normal levels of folic acid in their red blood cells.[3] Further research is needed to determine whether supplemental folic acid prevents a deficiency of the vitamin or indirectly reduces the beneficial effects of piroxicam.

Lithium (page 157)

Lithium is a mineral that is present in some supplements and is also used in large amounts to treat mood disorders such as bipolar disorder (manic depression). Blood levels of lithium may increase in people taking NSAIDs and lithium supplements together (compared with lithium alone),[4] possibly resulting in unwanted side effects such as diarrhea, nausea, muscle weakness, and lack of coordination. More research is needed to determine whether piroxicam specifically increases lithium blood levels. Until more is known, people should avoid lithium supplementation except when it is prescribed by a doctor.

Interactions with Herbs

White willow bark (Salix alba)

White willow bark contains salicin, which is related to **aspirin** (page 26). Both salicin and aspirin produce anti-inflammatory effects after they have been converted to salicylic acid in the body. Taking aspirin significantly lowers blood levels of piroxicam and increases the potential for adverse side effects.[5] Though no studies have investigated interactions between willow bark and piroxicam, people taking the drug should avoid the herb until more information is available.

Interactions with Foods and Other Compounds

Food

Taking piroxicam with a meal may delay the speed, but not the overall amount, of drug absorption.[6] Therefore, it may be taken with food if stomach upset occurs when taking the drug on an empty stomach.

POTASSIUM CHLORIDE

Common names: Apo-K, K-10, K-Dur, Kaochlor, Klor-Con, Klorvess, Roychlor, Slow-K

Potassium chloride is a prescription drug used to replace potassium in people with low blood levels of potassium, to prevent potassium depletion in specific diseases or resulting from specific drug therapies, and to help lower mild high blood pressure in some people. Potassium chloride is also available without prescription in some supplements and in salt substitutes found in grocery stores. While potassium depletion is a health risk, high levels of potassium are also associated with health risks. Potassium-containing drugs should be used only under medical supervision. The potassium found in fruit is both safe and healthful for most people, except those taking potassium-sparing diuretic drugs (page 94) and individuals with kidney failure.

Summary of Interactions for Potassium Chloride

In some cases, an herb or supplement may appear in more than one category, which may seem contradictory. For clarification, read the full article for details about the summarized interactions.

ⓘ Check: Other	Digitalis Salt substitutes
Depletion or interference	None known
Side effect reduction/prevention	None known
Supportive interaction	None known
Reduced drug absorption/bioavailability	None known
Adverse interaction	None known

Interactions with Dietary Supplements
Salt substitutes

Salt substitutes (No Salt, Salt Substitute, Lite Salt, and others) contain potassium chloride in place of sodium chloride. They are used by people on sodium-restricted diets. When used in moderation, they are a more healthful choice for many people compared with using regular table salt. However, people taking potassium chloride drug products should consult with their prescribing doctor before using salt substitutes[1] or even eating large amounts of high-potassium foods (primarily fruit).

Interactions with Herbs
Digitalis (Digitalis lanata, Digitalis purpurea)

Digitalis refers to a family of plants commonly called foxglove that contain digitalis glycosides, chemicals with actions and toxicities similar to the prescription drug **digoxin** (page 90). Low serum potassium increases the risk of digitalis toxicity.[2] People using digitalis-containing products should have their potassium status monitored by the healthcare professional overseeing the digitalis therapy.

Interactions with Foods and Other Compounds
Food

Potassium chloride drugs should be taken after meals to avoid stomach upset.[3] Potassium-containing salt substitutes, however, are meant to be taken with food. Tablets should be swallowed whole and chewing or crushing should be avoided.[4] Liquid, powder, and ef-

fervescent potassium chloride products may be dissolved in a glass of cold water or juice to mask the unpleasant flavor.[5]

PRAMIPEXOLE

Common names: Mirapexin, Mirapex

Pramipexole is used to treat the signs and symptoms of Parkinson's disease.

Summary of Interactions for Pramipexole

In some cases, an herb or supplement may appear in more than one category, which may seem contradictory. For clarification, read the full article for details about the summarized interactions.

⊘ Avoid: Adverse interaction	Alcohol
Depletion or interference	None known
Side effect reduction/prevention	None known
Supportive interaction	None known
Reduced drug absorption/bioavailability	None known

Interaction with Food and Other Compounds
Alcohol

Drinking alcoholic beverages with pramipexole can increase the amount of drowsiness caused by the drug.[1] Consequently, people taking pramipexole should avoid drinking alcohol, especially when they must stay alert.

PRAVASTATIN

Common names: Pravachol

Pravastatin is a member of the HMG-CoA reductase inhibitor family of drugs, also called "statins," such as **lovastatin** (page 163) and **simvastatin** (page 239). Pravastatin blocks a key step in the body's production of cholesterol and is used to lower cholesterol levels in people with hypercholesterolemia (high cholesterol).

Summary of Interactions for Pravastatin

In some cases, an herb or supplement may appear in more than one category, which may seem contradictory. For clarification, read the full article for details about the summarized interactions.

✓ May be Beneficial: Depletion or interference	Coenzyme Q₁₀
✓ May be Beneficial: Side effect reduction/prevention	Milk thistle*
✓ May be Beneficial: Supportive interaction	Fish oil (EPA)
⊘ Avoid: Adverse interaction	Red yeast rice*
ⓘ Check: Other	Vitamin A Vitamin B₃ (niacin)
Reduced drug absorption/bioavailability	None known

Interactions with Dietary Supplements

Coenzyme Q₁₀

In double-blind trials, treatment with pravastatin and other HMG-CoA reductase inhibitors has resulted in depleted blood levels of coenzyme Q_{10} (CoQ_{10}).[1, 2] Supplementation with 90–100 mg CoQ_{10} per day has been shown to prevent reductions in blood levels of CoQ_{10} due to **simvastatin** (page 239), another drug in the same category as pravastatin.[3, 4] However, some investigators have questioned whether it is worthwhile or necessary for individuals taking HMG-CoA reductase inhibitors to supplement with CoQ_{10}.[5] Until more is known, people taking pravastatin should ask a doctor about supplementation with 30–100 mg CoQ_{10} per day.

Fish oil

The omega-3 fatty acid EPA present in fish oil may improve the cholesterol and triglyceride-lowering effect of pravastatin. In a preliminary trial, people with high cholesterol who had been taking pravastatin for about three years were able to significantly lower their triglyceride levels and raise their levels of HDL ("good") cholesterol by supplementing with either 900 mg or 1,800 mg of EPA for three months in addition to pravastatin.[6] The authors of the study concluded that the combination of pravastatin and EPA may prevent coronary heart disease better than pravastatin alone.

Vitamin B₃ (niacin, nicotinic acid)

Niacin is a vitamin used to lower cholesterol. Sixteen people with diabetes and high cholesterol were given pravastatin plus niacin to lower cholesterol.[7] Niacin was added over a two week period, to a maximum amount of 500 mg three times per day. The combination of pravastatin plus niacin was continued for four weeks. Compared with pravastatin, niacin plus pravastatin resulted in significantly reduced cholesterol levels. Others have also shown that the combination of pravastatin and niacin is more effective in lowering cholesterol levels than is pravastatin alone.[8] However, large amounts of niacin taken with pravastatin might cause serious muscle disorders (myopathy or rhabdomyolysis).[9] Individuals taking pravastatin should consult a doctor before taking niacin.

Red yeast rice (Monascus purpureas)

A supplement containing red yeast rice (*Monascus purpureas*) (Cholestin) has been shown to effectively lower cholesterol and triglycerides in people with moderately elevated levels of these blood lipids.[10] This extract contains small amounts of naturally occurring HMG-CoA reductase inhibitors such as **lovastatin** (page 163) and should not be used by people who are currently taking lovastatin or pravastatin.

Vitamin A

A study of 37 people with high cholesterol treated with diet and HMG-CoA reductase inhibitors found serum vitamin A levels increased over two years of therapy.[11] It remains unclear whether this moderate increase suggests that people taking lovastatin have a particular need to restrict vitamin A supplementation.

Interactions with Herbs

Milk thistle (Silybum marianum)

One of the possible side effects of pravastatin is liver toxicity. Although no clinical studies substantiate its use with pravastatin, a milk thistle extract standardized to 70–80% silymarin may reduce the potential liver toxicity of pravastatin. The suggested use is 200 mg of the extract three times daily.

Interactions with Foods and Other Compounds

Food

Pravastatin may be taken with or without food.[12]

Grapefruit juice

While grapefruit juice is known to increase levels of **lovastatin** (page 163)[13] and some other statin drugs, this interaction does not occur between grapefruit juice and pravastatin.[14] It appears, therefore, that people taking pravastatin can safely consume grapefruit or grapefruit juice.

PRAZOSIN

Common names: Alti-Prazosin, Apo-Prazo, Minipress, Novo-Prazin, Nu-Prazo

Prazosin is a member of the alpha blocker family of drugs used to lower blood pressure in people with hypertension. Prazosin is also used to treat some instances of heart failure.

Summary of Interactions for Prazosin

In some cases, an herb or supplement may appear in more than one category, which may seem contradictory. For clarification, read the full article for details about the summarized interactions.

Depletion or interference	None known
Side effect reduction/prevention	None known
Supportive interaction	None known
Reduced drug absorption/bioavailability	None known
Adverse interaction	None known

Interactions with Foods and Other Compounds

Food
Prazosin may be taken with or without food.[1]

PREMIQUE

Contains the following ingredients:
Conjugated estrogens (page 109)
Medroxyprogesterone (page 167)

PREMIUMS

Contains the following ingredients:
Aluminium
Calcium
Magnesium
Peppermint oil

PREMPAK-C

Contains the following ingredients:
Conjugated estrogens (page 109)
Norgestrel

PREMPRO

Contains the following ingredients:
Conjugated estrogens (page 109)
Medroxyprogesterone (page 167)

PRESTIM

Contains the following ingredients:
Bendroflumethiazide
Timolol (page 263)

PRIMATENE DUAL ACTION

Contains the following ingredients:
Ephedrine (page 104)
Guaifenesin (page 133)
Theophylline (page 256)

PRINIZIDE

Contains the following ingredients:
Hydrochlorothiazide
Lisinopril (page 156)

PROCHLORPERAZINE

Common names: Buccastem, Compazine, Stemetil

Prochlorperazine is used to treat severe nausea and vomiting. It is also used to treat symptoms of psychosis, such as delusions, hallucinations, disorganized thinking and speech, and bizarre behavior. Prochlorperazine is in a class of drugs known as phenothiazines.

Summary of Interactions for Prochlorperazine

In some cases, an herb or supplement may appear in more than one category, which may seem contradictory. For clarification, read the full article for details about the summarized interactions.

⊘ Avoid: Reduced drug absorption/ bioavailability	**Antacids** (page 18)
⊘ Avoid: Adverse interaction	Alcohol Bacopa **Lithium** (page 157) (prescription) Lithium (supplements)
Depletion or interference	None known
Side effect reduction/prevention	None known
Supportive interaction	None known

Interactions with Dietary Supplements
Lithium (page 157)
Lithium is a mineral that may be present in some supplements and is also used in large amounts to treat mood disorders, such as bipolar disorder. Taking lithium at the same time as phenothiazines may result in drug side effects such as disorientation and unconsciousness.[1] Though no studies have investigated whether the small amount of lithium available in supplements might interact with prochlorperazine to cause similar effects, people taking the drug should exercise caution when supplementing with lithium.

Interactions with Herbs
Bacopa
An animal study found that the effects of chlorpromazine, a drug similar to (perphenazine, prochlorperazine, thioridazine), were enhanced when a bacopa extract was given along with it.[2] Until more is known, people taking medications from this family of drugs (called phenothiazines) should not take bacopa.

Interactions with Foods and Other Compounds
Alcohol
Taking prochlorperazine may increase or prolong the effects of alcohol, such as drowsiness, dizziness, and poor coordination.[3] Therefore, people taking prochlorperazine should avoid drinking alcohol, especially when they must stay alert.

Antacids (page 18)
Many antacid products contain **aluminum hydroxide** (page 10), which reduces the absorption of phenothiazine drugs.[4] Though no studies are available that confirm an interaction between prochloroperazine and antacids, people who are using antacids should take them an hour before or two hours after the drug.

PROMETHAZINE

Common names: Phenergan Nighttime, Phenergan, Q-Mazine, Sominex

Combination drugs: Phenergan VC, Phenergan VC with Codeine, Phenergan with Codeine

Promethazine is an antihistamine used to relieve allergic rhinitis (seasonal allergy) symptoms including sneezing, runny nose, itching, and watery eyes and itching and swelling associated with uncomplicated allergic skin reactions. It is also used as a sleep aid for surgical procedures and to prevent/treat motion sickness, nausea, and vomiting. Promethazine is available as a nonprescription product alone and in a combination product to treat symptoms of allergy, colds, and upper respiratory infections. It is also available in prescription products with **codeine** (page 75), to treat coughs associated with colds and upper respiratory infections.

Summary of Interactions for Promethazine
In some cases, an herb or supplement may appear in more than one category, which may seem contradictory. For clarification, read the full article for details about the summarized interactions.

⊘ Avoid: Adverse interaction	Henbane*
Depletion or interference	None known
Side effect reduction/prevention	None known
Supportive interaction	None known
Reduced drug absorption/bioavailability	None known

Interactions with Herbs
Henbane (Hyoscyamus niger)
Antihistamines, including promethazine, can cause "anticholinergic" side effects such as dryness of mouth and heart palpitations. Henbane also has anticholinergic activity and side effects. Therefore, use with promethazine could increase the risk of anticholinergic side effects,[1] though apparently no interactions have yet been reported with promethazine and henbane. Henbane should not be taken except by prescription from a physician trained in its use, as it is extremely toxic.

Interactions with Foods and Other Compounds
Alcohol
Promethazine causes drowsiness.[2] Alcohol may intensify this effect and increase the risk of accidental injury.[3] To prevent problems, people taking promethazine or promethazine-containing products should avoid alcohol.

PROPACET 100

Contains the following ingredients:
  Acetaminophen (page 3)
  Propoxyphene (page 224)

PROPAFENONE

Common names: Arythmol, Rythmol

Propafenone is used to treat and prevent certain types of heart arrhythmia. At the time of this writing, no evidence of nutrient or herb interactions involving propafenone was found in the medical literature.

Summary of Interactions for Propafenone

In some cases, an herb or supplement may appear in more than one category, which may seem contradictory. For clarification, read the full article for details about the summarized interactions.

Depletion or interference	None known
Side effect reduction/prevention	None known
Supportive interaction	None known
Reduced drug absorption/bioavailability	None known
Adverse interaction	None known

PROPOXYPHENE

Common names: Darvon, Darvon-N, Dextropropoxyphene, Doloxene

Combination drugs: Co-Proxamol, Coalgesic, Darvocet N, Darvon Compound, Distalgesic, Propacet 100, Wygesic

Propoxyphene is a narcotic analgesic used to relieve mild to moderate pain. Propoxyphene is available alone and in combination with other drugs.

Summary of Interactions for Propoxyphene

In some cases, an herb or supplement may appear in more than one category, which may seem contradictory. For clarification, read the full article for details about the summarized interactions.

ⓘ Check: Other	Fiber
Depletion or interference	None known
Side effect reduction/prevention	None known
Supportive interaction	None known
Reduced drug absorption/bioavailability	None known
Adverse interaction	None known

Interactions with Foods and Other Compounds

Food

Propoxyphene may cause gastrointestinal (GI) upset. Propoxyphene-containing products may be taken with food to reduce or prevent GI upset.[1] A common side effect of narcotic analgesics is constipation.[2] Increasing dietary fiber (especially vegetables and whole-grain foods) and water intake can ease constipation.

Alcohol

Propoxyphene may cause drowsiness, dizziness, or blurred vision. Alcohol may intensify these effects and increase the risk of accidental injury.[3] To prevent problems, people taking propoxyphene should avoid alcohol.

PROPRANOLOL

Common names: Angilol, Apo-Propranolol, Apsolol, Bedranol SR, Berkolol, Beta Prograne, Betachron, Cardinol, Half Beta Prograne, Half-Inderal, Inderal-LA, Inderal, Lopranol LA, Nu-Propranolol, Probeta LA, Propanix SR, Propanix

Combination drugs: Inderetic, Inderex, Inderide

Propranolol is a beta-blocker drug. Propranolol is used to treat or prevent some heart conditions, reduce the symptoms of angina pectoris (chest pain), lower blood pressure in people with hypertension, and improve survival after a heart attack. Propranolol is sometimes used to prevent migraine headaches, to reduce movement associated with essential tremor, and to reduce performance anxiety.

Summary of Interactions for Propranolol

In some cases, an herb or supplement may appear in more than one category, which may seem contradictory. For clarification, read the full article for details about the summarized interactions.

✓ May be Beneficial: Depletion or interference	Coenzyme Q$_{10}$*
✓ May be Beneficial: Side effect reduction/prevention	Coenzyme Q$_{10}$*
⊘ Avoid: Adverse interaction	High-potassium foods* Pleurisy root* Potassium supplements* Tobacco

ⓘ Check: Other	Pepper
Supportive interaction	None known
Reduced drug absorption/bioavailability	None known

Interactions with Dietary Supplements

Coenzyme Q₁₀

Propranolol inhibits enzymes dependent on coenzyme Q_{10} (CoQ_{10}). In one trial, propranolol-induced symptoms were reduced in people given 60 mg of CoQ_{10} per day.[1]

Potassium

Some beta-adrenergic blockers (called "nonselective" beta blockers) decrease the uptake of potassium from the blood into the cells,[2] leading to excess potassium in the blood, a potentially dangerous condition known as hyperkalemia.[3] People taking beta-blockers should therefore avoid taking potassium supplements, or eating large quantities of fruit (e.g., bananas), unless directed to do so by their doctor.

Interactions with Herbs

Pepper (Piper nigrum, Piper longum)

In a single-dose human study, piperine, a chemical found in black pepper and long pepper, was reported to increase blood levels of propranolol,[4] which could increase the activity and risk of side effects of the drug.

Pleurisy root

As pleurisy root and other plants in the Aesclepius genus contain cardiac glycosides, it is best to avoid use of pleurisy root with heart medications such as beta-blockers.[5]

Interactions with Foods and Other Compounds

Food

Food increases the absorption of propranolol.[6] Propranolol should be taken at the same time every day, always with or always without food. High-protein foods may interfere with propranolol metabolism, increasing propranolol blood levels and activity.[7]

Alcohol

Propranolol may cause drowsiness or dizziness.[8] Alcohol may intensify this action. To prevent accidental injury, people taking propranolol should avoid alcohol.

Tobacco

In a double-blind study of ten cigarette smokers with angina treated with propranolol for one week, angina episodes were significantly reduced during the non-smoking phase compared with the smoking phase.[9] People with angina taking propranolol who do not smoke should avoid starting. Those who smoke should consult with their prescribing doctor about quitting.

PSYLLIUM

Common names: Effer-syllium, Fiberall, Hydrocil Instant, Konsyl, Metamucil, Modane Bulk, Novo-Mucilax, Perdiem Fiber, Prodiem Plain, Reguloid, Serutan, Siblin, Syllact, V-Lax

Psyllium is a bulk laxative used for short-term treatment of constipation. It is also used to treat people with irritable bowel syndrome, diverticular disease, and hemorrhoids and to lower cholesterol in people with high cholesterol. Psyllium is available as nonprescription drug products and as herbal dietary supplement products.

Summary of Interactions for Psyllium

In some cases, an herb or supplement may appear in more than one category, which may seem contradictory. For clarification, read the full article for details about the summarized interactions.

Depletion or interference	None known
Side effect reduction/prevention	None known
Supportive interaction	None known
Reduced drug absorption/bioavailability	None known
Adverse interaction	None known

QUETIAPINE

Common names: Seroquel

Quetiapine is used to treat symptoms associated with psychiatric disorders, such as delusions, hallucinations, disorganized thinking and speech, and bizarre behavior. It is in a class of antipsychotic drugs known as dibenzapines.

Summary of Interactions for Quetiapine

In some cases, an herb or supplement may appear in more than one category, which may seem contradictory.

Quetiapine

For clarification, read the full article for details about the summarized interactions.

✓ May be Beneficial: Supportive interaction	Food
⊘ Avoid: Adverse interaction	Alcohol
Depletion or interference	None known
Side effect reduction/prevention	None known
Reduced drug absorption/bioavailability	None known

Interaction with Food and Other Compounds

Food

Taking quetiapine with food increases both the absorption and the maximum blood concentration of the drug.[1] Problems may arise when individuals switch from taking quetiapine with a meal to taking it on an empty stomach and vice versa. Therefore, people should consistently take quetiapine with a meal to enhance drug actions and to avoid potential problems.

Alcohol

Quetiapine aggravates the adverse effect of alcohol on mental and motor skills, which might have serious consequences.[2] Therefore, people taking quetiapine should avoid drinking alcohol, especially when they must stay alert.

QUINAPRIL

Common names: Accupril, Accupro

Combination drug: Accuretic

Quinapril is an **angiotensin-converting enzyme (ACE) inhibitor** (page 17), a family of drugs used to treat high blood pressure and some types of heart failure.

Summary of Interactions for Quinapril

In some cases, an herb or supplement may appear in more than one category, which may seem contradictory. For clarification, read the full article for details about the summarized interactions.

✓ May be Beneficial: Depletion or interference	Zinc*
✓ May be Beneficial: Side effect reduction/prevention	Iron

⊘ Avoid: Adverse interaction	High-potassium foods* Potassium supplements* Salt substitutes*
Supportive interaction	None known
Reduced drug absorption/bioavailability	None known

Interactions with Dietary Supplements

Potassium

An uncommon yet potentially serious side effect of taking ACE inhibitors is increased blood potassium levels.[1, 2, 3] This problem is more likely to occur in people with advanced kidney disease. Taking potassium supplements,[4] potassium-containing salt substitutes (No Salt, Morton Salt Substitute, and others),[5, 6, 7] or large amounts of high-potassium foods at the same time as taking ACE inhibitors could cause life-threatening problems.[8] Therefore, people should consult their healthcare practitioner before supplementing additional potassium and should have their blood levels of potassium checked periodically while taking ACE inhibitors.

Zinc

In a study of 34 people with hypertension, six months of **captopril** (page 47) or **enalapril** (page 103) (ACE inhibitors related to quinapril) treatment led to decreased zinc levels in certain white blood cells,[9] raising concerns about possible ACE inhibitor–induced zinc depletion.

While zinc depletion has not been reported with quinapril, until more is known, it makes sense for people taking quinapril long term to consider, as a precaution, taking a zinc supplement or a multimineral tablet containing zinc. (Such multiminerals usually contain no more than 99 mg of potassium, probably not enough to trigger the above-mentioned interaction.) Supplements containing zinc should also contain copper, to protect against a zinc-induced copper deficiency.

Iron

In a double-blind study of patients who had developed a cough attributed to an ACE inhibitor, supplementation with iron (in the form of 256 mg of ferrous sulfate per day) for four weeks reduced the severity of the cough by a statistically significant 45%, compared with a nonsignificant 8% improvement in the placebo group.[10]

Interactions with Foods and Other Compounds
Food
High-fat meals may reduce quinapril absorption;[11] otherwise, quinapril may be taken with or without food.[12]

QUINIDINE

Common names: Kinidin Durules, Quinaglute, Quinidex, Quinora

Quinidine is used to treat and prevent certain forms of heart arrhythmia.

Summary of Interactions for Quinidine
In some cases, an herb or supplement may appear in more than one category, which may seem contradictory. For clarification, read the full article for details about the summarized interactions.

✓	May be Beneficial: Side effect reduction/prevention	Beta-carotene Magnesium Potassium
✓	May be Beneficial: Supportive interaction	Food
⊘	Avoid: Reduced drug absorption/ bioavailability	High-salt diet
⊘	Avoid: Adverse interaction	Food Grapefruit juice Low-salt diet **Sodium bicarbonate** (page 240)
	Depletion or interference	None known

Interactions with Dietary Supplements
Potassium and magnesium
People taking **potassium-depleting diuretics** (page 94) may develop low potassium and magnesium blood levels. Prolonged diarrhea and vomiting might also result in low blood potassium levels. People with low potassium or magnesium blood levels who take quinidine might develop serious drug side effects.[1] Therefore, people taking quinidine should have their blood potassium and magnesium levels checked regularly and might need to supplement with both minerals, especially when taking potassium-depleting diuretics.

Beta-carotene
Some people taking quinidine develop sensitivity to ultraviolet radiation from the sun. In a preliminary study, three people with quinidine-induced skin inflammation were able to tolerate intense sun exposure without recurrence of the rash after supplementing with 90–180 mg of beta-carotene each day.[2] Further research is needed to confirm that people taking quinidine can prevent side effects by supplementing with beta-carotene.

Interaction with Foods and Other Compounds
Grapefruit juice
Drinking grapefruit juice together with quinidine increases the amount of time that the drug remains in the body,[3] which might increase the likelihood of side effects and toxicity. Therefore, based on currently available information, people taking quinidine should avoid drinking grapefruit juice or eating grapefruit.

Salt
One controlled study showed that people consuming a high-salt diet had dramatically lower quinidine blood levels compared with people on a low-salt diet.[4] Problems might occur when people switch from a high-salt diet to a low-salt diet and vice versa. Therefore, people taking quinidine should notify their health practitioner before changing their salt intake.

Food
Taking quinidine with food greatly increases the speed and extent of absorption of the drug.[5] Serious problems might occur when people switch from taking quinidine with a meal to taking it on an empty stomach and vice versa. Therefore, quinidine should be consistently taken with a meal to enhance drug action and to avoid potential problems.

Sodium bicarbonate (page 240)
Sodium bicarbonate reduces the amount of quinidine eliminated from the body, which might result in increased drug side effects and toxicity.[6] Therefore, people taking quinidine should avoid using antacids or toothpaste that contain sodium bicarbonate.

QUININE SULFATE

Common names: Quinamm, Quinine Sulphate

Quinine can be used to treat malaria; however, it is most often used to treat leg cramps that occur at night.

Summary of Interactions for Quinine Sulfate

In some cases, an herb or supplement may appear in more than one category, which may seem contradictory. For clarification, read the full article for details about the summarized interactions.

Depletion or interference	None known
Side effect reduction/prevention	None known
Supportive interaction	None known
Reduced drug absorption/bioavailability	None known
Adverse interaction	None known

QUINOCORT

Contains the following ingredients:
    Hydrocortisone
    Hydroxyquinolone

QUINOLONES

Common names: Alatrofloxacin, Avelox, Cinobac, Cinoxacin, Enoxacin, Gatifloxacin, Lomefloxacin, Maxaquin, Mictral, Nalidixic Acid, Negram, Norfloxacin, Noroxin, Penetrex, Sparfloxacin, Tequin, Trovafloxacin, Trovan, Unitor, Uriben, Zagam

Quinolones, including fluoroquinolones, are a family of **antibiotics** (page 19) used to treat a broad spectrum of bacterial infections occurring in the body. Each drug within the family kills specific bacteria; therefore, healthcare practitioners prescribe quinolones based on the individual's current needs.

There are interactions that are common to **antibacterial drugs** (page 19) in general and interactions involving a specific quinolone. For the latter interactions, refer to the highlighted drugs listed below.

- Cinoxacin (Cinobac)
- **Ciprofloxacin** (page 62) (Cipro)
- Enoxacin (Penetrex)
- Gatifloxacin (Tequin)
- **Levofloxacin** (page 155) (Levaquin)
- Lomefloxacin (Maxaquin)
- Moxifloxacin (Avelox)
- Nalidixic acid (NegGram)
- Norfloxacin (Noroxin)
- **Ofloxacin** (page 195) (Floxin)
- Sparfloxacin (Zagam)
- Trovafloxacin and Alatrofloxacin (Trovan)

Summary of Interactions for Quinolones

In some cases, an herb or supplement may appear in more than one category, which may seem contradictory. For clarification, read the full article for details about the summarized interactions.

✓	May be Beneficial: Depletion or interference	Vitamin K*
✓	May be Beneficial: Side effect reduction/prevention	Bifidobacterium longum* Lactobacillus acidophilus* Lactobacillus casei* Saccharomyces boulardii* Saccharomyces cerevisiae* Vitamin K*
✓	May be Beneficial: Supportive interaction	Saccharomyces boulardii*
⊘	Avoid: Adverse interaction	Calcium Magnesium
	Reduced drug absorption/bioavailability	None known

Interactions common to many, if not all, Quinolones are described in this article. Interactions reported for only one or several drugs in this class may not be listed in this article. Some drugs listed in this article are linked to articles specific to that respective drug; please refer to those individual drug articles. The information in this article may not necessarily apply to drugs in this class for which no separate article exists. If you are taking a Quinolone for which no separate article exists, talk with your doctor or pharmacist.

Interactions with Dietary Supplements

Calcium

Calcium has been shown to interfere substantially with the absorption of quinolones.[1] Separating quinolones from calcium by at least four hours is recommended.

Magnesium

Magnesium has been shown to interfere substantially with the absorption of quinolones.[2] Separating quinolones from magnesium by at least four hours is recommended.

Probiotics

A common side effect of antibiotics is diarrhea, which may be caused by the elimination of beneficial bacteria normally found in the colon. Controlled studies have shown that taking probiotic microorganisms—such as *Lactobacillus casei, Lactobacillus acidophilus, Bifidobacterium longum*, or *Saccharomyces boulardii*—helps prevent antibiotic-induced diarrhea.[3]

The diarrhea experienced by some people who take antibiotics also might be due to an overgrowth of the bacterium *Clostridium difficile*, which causes a disease known as pseudomembranous colitis. Controlled studies have shown that supplementation with harmless yeast—such as *Saccharomyces boulardii*[4] or *Saccharomyces cerevisiae* (baker's or brewer's yeast)[5]—helps prevent recurrence of this infection. In one study, taking 500 mg of *Saccharomyces boulardii* twice daily enhanced the effectiveness of the antibiotic vancomycin in preventing recurrent clostridium infection.[6] Therefore, people taking antibiotics who later develop diarrhea might benefit from supplementing with saccharomyces organisms.

Treatment with antibiotics also commonly leads to an overgrowth of yeast *(Candida albicans)* in the vagina (candida vaginitis) and the intestines (sometimes referred to as "dysbiosis"). Controlled studies have shown that *Lactobacillus acidophilus* might prevent candida vaginitis.[7]

Vitamin K
Several cases of excessive bleeding have been reported in people who take antibiotics.[8, 9, 10, 11] This side effect may be the result of reduced vitamin K activity and/or reduced vitamin K production by bacteria in the colon. One study showed that people who had taken broad-spectrum antibiotics had lower liver concentrations of vitamin K_2 (menaquinone), though vitamin K_1 (phylloquinone) levels remained normal.[12] Several antibiotics appear to exert a strong effect on vitamin K activity, while others may not have any effect. Therefore, one should refer to a specific antibiotic for information on whether it interacts with vitamin K. Doctors of natural medicine sometimes recommend vitamin K supplementation to people taking antibiotics. Additional research is needed to determine whether the amount of vitamin K_1 found in some multivitamins is sufficient to prevent antibiotic-induced bleeding. Moreover, most multivitamins do not contain vitamin K.

RALOXIFENE

Common names: Evista

Raloxifene is a type of drug called a selective estrogen receptor modulator (SERM). It is used to prevent osteoporosis in women after menopause.

Summary of Interactions for Raloxifene
In some cases, an herb or supplement may appear in more than one category, which may seem contradictory.

For clarification, read the full article for details about the summarized interactions.

✓	May be Beneficial: Depletion or interference	Phytoestrogens
	Side effect reduction/prevention	None known
	Supportive interaction	None* known
	Reduced drug absorption/bioavailability	None known
	Adverse interaction	None known

Interactions with Herbs
Formononetin
Some chemicals called phytoestrogens, found naturally in plants, have estrogen-like activity; and some people use these phytoestrogens from dietary sources or from supplements to prevent or treat hormone-related health problems. In test tube studies, the estrogenic activity of one phytoestrogen, formononetin, was blocked by raloxifene.[1] Further research is necessary to determine the overall effect of raloxifene on formononetin and other phytoestrogens in humans.

RAMIPRIL

Common names: Altace, Tritace

Combination drug: Triapin

Ramipril is an **angiotensin-converting enzyme (ACE) inhibitor** (page 17), a family of drugs used to treat high blood pressure and some types of heart failure.

Summary of Interactions for Ramipril
In some cases, an herb or supplement may appear in more than one category, which may seem contradictory. For clarification, read the full article for details about the summarized interactions.

✓	May be Beneficial: Depletion or interference	Zinc*
✓	May be Beneficial: Side effect reduction/prevention	Iron
🚫	Avoid: Adverse interaction	High-potassium foods* Potassium supplements* Salt substitutes*
	Supportive interaction	None known
	Reduced drug absorption/bioavailability	None known

Ramipril

Interactions with Dietary Supplements
Potassium

An uncommon yet potentially serious side effect of taking ACE inhibitors is increased blood potassium levels.[1, 2, 3] This problem is more likely to occur in people with advanced kidney disease. Taking potassium supplements,[4] potassium-containing salt substitutes (No Salt, Morton Salt Substitute, and others),[5, 6, 7] or large amounts of high-potassium foods at the same time as taking ACE inhibitors could cause life-threatening problems.[8] Therefore, people should consult their healthcare practitioner before supplementing additional potassium and should have their blood levels of potassium checked periodically while taking ACE inhibitors.

Zinc

In a study of 34 people with hypertension, six months of **captopril** (page 47) or **enalapril** (page 103) (ACE inhibitors related to ramipril) treatment led to decreased zinc levels in certain white blood cells,[9] raising concerns about possible ACE inhibitor–induced zinc depletion.

While zinc depletion has not been reported with ramipril, until more is known, it makes sense for people taking ramipril long term to consider, as a precaution, taking a zinc supplement or a multimineral tablet containing zinc. (Such multiminerals usually contain no more than 99 mg of potassium, probably not enough to trigger the above-mentioned interaction.) Supplements containing zinc should also contain copper, to protect against a zinc-induced copper deficiency.

Iron

In a double-blind study of patients who had developed a cough attributed to an ACE inhibitor, supplementation with iron (in the form of 256 mg of ferrous sulfate per day) for four weeks reduced the severity of the cough by a statistically significant 45%, compared with a nonsignificant 8% improvement in the placebo group.[10]

Interactions with Foods and Other Compounds
Food

Food slows the rate of ramipril absorption but not the total amount of drug absorbed.[11]

RANITIDINE

Common names: Alti-Ranitidine, Apo-Ranitidine, Gen-Ranitidine, Novo-Ranidine, Nu-Ranit, Rantec, Zaedoc, Zantac

Ranitidine is a member of the H-2 (histamine blocker) family of drugs, which prevents the release of acid into the stomach. Ranitidine is used to treat stomach and duodenal ulcers, gastroesophageal reflux disease, erosive esophagitis, and Zollinger-Ellison syndrome. Ranitidine is available as a prescription drug and also as a nonprescription over-the-counter product for relief of heartburn.

Summary of Interactions for Ranitidine

In some cases, an herb or supplement may appear in more than one category, which may seem contradictory. For clarification, read the full article for details about the summarized interactions.

✓ May be Beneficial: Depletion or interference	Folic acid Iron Vitamin B$_{12}$*
🚫 Avoid: Reduced drug absorption/ bioavailability	**Magnesium hydroxide** (page 166) Tobacco
Side effect reduction/prevention	None known
Supportive interaction	None known
Adverse interaction	None known

Interactions with Dietary Supplements
Folic acid

Folic acid is needed by the body to utilize vitamin B$_{12}$. Antacids, including ranitidine, inhibit folic acid absorption.[1] People taking antacids are advised to supplement with folic acid.

Iron

Stomach acid may facilitate iron absorption. H-2 blocker drugs reduce stomach acid and are associated with decreased dietary iron absorption.[2] People with ulcers may also be iron deficient due to blood loss and benefit from iron supplementation. Iron levels in the blood can be checked with lab tests.

Magnesium

In healthy volunteers, a **magnesium hydroxide** (page 166)/**aluminum hydroxide** (page 10) antacid, taken with ranitidine, decreased ranitidine absorption by 20%–25%.[3] It was unclear from this study if magnesium or the specific form of magnesium as magnesium hydroxide was part of the problem. It is not known if other forms of magnesium would cause this problem. People can avoid this interaction by taking ranitidine two hours before or after any aluminum/magnesium-containing **antacids** (page 18), including magnesium hydroxide found in some vitamin/mineral supplements.

Vitamin B₁₂

Vitamin B₁₂
Stomach acid is needed to release vitamin B_{12} from food so it can be absorbed by the body. H-2 blocker drugs reduce stomach acid and are associated with decreased dietary vitamin B_{12} absorption.[4] The vitamin B_{12} found in supplements is available to the body without the need for stomach acid. Lab tests can determine vitamin B_{12} levels.

Interactions with Foods and Other Compounds

Food
Ranitidine may be taken with or without food.[5]

Tobacco (Nicotiana species)
A study of 18 healthy people found smoking decreased the acid blocking effects of ranitidine.[6]

RENNIE

Contains the following ingredients:
   Calcium
   Magnesium

RENNIE DEFLATINE

Contains the following ingredients:
   Calcium
   Dimethicone
   Magnesium

REPAGLINIDE

Common names: Gluconorm, NovoNorm, Prandin

Repaglinide is used to treat individuals with type 2 (non-insulin-dependent) diabetes mellitus; it is in the meglitinide class of anti-diabetic drugs. It may be used as an adjunct to diet and exercise either alone or in combination with other anti-diabetic medications.

Summary of Interactions for Repaglinide

In some cases, an herb or supplement may appear in more than one category, which may seem contradictory. For clarification, read the full article for details about the summarized interactions.

⊘ Avoid: Adverse interaction	*Ginkgo biloba* Willow*
ⓘ Check: Other	Vitamin B₃
Depletion or interference	None known
Side effect reduction/prevention	None known
Supportive interaction	None known
Reduced drug absorption/bioavailability	None known

Interactions with Dietary Supplements

Vitamin B₃ (niacin)
Supplementation with large amounts of niacin (also called nicotinic acid) can increase blood glucose levels in diabetics, which might interfere with the blood-sugar-lowering effects of repaglinide.[1] The form of vitamin B_3 known as niacinamide does not have this effect. People who start or stop supplementing niacin while on repaglinide should carefully monitor their blood sugar levels and consult their prescribing doctor about making adjustments in the daily amount of drug taken.

Interactions with Herbs

White willow bark (Salix alba)
White willow bark contains salicin, which is related to **aspirin** (page 26). Both salicin and aspirin produce anti-inflammatory effects after they have been converted to salicylic acid in the body. Taking aspirin together with repaglinide enhances the blood-sugar-lowering effects of the drug,[2] which might result in unwanted side effects. Controlled research is needed to determine whether taking willow bark together with repaglinide might produce similar effects.

Ginkgo biloba
In a preliminary trial, administration of *Ginkgo biloba* extract (120 mg per day) for three months to patients with type 2 diabetes who were taking oral anti-diabetes medication resulted in a significant worsening of glucose tolerance. Ginkgo did not impair glucose tolerance in individuals whose diabetes was controlled by diet.[3] Individuals taking oral anti-diabetes medication should consult a doctor before taking *Ginkgo biloba*.

Interactions with Foods and Other Compounds

Food
Taking repaglinide with food can result in decreased absorption of the drug.[4] Consequently, to achieve the best results, repaglinide should be taken on an empty stomach.

RIFAMATE

Contains the following ingredients:
Isoniazid (page 146)
Rifampin

RIMACTANE

Contains the following ingredients:
Isoniazid (page 146)
Rifampin

RISEDRONATE

Common names: Actonel

Risedronate is used to treat Paget's disease of the bone, and is in a family of drugs known as bisphosphonates.

Summary of Interactions for Risedronate

In some cases, an herb or supplement may appear in more than one category, which may seem contradictory. For clarification, read the full article for details about the summarized interactions.

✓	May be Beneficial: Depletion or interference	Calcium*
⊘	Avoid: Reduced drug absorption/bioavailability	**Antacids** (page 18) Calcium Food Iron Magnesium Zinc (absorption) Zinc (action)
	Side effect reduction/prevention	None known
	Supportive interaction	None known
	Adverse interaction	None known

Interactions with Dietary Supplements
Calcium and vitamin D
Short-term treatment with risedronate in people with hyperparathydoidism—a disorder characterized by high blood levels of calcium—resulted in lower calcium blood levels.[1] Additional research is needed to determine whether people taking risedronate for Paget's dis-

ease might develop low blood calcium levels. As a precaution, people with Paget's disease should take supplemental calcium and vitamin D if dietary intake is inadequate. However, taking risedronate at the same time as calcium supplements reduces absorption of the drug.[2] Therefore, people taking risedronate for Paget's disease should take calcium supplements an hour before or two hours after taking the drug.

Minerals
Taking risedronate at the same time as iron, zinc, or magnesium may reduce the amount of drug absorbed.[3] Therefore, people taking risedronate who wish to supplement with these minerals should take them an hour before or two hours after the drug.

Interactions with Foods and Other Compounds
Antacids (page 18)
Taking risedronate at the same time as antacids containing calcium or magnesium may reduce absorption of the drug. Therefore, people taking risedronate should take calcium- or magnesium-containing antacids an hour before or two hours after the drug.

Food
One controlled study showed that taking risedronate either a half an hour before or two hours after a meal dramatically reduced absorption of the drug, compared with taking the drug one hour before or four hours after a meal.[4] Consequently, people should take risedronate one hour before a meal or 4 hours after a meal, as long as the latter is at least one hour before the next meal.

RISPERIDONE

Common names: Risperdal

Risperidone is used to manage symptoms associated with psychotic disorders, especially schizophrenia.

Summary of Interactions for Risperidone

In some cases, an herb or supplement may appear in more than one category, which may seem contradictory. For clarification, read the full article for details about the summarized interactions.

✓	May be Beneficial: Side effect reduction/prevention	Vitamin B$_6$ Vitamin E
✓	May be Beneficial: Supportive interaction	Glycine

ⓘ Check: Other	Licorice White Peony
Depletion or interference	None known
Reduced drug absorption/bioavailability	None known
Adverse interaction	None known

Interactions with Dietary Supplements

Vitamin E and vitamin B6

Vitamin E along with vitamin B_6 was used to treat a side effect of risperidone called neuroleptic malignant syndrome in a 74-year-old woman, and results were encouraging.[1] However, whether vitamin E and vitamin B_6 supplementation might help prevent this condition in people taking risperidone is unknown.

Glycine

In a small double-blind study, people with schizophrenia being treated with risperidone experienced an improvement in their symptoms when glycine was added to their treatment regimen.[2] The initial amount of glycine used was 4 grams per day; this was increased gradually over a period of 10 to 17 days to a maximum of 0.8 grams per 2.2 pounds of body weight per day.

Lithium (page 157)

Lithium is a mineral present in large amounts in some medications, and may be included in some mineral supplements. The combination of lithium and risperidone has produced unwanted side effects such as delirium, confusion, and fever.[3, 4] Smaller amounts of lithium are available in some nutritional supplements, but it is not known whether these amounts are enough to cause a problem in individuals taking risperidone.

Interactions with Herbs

Licorice (Glycyrrhiza radix) and white peony (Paeonia radix)

An Oriental herb formula containing *Glycyrrhiza radix* (licorice root) and *Paeonia radix* (white peony root) successfully restored menses in a 28-year-old woman who had developed amenorrhea (lack of menstruation) while taking risperidone.[5] Discontinuation of these herbs while the woman continued taking risperidone again led to disruption of her menses. Controlled research is needed to determine whether supplementation with licorice and peony might help prevent amenorrhea in women taking risperidone.

Interactions with Foods and Other Compounds

Food

Risperidone oral solution should be mixed in half a glass of water, coffee, orange juice, or low-fat milk and immediately consumed.[6] It should not be mixed with cola or tea.[7]

Alcohol

Alcohol increases the breakdown of many antipsychotic drugs.[8] More research is necessary to determine if alcohol consumption might lower blood levels of risperidone.

ROBITUSSIN AC

Contains the following ingredients:
   Codeine (page 75)
   Guaifenesin (page 133)

ROBITUSSIN CF

Contains the following ingredients:
   Dextromethorphan (page 87)
   Guaifenesin (page 133)
   Phenylpropanolamine (page 218)

ROBITUSSIN DM

Contains the following ingredients:
   Dextromethorphan (page 87)
   Guaifenesin (page 133)

ROSIGLITAZONE

Common names: Avandia, Pioglitazone

Rosiglitazone is used in association with diet control, weight loss, and exercise to treat non-insulin-dependent (type 2) diabetes. At the time of this writing, no evidence of nutrient or herb interactions involving rosiglitazone was found in the medical literature.

Summary of Interactions for Rosiglitazone

In some cases, an herb or supplement may appear in more than one category, which may seem contradictory. For clarification, read the full article for details about the summarized interactions.

Rosiglitazone

Depletion or interference	None known
Side effect reduction/prevention	None known
Supportive interaction	None known
Reduced drug absorption/bioavailability	None known
Adverse interaction	None known

ROSUVASTATIN

Common names: Crestor

Rosuvastatin is used along with dietary changes to reduce cholesterol and fat levels in the blood, and to increase HDL ("good") cholesterol levels. It belongs to a class of drugs called HMG-CoA reductase inhibitors.

Summary of Interactions for Rosuvastatin

In some cases, an herb or supplement may appear in more than one category, which may seem contradictory. For clarification, read the full article for details about the summarized interactions.

✓ May be Beneficial: Supportive interaction	Niacin
⊘ Avoid: Adverse interaction	Niacin*
Depletion or interference	None known
Side effect reduction/prevention	None known
Reduced drug absorption/bioavailability	None known

Interactions with Dietary Supplements
Niacin
A recent blinded study showed that individuals taking both rosuvastatin and niacin had a greater increase in HDL ("good") cholesterol and apolipoprotein A-I than did those taking rosuvastatin alone.[1] People taking rosuvastatin might benefit from taking niacin, though they should consult with their healthcare provider before starting the supplement. When taken with niacin, some statin drugs may become more toxic so there is a possibility of an adverse interaction.

ROTER

Contains the following ingredients:
Bismuth (page 40)
Frangula

Magnesium
Sodium bicarbonate (page 240)

ROXICET

Contains the following ingredients:
Acetaminophen (page 3)
Oxycodone (page 205)

ROXIPRIN

Contains the following ingredients:
Aspirin (page 26)
Oxycodone (page 205)

SALMETEROL

Common names: Serevent

Combination drug: Seretide

Salmeterol is a member of the drug family known as long-acting, beta-adrenergic bronchodilators. It is inhaled by mouth, into the lungs, to treat asthma and prevent bronchospasm. Salmeterol is also used to prevent exercise-induced bronchospasm.

Summary of Interactions for Salmeterol

In some cases, an herb or supplement may appear in more than one category, which may seem contradictory. For clarification, read the full article for details about the summarized interactions.

✓ May be Beneficial: Supportive interaction	Coleus*
Depletion or interference	None known
Side effect reduction/prevention	None known
Reduced drug absorption/bioavailability	None known
Adverse interaction	None known

Interactions with Herbs
Coleus (Coleus forskohlii)
A test tube study demonstrated that the bronchodilating effects of salbutamol, another beta-adrenergic bronchodilator drug, were significantly increased by the addition of forskolin, the active component of the herb *Coleus forskohlii*.[1] The results of this preliminary research

suggest that the combination of forskolin and beta-agonists might provide an alternative to raising the doses of the beta-agonist drugs as they lose effectiveness. Until more is known, coleus should not be combined with salmeterol without the supervision of a doctor.

SALSALATE

Common names: Amigesic, Disalcid, Marthritic, Mono Gesic, Salflex, Salicylic acid, Salsitab

Combination drug: Diprosalic

Salsalate is used to treat rheumatoid arthritis and osteoarthritis and is in a class of medications known as **nonsteroidal anti-inflammatory drugs** (page 193) (NSAIDs).

Summary of Interactions for Salsalate

In some cases, an herb or supplement may appear in more than one category, which may seem contradictory. For clarification, read the full article for details about the summarized interactions.

✓ May be Beneficial: Depletion or interference	Folic acid* Potassium* Vitamin C*
⊘ Avoid: Adverse interaction	**Lithium** (page 157)* White willow*
Side effect reduction/prevention	None known
Supportive interaction	None known
Reduced drug absorption/bioavailability	None known

Interactions with Dietary Supplements
Folic acid
Salsalate and **aspirin** (page 26) produce anti-inflammatory effects after they are converted in the body to salicylic acid. Studies have shown that aspirin can reduce the amount of folic acid in the blood,[1] though it is not known whether this change is significant. Controlled studies are needed to determine whether people taking salsalate are at risk for folic acid deficiency.

Lithium (page 157)
Lithium is a mineral that may be present in some supplements and is also used in large amounts to treat mood disorders such as manic-depression (bipolar disorder). Most NSAIDs inhibit the excretion of lithium from the body, resulting in higher blood levels of the mineral, though **sulindac** (page 249) may have an opposite effect.[2] Since major changes in lithium blood levels can produce unwanted side effects or interfere with its efficacy, NSAIDs should be used with caution, and only under medical supervision, in people taking lithium supplements.

Potassium
Salsalate and **aspirin** (page 26) are rapidly converted in the body to salicylic acid. Taking large amounts of aspirin can result in lower than normal blood levels of potassium,[3] though it is not known whether this change is significant. Controlled studies are needed to determine whether people taking salsalate are at risk for potassium deficiency.

Vitamin C
Salsalate and **aspirin** (page 26) are rapidly converted in the body to salicylic acid. Controlled studies show that taking aspirin increases the elimination of vitamin C from the body and lowers blood levels.[4] Further controlled research is needed to determine whether salsalate specifically reduces vitamin C levels and whether people taking the drug are at risk for vitamin C deficiency.

Interactions with Herbs
White willow bark (Salix alba)
White willow bark contains salicin, which is related to **aspirin** (page 26). Salsalate, salicin, and aspirin produce anti-inflammatory effects after they have been converted to salicylic acid in the body. Taking aspirin at the same time as other salicylate drugs can result in adverse effects, such as ringing in the ears, dizziness, headache, confusion, and diarrhea.[5] Though there are no studies specifically investigating an interaction between willow bark and salsalate, people taking salsalate should probably avoid using the herb until more information is available.

Interactions with Foods and Other Compounds
Food
Taking salsalate with food can slow the speed of absorption but not the overall amount of drug absorbed;[6] therefore, it can be taken with a meal, if needed, to avoid stomach upset.

SECRADEX

Contains the following ingredients:
Acebutolol (page 3)
Hydrochlorothiazide

SELEGILINE

Common names: Carbex, Centrapryl, Eldepryl, Zelpar

Selegiline is used together with **levodopa** (page 154) and **carbidopa** (page 48) to treat symptoms of Parkinson's disease.

Summary of Interactions for Selegiline

In some cases, an herb or supplement may appear in more than one category, which may seem contradictory. For clarification, read the full article for details about the summarized interactions.

✓ May be Beneficial: Supportive interaction	5-HTP Food L-Tryptophan
⊘ Avoid: Adverse interaction	Ephedra Tyramine
Depletion or interference	None known
Side effect reduction/prevention	None known
Reduced drug absorption/bioavailability	None known

Interactions with Dietary Supplements

L-tryptophan and 5-HTP

Both L-tryptophan and 5-HTP have been used to treat depression. One controlled study showed that taking selegiline at the same time as 5-HTP enhanced the antidepressant effect when compared with 5-HTP alone.[1] Further research is needed to determine whether taking selegiline and 5-HTP together might result in unwanted side effects.

Interactions with Herbs

Ephedra

Ephedrine is an active ingredient found in ephedra, an herb that until 2004 was used in cold remedies and herbal weight loss products. One individual taking selegiline together with ephedrine experienced a serious side effect known as hypertensive crisis, in which blood pressure can reach dangerous levels.[2] Though no studies have investigated whether the herb ephedra might result in similar effects, the current evidence suggests that people taking selegiline should avoid all products that contain ephedra.

Interactions with Foods and Other Compounds

Food

Taking selegiline with food dramatically increases the absorption of the drug.[3] Problems might occur when in-

dividuals switch from taking selegiline with food to taking it on an empty stomach and vice versa. Therefore, people should consistently take selegiline with a meal to enhance the effects of the drug and to avoid problems.

Tyramine-containing foods

Rarely, people taking selegiline might experience a rapid rise in blood pressure and a severe throbbing headache when the drug is taken with foods that contain tyramine, such as cheese (especially aged); sour cream; yogurt; alcoholic beverages; meat, fish, and poultry; a variety of fruits and vegetables, including avocados, figs, and eggplant; fava beans; some soups; and chocolate.[4] One study showed that taking 30 mg of selegiline each day greatly increases tyramine sensitivity.[5] It has therefore been suggested that people taking 30 mg or more of selegiline per day should consume a tyramine-free diet.

SENNA

Common names: Black-Draught, Fletcher's Castoria, Gentlax, Glysennid, Manevac, PMS-Sennosides, Riva-Senna, Senexon, Senna Lax, Senna-Gen, Sennatab, Senokot, Senolax, X-Prep

Senna is a laxative used for short-term treatment of constipation. It is available as nonprescription drugs and as herbal products.

Summary of Interactions for Senna

In some cases, an herb or supplement may appear in more than one category, which may seem contradictory. For clarification, read the full article for details about the summarized interactions.

ⓘ Check: Other	Digitalis Potassium Sodium
Depletion or interference	None known
Side effect reduction/prevention	None known
Supportive interaction	None known
Reduced drug absorption/bioavailability	None known
Adverse interaction	None known

Interactions with Dietary Supplements

Sodium and potassium

Overuse or misuse of laxatives, including senna, can cause water, sodium, and potassium depletion.[1] To avoid depletion problems, people should limit laxative use, including senna, to one week or less.[2]

Interactions with Herbs

Digitalis (Digitalis lanata, Digitalis purpurea)

Digitalis refers to a family of plants commonly called foxglove that contain digitalis glycosides, chemicals with actions and toxicities similar to the prescription drug **digoxin** (page 90). While the interaction has not been reported, overuse or misuse of senna (leading to potassium loss) may increase digitalis effects and risk of side effects.[3] Senna and digitalis-containing products should be used only under the direct supervision of a doctor trained in their use.

SERETIDE

Contains the following ingredients:
  Fluticasone
  Salmeterol (page 234)

SERTRALINE

Common names: Lustral, Zoloft

Sertraline is a member of the selective serotonin reuptake inhibitor (SSRI) family of drugs used to treat people with depression.

Summary of Interactions for Sertraline

In some cases, an herb or supplement may appear in more than one category, which may seem contradictory. For clarification, read the full article for details about the summarized interactions.

✓ May be Beneficial: Depletion or interference	Sodium
✓ May be Beneficial: Side effect reduction/prevention	Ginkgo biloba*
✓ May be Beneficial: Supportive interaction	Chromium*
⊘ Avoid: Adverse interaction	5-Hydroxytryptophan (5-HTP) L-tryptophan St. John's wort*
Reduced drug absorption/bioavailability	None known

Interactions with Dietary Supplements

Chromium

There have been five case reports of chromium supplementation (200–400 mcg per day) significantly improving mood in people with a type of depression called dysthymic disorder who were also taking sertraline.[1] These case reports, while clearly limited and preliminary in scope, warrant a controlled trial to better understand the benefits, if any, of chromium supplementation in people taking this drug.

5-hydroxytryptophan (5-HTP) and L-tryptophan

Sertraline increases serotonin activity in the brain. 5-HTP and L-tryptophan are converted to serotonin in the brain, and taking either of these compounds with sertraline may increase sertraline-induced side effects.

In one report, dietary supplements of L-tryptophan (available only by prescriptions from special compounding pharmacists) taken with paroxetine (a drug similar to sertraline) caused headache, sweating, dizziness, agitation, restlessness, nausea, vomiting, and other symptoms.[2] On the other hand, the combination of 45 mg DL-tryptophan (a synthetic variation of L-tryptophan) per pound of body weight (a relatively high dose) with zimelidine, a drug with a similar action to sertraline, did not cause these side effects in another trial.[3] Some doctors have used small amounts of L-tryptophan in combination with SSRIs, to increase the effectiveness of the latter. However, because of the potential for side effects, 5-HTP and L-tryptophan should never be taken in combination with sertraline or other SSRIs, unless the combination is being closely monitored by a doctor. Foods rich in L-tryptophan do not appear to interact with sertraline or other SSRIs.

Sodium

SSRI drugs, including sertraline, have been reported to cause sodium depletion.[4, 5, 6] The risk for SSRI-induced sodium depletion appears to be increased during the first few weeks of treatment in women, the elderly, and patients also using **diuretics** (page 94). Doctors prescribing SSRI drugs, including sertraline, should monitor their patients for signs of sodium depletion.

Interactions with Herbs

Ginkgo biloba

In three men and two women treated with **fluoxetine** (page 120) or **sertraline** (page 237) (SSRI drugs closely related to paroxetine) for depression who experienced sexual dysfunction, addition of *Ginkgo biloba* extract (GBE) in the amount of 240 mg per day effectively reversed the sexual dysfunction.[7] This makes sense because ginkgo has been reported to help men with some forms of erectile dysfunction.[8]

St. John's wort (Hypericum perforatum)

One report described a case of serotonin syndrome in a patient who took St. John's wort and **trazodone** (page

267), a weak SSRI drug.[9] The patient reportedly experienced mental confusion, muscle twitching, sweating, flushing, and ataxia. In another case, a patient experienced grogginess, lethargy, nausea, weakness, and fatigue after taking one dose of **paroxetine** (page 208) (Paxil, another SSRI drug) after ten days of St. John's wort use.[10]

Interactions with Foods and Other Compounds

Food
Results of two nonblinded randomized studies in healthy people suggest sertraline may be taken with or without food.[11]

Alcohol
SSRI drugs, including sertraline, may cause dizziness or drowsiness.[12] Alcohol may intensify these effects and increase the risk of accidental injury. Alcohol should be avoided during sertraline therapy.

SIBUTRAMINE

Common names: Meridia

Sibutramine is used for the management of obesity, including weight loss and maintenance of weight loss, and should be used in association with a reduced calorie diet.

Summary of Interactions for Sibutramine

In some cases, an herb or supplement may appear in more than one category, which may seem contradictory. For clarification, read the full article for details about the summarized interactions.

⊘ Avoid: Adverse interaction	5-HTP
	Alcohol
	Ephedra
	L-tryptophan
Depletion or interference	None known
Side effect reduction/prevention	None known
Supportive interaction	None known
Reduced drug absorption/bioavailability	None known

Interaction with Dietary Supplements

L-tryptophan and 5-HTP
The amino acids L-tryptophan and 5-hydroxytryptophan (5-HTP) are occasionally used to treat mental depression. Taking sibutramine with L-tryptophan or 5-HTP might result in a rare, but serious group of symptoms known as "serotonin syndrome."[1] Symptoms associated with serotonin syndrome may include confusion, anxiety, muscle weakness, incoordination, and vomiting. Therefore, individuals taking sibutramine should avoid supplementing with L-tryptophan and 5-HTP.

Interaction with Herbs

Ephedra
One side effect of sibutramine is high blood pressure. Ephedra, an herb that until 2004 was used in cold remedies and herbal weight loss products, contains **ephedrine** (page 104), which can also increase blood pressure. Though no studies have investigated whether taking sibutramine together with ephedra might produce an adverse interaction, currently available evidence suggests that this combination should be used with caution.[2]

Interaction with Food and Other Compounds

Alcohol
Though one controlled study showed that drinking alcoholic beverages while taking sibutramine produced no clinically important interaction, it is nevertheless recommended that individuals taking the drug should avoid drinking alcohol.[3]

SILDENAFIL

Common names: Viagra

Sildenafil is a drug used to treat erectile dysfunction (ED), commonly known as impotence, in men.

In one study, ingestion of 250 ml (approximately one cup) of grapefruit juice one hour before and together with sildenafil increased the total amount of sildenafil absorbed by 23%, but tended to delay the absorption of the drug.[1] The authors of this study recommended that sildenafil and grapefruit juice not be taken together.

Summary of Interactions for Sildenafil

In some cases, an herb or supplement may appear in more than one category, which may seem contradictory. For clarification, read the full article for details about the summarized interactions.

⊘ Avoid: Adverse interaction	Grapefruit juice
Depletion or interference	None known
Side effect reduction/prevention	None known
Supportive interaction	None known
Reduced drug absorption/bioavailability	None known

SIMECO

Contains the following ingredients:
    Aluminium
    Dimethicone
    Magnesium

SIMETHICONE

Common names: Activated Polymethylsiloxane, Baby's Own Infant Drops, Dentinox Colic Drops, Gas-X, Infacol, Mylicon, Ovol, Phazyme, Setlers Wind-eze, Simethicone, SonoRX, Windcheaters, Woodard's Colic Drops

Combination drugs: Advanced Formula Di-Gel Tablets, Tempo Tablets

Simethicone is a nonprescription drug used for short-term relief of excess gas in the gastrointestinal (GI) tract. It is also used to relieve symptoms of infant colic. Simethicone is available as a nonprescription product alone and in combination with nonprescription **antacids** (page 18), for relief of stomach upset.

Summary of Interactions for Simethicone

In some cases, an herb or supplement may appear in more than one category, which may seem contradictory. For clarification, read the full article for details about the summarized interactions.

Depletion or interference	None known
Side effect reduction/prevention	None known
Supportive interaction	None known
Reduced drug absorption/bioavailability	None known
Adverse interaction	None known

SIMVASTATIN

Common names: Zocor

Simvastatin is a member of the HMG-CoA reductase inhibitor family of drugs that blocks the body's production of cholesterol. Simvastatin is used to lower elevated cholesterol and to reduce the risk of heart attack and death.

Summary of Interactions for Simvastatin

In some cases, an herb or supplement may appear in more than one category, which may seem contradictory. For clarification, read the full article for details about the summarized interactions.

✔	May be Beneficial: Depletion or interference	Coenzyme Q_{10}
✔	May be Beneficial: Supportive interaction	Fish oil (EPA)
⊘	Avoid: Adverse interaction	Grapefruit or grapefruit juice Vitamin A*
ⓘ	Check: Other	Vitamin B_3 (niacin) Vitamin E*
	Side effect reduction/prevention	None known
	Reduced drug absorption/bioavailability	None known

Interactions with Dietary Supplements

Coenzyme Q_{10}

In patients with high cholesterol, simvastatin therapy results in decreased serum coenzyme Q_{10} (CoQ_{10}) levels.[1, 2] Several trials, including double-blind trials, have confirmed this effect of simvastatin and other HMG-CoA reductase inhibitors, such as **lovastatin** (page 163) and **pravastatin** (page 220).[3, 4, 5] Supplementation with 100 mg[6] per day or 10 mg three times daily[7] of CoQ_{10} has been shown to prevent reductions in blood levels of CoQ_{10} due to simvastatin. In the latter study, people taking CoQ_{10} along with simvastatin increased their blood CoQ_{10} concentration by 63%. Many doctors recommend that people taking HMG-CoA reductase inhibitor drugs such as simvastatin also supplement with approximately 100 mg CoQ_{10} per day, although lower amounts, such as 10–30 mg per day might conceivably be effective in preventing the decline in CoQ_{10} levels.

Fish oil (EPA)

The omega-3 fatty acid EPA, present in fish oil, may improve the cholesterol- and triglyceride-lowering effect of simvastatin. In a preliminary trial, people with high cholesterol who had been taking simvastatin for about three years were able to significantly lower their triglyceride levels and raise their levels of HDL ("good") cholesterol by supplementing with either 900 mg or 1800 mg of EPA for three months in addition to simvastatin.[8] The authors of the study concluded that the combination of simvastatin and EPA may prevent coronary heart disease better than simvastatin alone.

Simvastatin

Vitamin B₃ (niacin)

Niacin is the form of vitamin B_3 used to lower cholesterol. Taking large amounts of niacin along with HMG-CoA reductase inhibitors may cause muscle disorders (myopathy) that can become serious (rhabdomyolysis).[9, 10] Such problems appear to be uncommon.[11, 12] Moreover, concurrent use of niacin has been reported to enhance the cholesterol-lowering effect of HMG-CoA reductase inhibitors.[13, 14] Individuals taking simvastatin should consult a doctor before taking niacin.

Vitamin A

A study of 37 people with high cholesterol treated with diet and HMG-CoA reductase inhibitors found blood vitamin A levels increased over two years of therapy.[15] Until more is known, people taking HMG-CoA reductase inhibitors, including simvastatin, should have blood levels of vitamin A monitored if they intend to supplement vitamin A.

Vitamin E

In a study of seven patients with hypercholesterolemia, eight weeks of simvastatin plus vitamin E 300 IU improved markers of blood vessel elasticity more than simvastatin alone.[16]

Antioxidants

In another study, daily supplementation with a combination of antioxidants (800 IU of vitamin E, 1,000 mg of vitamin C, 25 mg of beta-carotene, and 100 mcg of selenium) blocked the beneficial effect of simvastatin-plus-niacin on HDL cholesterol levels.[17] Although there is evidence that some or all of these nutrients may help prevent heart disease, individuals taking simvastatin who wish to take antioxidants should discuss the use of these supplements with their doctor.

Interactions with Foods and Other Compounds

Food

Simvastatin may be taken with or without food.[18]

Grapefruit or grapefruit juice

Grapefruit contains substances that may inhibit the body's ability to break down simvastatin; consuming grapefruit or grapefruit juice might therefore increase the potential toxicity of the drug. In a study of healthy volunteers, ingesting 200 ml of grapefruit juice along with simvastatin increased blood levels of the drug, compared with taking simvastatin with water.[19] There is one case report of a woman developing severe muscle damage from simvastatin after she began eating one grapefruit per day.[20] Although there have been no reports of a grapefruit–simvastatin interaction, to be on the safe side, people taking simvastatin should not eat grapefruit or drink grapefruit juice.

SODIUM BICARBONATE

Common names: Soda Mint Tablets, Sodium Bicarbonate Compound Tablets BP

Combination drugs: Alka-Seltzer, Birley, Bismag, Bisodol Extra Strong Mint Tablets, Bisodol Heartburn Relief Tablets, Bisodol Indigestion Relief Powder, Bisodol Indigestion Relief Tablets, Bisodol Wind Relief Tablets, Boots Indigestion Tablets, De Witt's Antacid Powder, Gaviscon 250 Tablets, Opas, Roter

Sodium bicarbonate (baking soda) is used as an **antacid** (page 18) for short-term relief of stomach upset, to correct acidosis in kidney disorders, to make the urine alkaline during bladder infections, and to minimize uric acid crystallization during gout treatment. A prescription sodium bicarbonate product is given by injection to treat metabolic acidosis and some drug intoxications. Sodium bicarbonate is available as a nonprescription drug alone (sodium bicarbonate tablets) or in combination with other nonprescription drugs for short-term treatment of various conditions to treat fever and mild to moderate pain.

Summary of Interactions for Sodium Bicarbonate

In some cases, an herb or supplement may appear in more than one category, which may seem contradictory. For clarification, read the full article for details about the summarized interactions.

✓ May be Beneficial: Depletion or interference	Folic acid Iron*
Side effect reduction/prevention	None known
Supportive interaction	None known
Reduced drug absorption/bioavailability	None known
Adverse interaction	None known

Interactions with Dietary Supplements

Folic acid

Folic acid is needed by the body to utilize vitamin B_{12}. Antacids, including sodium bicarbonate, inhibit folic acid absorption.[1] People taking antacids are advised to supplement with folic acid.

Iron

In a study of nine healthy people, sodium bicarbonate administered with 10 mg of iron led to lower iron levels compared to iron administered alone.[2] This interaction may be avoided by taking sodium bicarbonate-containing products two hours before or after iron-containing supplements.

SODIUM FLUORIDE

Common names: En-De-Kay Fluotabs, Fluor-A-Day, Fluorigard, Fluorinse, Fluoritab, Fluorodex, Fluotic, Flura-Drops, Flura-Tab, Karidium, Luride, Pedi-Dent, Pediaflor, PreviDent

Sodium fluoride is used to prevent dental cavities and might be effective in the treatment of osteoporosis.

Summary of Interactions for Sodium Fluoride

In some cases, an herb or supplement may appear in more than one category, which may seem contradictory. For clarification, read the full article for details about the summarized interactions.

✓	May be Beneficial: Depletion or interference	Zinc
✓	May be Beneficial: Supportive interaction	Vitamin D Vitamin E
ⓘ	Check: Other	Calcium
	Side effect reduction/prevention	None known
	Reduced drug absorption/bioavailability	None known
	Adverse interaction	None known

Interactions with Dietary Supplements

Calcium

Research shows that calcium from leg bones may be transferred to bones in the spine causing stress fractures when fluoride is taken alone. However, supplementing with 1,500 mg of calcium each day together with slow-release forms of fluoride increases the bone density of the lumbar spine without causing fractures.[1] Therefore, people taking sodium fluoride to treat osteoporosis should probably supplement with calcium to prevent this adverse effect. However, taking fluoride and calcium at the same time significantly reduces the absorption of fluoride;[2] consequently, they should be taken at least an hour apart.

Vitamin D

Collagen is a protein that is used in many areas of the body for structural support. One test tube study showed that the active form of vitamin D, 1,25 dihydroxycholecalciferol, increased the production of a certain type of collagen when it was combined with fluoride.[3] Controlled research is needed to determine whether taking 1,25 dihydroxycholecalciferol with sodium fluoride might promote beneficial collagen growth.

Zinc

Individuals who are bedridden for long periods may become deficient in zinc, which can affect the strength of bone that is formed. In a controlled study of healthy adults who were confined to bed, fluoride supplementation prevented zinc loss from the body.[4] Bedridden individuals should consult a qualified healthcare practitioner for guidance in using fluoride to prevent zinc deficiency.

Vitamin E

Vitamin E increases the resistance of tooth enamel to acids that cause cavities, and test tube studies show that fluoride, when added to vitamin E, enhances this effect.[5] Controlled research is needed to determine whether people might develop fewer cavities when taking vitamin E and fluoride together.

Interactions with Foods and Other Compounds

Food

Taking sodium fluoride with food[6] or dairy products[7] reduces the absorption of the mineral. Therefore, sodium fluoride should be taken an hour before or two hours after a meal, or any snack containing milk, ice cream, yogurt, or cheese.

Tea

Many compounds in tea, such as tannin, catechin, and **caffeine** (page 44), can increase the resistance of tooth enamel to acids that cause cavities, and test tube studies show that fluoride, when added to these compounds, enhances this effect.[8] Controlled research is needed to determine whether drinking tea might further reduce the number of cavities in people taking fluoride.

SOMA COMPOUND

Contains the following ingredients:
Aspirin (page 26)
Carisoprodol (page 50)

SOMA COMPOUND WITH CODEINE

Contains the following ingredients:
Aspirin (page 26)
Carisoprodol (page 50)
Codeine (page 75)

SOTALOL

Common names: Beta-Cardone, Betapace, Sotacor

Sotalol is used to treat certain types of heart arrhythmia, and is in a family of drugs known as **beta-adrenergic blockers** (page 37).

Summary of Interactions for Sotalol

In some cases, an herb or supplement may appear in more than one category, which may seem contradictory. For clarification, read the full article for details about the summarized interactions.

✓	May be Beneficial: Side effect reduction/prevention	Magnesium
⊘	Avoid: Reduced drug absorption/ bioavailability	**Antacids** (page 18) Calcium supplements Food Milk
⊘	Avoid: Adverse interaction	High-potassium foods* Pleurisy root* Potassium (low) Potassium supplements*
	Depletion or interference	None known
	Supportive interaction	None known

Interactions with Dietary Supplements
Calcium
One controlled study showed that taking sotalol with a calcium gluconate solution dramatically reduces the absorption of the drug.[1] Consequently, people who take a calcium supplement should take sotalol an hour before or two hours after the calcium.

Magnesium
Two individuals taking sotalol developed a side effect of the drug (a heart arrhythmia known as torsades de pointes) which was effectively treated with intravenous magnesium.[2, 3] Additional research is needed to determine whether people taking sotalol might be able to prevent this side effect by taking supplemental magnesium.

Potassium
People with prolonged diarrhea and vomiting, as well as those taking **potassium-depleting diuretics** (page 94), might develop low blood potassium levels. Individuals with low blood potassium levels who take sotalol have an increased risk of developing a serious heart arrhythmia and fainting. Therefore, people taking sotalol should have their blood potassium levels checked regularly and may need to supplement with potassium, especially when taking potassium-depleting diuretics.

Some beta-adrenergic blockers (called "nonselective" beta blockers) decrease the uptake of potassium from the blood into the cells,[4] leading to excess potassium in the blood, a potentially dangerous condition known as hyperkalemia.[5] People taking beta-blockers should therefore avoid taking potassium supplements, or eating large quantities of fruit (e.g., bananas), unless directed to do so by their doctor.

Interactions with Herbs
Pleurisy root
As pleurisy root and other plants in the *Aesclepius* genus contain cardiac glycosides, it is best to avoid use of pleurisy root with heart medications such as beta-blockers.[6]

Interactions with Foods and Other Compounds
Food
Taking sotalol with food gretly reduces the absorption of the drug.[7] One study showed that taking sotalol with milk also decreases absorption.[8] Therefore, sotalol should be taken an hour before or two hours after a meal or milk.

Antacids (page 18)
Taking sotalol within two hours of antacids containing aluminum oxide and **magnesium hydroxide** (page 166) dramatically reduces the absorption of the drug. Antacids that contain calcium carbonate might also reduce absorption.[9] Consequently, if antacids are being used, sotalol should be taken one hour before or two hours after the antacids.

SOVOL

Contains the following ingredients:
    Aluminium
    Dimethicone
    Magnesium

SPIRONOLACTONE

Common names: Aldactone, Laractone, Novo-Spiroton, Spiroctan, Spirolone

Combination drug: Aldactazide

Spironolactone is a potassium-sparing **diuretic** (page 94). Diuretics cause water loss and are used to treat a variety of conditions, including high blood pressure, heart failure, and diseases of the kidneys and liver. Spironolactone is available as a single agent and in a combination drug product.

Summary of Interactions for Spironolactone

In some cases, an herb or supplement may appear in more than one category, which may seem contradictory. For clarification, read the full article for details about the summarized interactions.

⊘ Avoid: Adverse interaction	Buchu
	Cleavers
	Dandelion
	Gravel root
	Horsetail
	Juniper
	Magnesium*
	Potassium
	Uva ursi
ⓘ Check: Other	Sodium
Depletion or interference	None known
Side effect reduction/prevention	None known
Supportive interaction	None known
Reduced drug absorption/bioavailability	None known

Interactions with Dietary Supplements
Folic acid
One study showed that people taking diuretics for more than six months had dramatically lower blood levels of folic acid and higher levels of homocysteine compared with individuals not taking diuretics.[1] Homocysteine, a toxic amino acid by-product, has been associated with atherosclerosis. Folic acid is also an important cause of elevated homocysteine levels. Until further information is available, people taking diuretics for longer than six months should probably supplement with folic acid.

Magnesium
Preliminary research in animals suggests that **amiloride** (page 11), a drug similar to spironolactone, may in-

hibit the urinary excretion of magnesium.[2] It is unknown if this same effect would occur in humans or with spironolactone. Persons taking more than 300 mg of magnesium per day and spironolactone should consult with a doctor as this combination may lead to potentially dangerous increases in the level of magnesium in the body. The combination of spironolactone and hydrochlorothiazide would likely eliminate this problem, as hydrochlorothiazide may deplete magnesium.

Potassium
As a potassium-sparing diuretic, spironolactone reduces urinary loss of potassium, which can lead to elevated potassium levels.[3] People taking spironolactone should avoid potassium supplements, potassium-containing salt substitutes (Morton Salt Substitute, No Salt, Lite Salt, and others), and even high-potassium foods (primarily fruit). Doctors should monitor potassium blood levels in patients taking spironolactone to prevent problems associated with elevated potassium levels.

Sodium
Diuretics (page 94), including spironolactone, cause increased loss of sodium in the urine. By removing sodium from the body, diuretics also cause water to leave the body. This reduction of body water is the purpose of taking diuretics. Therefore, there is usually no reason to replace lost sodium, although strict limitation of salt intake in combination with the actions of diuretics can sometimes cause excessive sodium depletion. On the other hand, people who restrict sodium intake and in the process reduce blood pressure may need to have their dose of diuretics lowered. People taking spironolactone should talk with their prescribing doctor before severely restricting salt.

Interactions with Herbs
Diuretic herbs
Herbs that have a diuretic effect should be avoided when taking diuretic medications, as they may increase the effect of these drugs and lead to possible cardiovascular side effects. These herbs include dandelion, uva ursi, juniper, buchu, cleavers, horsetail, and gravel root.[4]

Interactions with Foods and Other Compounds
Food
Food can increase absorption of spironolactone.[5] Spironolactone should be taken at the same time and

always with food or always without food, every day for best results. People with questions about spironolactone and food should ask their prescribing doctor or pharmacist.

STANOZOLOL

Common names: Stromba, Winstrol

Stanozolol is a synthetic anabolic steroid related to the natural hormone testosterone. Stanozolol is used to treat hereditary angioedema (episodic swelling of areas of the body).

Summary of Interactions for Stanozolol

In some cases, an herb or supplement may appear in more than one category, which may seem contradictory. For clarification, read the full article for details about the summarized interactions.

✓ May be Beneficial: Depletion or interference	Iron*
Side effect reduction/prevention	None known
Supportive interaction	None known
Reduced drug absorption/bioavailability	None known
Adverse interaction	None known

Interactions with Dietary Supplements
Iron

Stanozolol was associated with iron depletion in a group of 16 people.[1] The results suggest that people taking this drug on a regular basis have their iron status monitored by the prescribing doctor. There is insufficient information to recommend routine iron supplementation during stanozolol treatment.

STAVUDINE

Common names: d4T, Stavudine, Zerit

Stavudine is used to treat human immunodeficiency virus (HIV) infections. It is in a class of drugs known as antivirals.

Summary of Interactions for Stavudine

In some cases, an herb or supplement may appear in more than one category, which may seem contradictory.

For clarification, read the full article for details about the summarized interactions.

✓ May be Beneficial: Depletion or interference	Acetyl-L-carnitine
✓ May be Beneficial: Side effect reduction/prevention	Acetyl-L-carnitine Vitamin B₁*
Supportive interaction	None known
Reduced drug absorption/bioavailability	None known
Adverse interaction	None known

Interactions with Dietary Supplements
Vitamin B₁ (thiamine)

A 30-year-old woman who was taking stavudine developed a rare side effect called lactic acidosis, which was successfully treated with intravenous thiamine.[1] Controlled studies are needed to determine whether lactic acidosis might be prevented if people taking stavudine supplement with vitamin B₁. Until more information is available, some health practitioners may recommend supplemental vitamin B₁ to individuals taking stavudine.

Acetyl-L-carnitine

Severe peripheral neuropathy (painful sensations due to nerve damage in the hands and feet) often develops in people taking stavudine or other drugs in its class. People with peripheral neuropathy who were taking one of these drugs were found to be deficient in acetyl-L-carnitine.[2] In a preliminary trial, supplementing with 1,500 mg of acetyl-L-carnitine twice a day resulted in improvement in the neuropathy after six months in people taking stavudine or related drugs.[3]

SUCRALFATE

Common names: Antipepsin, Apo-Sucralfate, Carafate, Novo-Sucralate, Nu-Sucralfate, Sulcrate

Sucralfate is used to treat intestinal ulcers, and it is a type of drug known as a polysaccharide antipeptic.

Summary of Interactions for Sucralfate

In some cases, an herb or supplement may appear in more than one category, which may seem contradictory. For clarification, read the full article for details about the summarized interactions.

✓ May be Beneficial: Depletion or interference	Calcium Phosphorus	
Side effect reduction/prevention	None known	
Supportive interaction	None known	
Reduced drug absorption/bioavailability	None known	
Adverse interaction	None known	

Interactions with Dietary Supplements

Calcium

Slight increases in blood calcium levels may occur in people taking sucralfate, which could be aggravated by calcium supplementation.[1] Therefore, people taking calcium supplements and sucralfate should have their blood calcium levels monitored by their healthcare practitioner and may need to avoid calcium supplementation.

Phosphorus

People taking sucralfate may develop lower than normal blood levels of phosphorus.[2] A 42-year-old woman who took sucralfate for two weeks experienced bone pain that was caused by low phosphorus levels. The bone pain disappeared after she stopped taking the drug and began supplementing with phosphorus.[3] Individuals taking sucralfate should have their blood phosphorus levels monitored regularly by their healthcare practitioner and may need to take supplemental phosphorus.

SULFAMETHOXAZOLE

Common names: Gantanol, Sulphamethoxazole

Sulfamethoxazole is a member of the sulfonamide family of **antibiotics** (page 19). It is used for people with infections caused by a variety of bacteria and protozoa. The combination drug product **trimethoprim/sulfamethoxazole (TMP/SMX)** (page 273) is used to treat a wide variety of bacterial infections and some infections due to parasites.

Summary of Interactions for Sulfamethoxazole

In some cases, an herb or supplement may appear in more than one category, which may seem contradictory. For clarification, read the full article for details about the summarized interactions.

✓ May be Beneficial: Depletion or interference	Calcium* Folic acid* Magnesium* Vitamin B$_{12}$* Vitamin B$_6$* Vitamin K*	
✓ May be Beneficial: Side effect reduction/prevention	*Bifidobacterium longum** *Lactobacillus acidophilus** *Lactobacillus casei** *Saccharomyces boulardii** *Saccharomyces cerevisiae** Vitamin K*	
✓ May be Beneficial: Supportive interaction	*Saccharomyces boulardii**	
⊘ Avoid: Adverse interaction	PABA* Potassium	
Reduced drug absorption/bioavailability	None known	

Interactions with Dietary Supplements

Calcium, magnesium, vitamin B$_{12}$

Sulfonamides, including sulfamethoxazole, can decrease absorption of calcium, magnesium, and vitamin B$_{12}$.[1] This is generally not a problem when taking sulfamethoxazole for two weeks or less. People taking sulfamethoxazole for longer than two weeks should ask their doctor about nutrient monitoring and supplementation.

Folic acid, vitamin B$_6$, vitamin K

Sulfonamides, including sulfamethoxazole, can interfere with the activity of folic acid, vitamin B$_6$, and vitamin K.[2] This is generally not a problem when taking sulfamethoxazole for two weeks or less. People taking sulfamethoxazole for longer than two weeks should ask their doctor about nutrient monitoring and supplementation.

PABA (para-aminobenzoic acid)

PABA may interfere with the activity of sulfamethoxazole. PABA should not be taken with this drug until more is known.

Potassium

TMP/SMX (page 273) has been reported to elevate potassium and other constituents of blood (creatinine and BUN).[3] In particular, people with impaired kidney function should be closely monitored by their prescrib-

Sulfamethoxazole

ing doctor for these changes. People taking sulfamethoxazole or TMP/SMX should talk with their prescribing doctor before taking any potassium supplements or potassium-containing products, such as No Salt, Salt Substitute, Lite Salt, and even high-potassium foods (primarily fruit).

Probiotics

A common side effect of antibiotics is diarrhea, which may be caused by the elimination of beneficial bacteria normally found in the colon. Controlled studies have shown that taking probiotic microorganisms—such as *Lactobacillus casei, Lactobacillus acidophilus, Bifidobacterium longum,* or *Saccharomyces boulardii*—helps prevent antibiotic-induced diarrhea.[4]

The diarrhea experienced by some people who take antibiotics also might be due to an overgrowth of the bacterium *Clostridium difficile,* which causes a disease known as pseudomembranous colitis. Controlled studies have shown that supplementation with harmless yeast—such as *Saccharomyces boulardii*[5] or *Saccharomyces cerevisiae* (baker's or brewer's yeast)[6]—helps prevent recurrence of this infection. In one study, taking 500 mg of *Saccharomyces boulardii* twice daily enhanced the effectiveness of the antibiotic vancomycin in preventing recurrent clostridium infection.[7] Therefore, people taking antibiotics who later develop diarrhea might benefit from supplementing with saccharomyces organisms.

Treatment with antibiotics also commonly leads to an overgrowth of yeast *(Candida albicans)* in the vagina (candida vaginitis) and the intestines (sometimes referred to as "dysbiosis"). Controlled studies have shown that *Lactobacillus acidophilus* might prevent candida vaginitis.[8]

Vitamin K

Several cases of excessive bleeding have been reported in people who take antibiotics.[9, 10, 11, 12] This side effect may be the result of reduced vitamin K activity and/or reduced vitamin K production by bacteria in the colon. One study showed that people who had taken broad-spectrum antibiotics had lower liver concentrations of vitamin K_2 (menaquinone), though vitamin K_1 (phylloquinone) levels remained normal.[13] Several antibiotics appear to exert a strong effect on vitamin K activity, while others may not have any effect. Therefore, one should refer to a specific antibiotic for information on whether it interacts with vitamin K. Doctors of natural medicine sometimes recommend vitamin K supplementation to people taking antibiotics. Additional re-

search is needed to determine whether the amount of vitamin K_1 found in some multivitamins is sufficient to prevent antibiotic-induced bleeding. Moreover, most multivitamins do not contain vitamin K.

Interactions with Foods and Other Compounds

Food

Food may interfere with the absorption of sulfonamides, including sulfamethoxazole. It is best to take sulfamethoxazole on an empty stomach with a full glass of water.[14, 15]

SULFASALAZINE

Common names: Alti-Sulfasalazine, Azulfidine, S.A.S., Salazopyrin, Sulazine EC, Sulphasalazine

Sulfasalazine is a member of the sulfonamide drug family. It is used to treat people with ulcerative colitis, Crohn's disease, and rheumatoid arthritis.

Summary of Interactions for Sulfasalazine

In some cases, an herb or supplement may appear in more than one category, which may seem contradictory. For clarification, read the full article for details about the summarized interactions.

✓	May be Beneficial: Depletion or interference	Folic acid Vitamin K*
✓	May be Beneficial: Side effect reduction/prevention	*Bifidobacterium longum* *Lactobacillus acidophilus* *Lactobacillus casei* *Saccharomyces boulardii* *Saccharomyces cerevisiae* Vitamin K*
✓	May be Beneficial: Supportive interaction	*Saccharomyces boulardii**
⊘	Avoid: Reduced drug absorption/ bioavailability	Iron
⊘	Avoid: Adverse interaction	PABA*

Interactions with Dietary Supplements

Folic acid

Sulfasalazine decreases the absorption of folic acid.[1] Biochemical evidence of depletion of folic acid has been reported in people taking this drug,[2] although available evidence remains mixed.[3, 4]

Folic acid is needed for the normal healthy replication of cells. Perhaps as a result, there is evidence that folic acid can reverse precancerous changes in humans.[5] Ulcerative colitis, a disease commonly treated with sulfasalazine, is associated with an increased risk of colon cancer. Folate deficiency has also been linked to an increased risk for colon cancer.[6] It is plausible that some of the increased risk for colon cancer in people with ulcerative colitis may be related to folate depletion caused by sulfasalazine.

Folic acid supplementation may help protect against colon cancer.[7] One study found that people who have ulcerative colitis *and* who supplement with folic acid have a 55% lower risk of getting colon cancer, compared with ulcerative colitis patients who do not supplement with folic acid (although this dramatic association with protection did not quite reach statistical significance).[8] Researchers at the University of Chicago Medical Center reported a 62% lower risk of colon cancer in folic acid supplementers.[9] They suggested that the link between folic acid supplementation and protection from colon cancer may well be due to overcoming the folic acid deficiency induced by sulfasalazine.

Many doctors believe that it is important for all people taking sulfasalazine to supplement with folic acid. Folic acid in the amount of 800 mcg can be found in many multivitamins and B-complex vitamins. People wishing to supplement with more—typically 1,000 mcg per day—should consult their doctor.

Iron
Iron can bind with sulfasalazine, decreasing sulfasalazine absorption and possibly decreasing iron absorption.[10] This interaction can be minimized by taking iron-containing products two hours before or after sulfasalazine.

PABA (para-aminobenzoic acid)
PABA may interfere with the activity of sulfasalazine. PABA should not be taken with this drug until more is known.

Probiotics
A common side effect of antibiotics is diarrhea, which may be caused by the elimination of beneficial bacteria normally found in the colon. Controlled studies have shown that taking probiotic microorganisms—such as *Lactobacillus casei, Lactobacillus acidophilus, Bifidobac-*

terium longum, or *Saccharomyces boulardii*—helps prevent antibiotic-induced diarrhea.[11]

The diarrhea experienced by some people who take antibiotics also might be due to an overgrowth of the bacterium *Clostridium difficile,* which causes a disease known as pseudomembranous colitis. Controlled studies have shown that supplementation with harmless yeast—such as *Saccharomyces boulardii*[12] or *Saccharomyces cerevisiae* (baker's or brewer's yeast)[13]—helps prevent recurrence of this infection. In one study, taking 500 mg of *Saccharomyces boulardii* twice daily enhanced the effectiveness of the antibiotic vancomycin in preventing recurrent clostridium infection.[14] Therefore, people taking antibiotics who later develop diarrhea might benefit from supplementing with saccharomyces organisms.

Treatment with antibiotics also commonly leads to an overgrowth of yeast *(Candida albicans)* in the vagina (candida vaginitis) and the intestines (sometimes referred to as "dysbiosis"). Controlled studies have shown that *Lactobacillus acidophilus* might prevent candida vaginitis.[15]

Vitamin K
Several cases of excessive bleeding have been reported in people who take antibiotics.[16, 17, 18, 19] This side effect may be the result of reduced vitamin K activity and/or reduced vitamin K production by bacteria in the colon. One study showed that people who had taken broad-spectrum antibiotics had lower liver concentrations of vitamin K_2 (menaquinone), though vitamin K_1 (phylloquinone) levels remained normal.[20] Several antibiotics appear to exert a strong effect on vitamin K activity, while others may not have any effect. Therefore, one should refer to a specific antibiotic for information on whether it interacts with vitamin K. Doctors of natural medicine sometimes recommend vitamin K supplementation to people taking antibiotics. Additional research is needed to determine whether the amount of vitamin K_1 found in some multivitamins is sufficient to prevent antibiotic-induced bleeding. Moreover, most multivitamins do not contain vitamin K.

Interactions with Foods and Other Compounds
Food
Sulfasalazine is best taken after meals, and it is important to swallow the tablets whole to avoid inactivation by stomach acid.[21]

SULFONAMIDES

Common names: AK-Sulf, AVC, Bleph-10, Gantrisin, Kelfizine W, Silvadene, Silver Sulfadiazine, Sodium Sulamyd, Sodium Sulfacetamide, SSD, Sulfadiazine, Sulfametopyrazine, Sulfanilamide, Sulfisoxazole, Sultrin Triple Sulfa, Triple Sulfa

Sulfonamides are a family of **antibiotics** (page 19) used to treat a wide range of bacterial infections. They are available in oral forms, to treat infections throughout the body, as well as in vaginal and ophthalmic (eye) preparations that are applied to specific areas. Each drug within the family kills specific bacteria; therefore, healthcare practitioners prescribe sulfonamides based on the individual's current needs.

There are interactions that are common to **antibacterial drugs** (page 19) in general and interactions involving a specific sulfonamide. For the latter interactions, refer to the highlighted drugs listed below.

- Silver sulfadiazine (Silvadene, SSD)
- Sodium sulfacetamide (AK-Sulf, Bleph-10, Sodium Sulamyd)
- **Sulfamethoxazole** (page 245) (Gantanol)
- Sulfanilamide (AVC)
- **Sulfasalazine** (page 246) (Azulfidine)
- Sulfisoxazole (Gantrisin)
- **Trimethoprim and Sulfamethoxazole** (page 273) (Bactrim, Cotrim, Septra, Sulfatrim Pediatric)
- Triple Sulfa (Sultrin Triple Sulfa)

Summary of Interactions for Sulfonamides

In some cases, an herb or supplement may appear in more than one category, which may seem contradictory. For clarification, read the full article for details about the summarized interactions.

✓	May be Beneficial: Depletion or interference	Vitamin K*
✓	May be Beneficial: Side effect reduction/prevention	Bifidobacterium longum* Lactobacillus acidophilus* Lactobacillus casei* Saccharomyces boulardii* Saccharomyces cerevisiae* Vitamin K*

✓	May be Beneficial: Supportive interaction	Saccharomyces boulardii*
	Reduced drug absorption/bioavailability	None known
	Adverse interaction	None known

Interactions common to many, if not all, Sulfonamides are described in this article. Interactions reported for only one or several drugs in this class may not be listed in this article. Some drugs listed in this article are linked to articles specific to that respective drug; please refer to those individual drug articles. The information in this article may not necessarily apply to drugs in this class for which no separate article exists. If you are taking a Sulfonamide for which no separate article exists, talk with your doctor or pharmacist.

Interactions with Dietary Supplements

Probiotics

A common side effect of antibiotics is diarrhea, which may be caused by the elimination of beneficial bacteria normally found in the colon. Controlled studies have shown that taking probiotic microorganisms—such as *Lactobacillus casei, Lactobacillus acidophilus, Bifidobacterium longum,* or *Saccharomyces boulardii*—helps prevent antibiotic-induced diarrhea.[1]

The diarrhea experienced by some people who take antibiotics also might be due to an overgrowth of the bacterium *Clostridium difficile*, which causes a disease known as pseudomembranous colitis. Controlled studies have shown that supplementation with harmless yeast—such as *Saccharomyces boulardii*[2] or *Saccharomyces cerevisiae* (baker's or brewer's yeast)[3]—helps prevent recurrence of this infection. In one study, taking 500 mg of *Saccharomyces boulardii* twice daily enhanced the effectiveness of the antibiotic vancomycin in preventing recurrent clostridium infection.[4] Therefore, people taking antibiotics who later develop diarrhea might benefit from supplementing with saccharomyces organisms.

Treatment with antibiotics also commonly leads to an overgrowth of yeast *(Candida albicans)* in the vagina (candida vaginitis) and the intestines (sometimes referred to as "dysbiosis"). Controlled studies have shown that *Lactobacillus acidophilus* might prevent candida vaginitis.[5]

Vitamin K

Several cases of excessive bleeding have been reported in people who take antibiotics.[6, 7, 8, 9] This side effect may be the result of reduced vitamin K activity and/or reduced vitamin K production by bacteria in the colon. One study showed that people who had taken broad-spectrum antibiotics had lower liver concentrations of vitamin K_2 (menaquinone), though vitamin K_1 (phylloquinone) levels remained normal.[10] Several antibiotics appear to exert a strong effect on vitamin K activity, while others may not have any effect. Therefore, one should refer to a specific antibiotic for information on whether it interacts with vitamin K. Doctors of natural medicine sometimes recommend vitamin K supplementation to people taking antibiotics. Additional research is needed to determine whether the amount of vitamin K_1 found in some multivitamins is sufficient to prevent antibiotic-induced bleeding. Moreover, most multivitamins do not contain vitamin K.

SULINDAC

Common names: Apo-Sulin, Clinoril, Novo-Sulindac, Nu-Sulindac

Sulindac is used to treat rheumatoid arthritis, osteoarthritis and ankylosing spondylitis, a rheumatic disorder involving the spine and large joints. It also treats both acute painful shoulder and gouty arthritis. Sulindac is in a class of medications known as **nonsteroidal anti-inflammatory drugs** (page 193) (NSAIDs).

Summary of Interactions for Sulindac

In some cases, an herb or supplement may appear in more than one category, which may seem contradictory. For clarification, read the full article for details about the summarized interactions.

✓	May be Beneficial: Depletion or interference	Potassium*
⊘	Avoid: Adverse interaction	Alcohol **Lithium** (page 157)* White willow*
ⓘ	Check: Other	Folic acid*
	Side effect reduction/prevention	None known
	Supportive interaction	None known
	Reduced drug absorption/bioavailability	None known

Interactions with Dietary Supplements

Potassium

Four people who took sulindac developed high blood levels of potassium, which returned to normal within a few days after the drug was stopped.[1] Controlled research is needed to determine whether potassium supplements or a high potassium diet might aggravate this problem. Until more information is available, people taking sulindac and potassium supplements, potassium containing salt substitutes, or large amounts of fruits and vegetables should have potassium blood levels checked regularly by their doctor.

Folic acid

Sulindac blocks the activity of enzymes that depend on folic acid[2] and may, like aspirin, reduce the amount of folic acid in red blood cells.[3] Further research is needed to determine whether supplementing folic acid changes the effects of sulindac therapy or prevents a deficiency of this vitamin in the body.

Lithium (page 157)

Lithium is a mineral that may be present in some supplements and is also used in large amounts to treat mood disorders such as manic-depression (bipolar disorder). Most NSAIDs inhibit the excretion of lithium from the body, resulting in higher blood levels of the mineral, though sulindac may have an opposite effect.[4] Since major changes in lithium blood levels can produce unwanted side effects or interfere with its efficacy, NSAIDs should be used with caution, and only under medical supervision, in people taking lithium supplements.

Interactions with Herbs

White willow bark (Salix alba)

White willow bark contains salicin, which is related to **aspirin** (page 26). Both salicin and aspirin produce anti-inflammatory effects after they have been converted to salicylic acid in the body. The administration of salicylates like aspirin to individuals taking oral NSAIDs may result in reduced blood levels of NSAIDs.[5] Though no studies have investigated interactions between white willow bark and NSAIDs, people taking NSAIDs should avoid the herb until more information is available.

Interactions with Foods and Other Compounds

Green tea

Current research is exploring the possibility sulindac and other NSAIDs might inhibit cancer growth.[6, 7] Test tube studies have shown catechins, which are compounds found in green tea, significantly enhance the ability of sulindac to cause the death of and inhibit the growth of lung cancer cells.[8] Controlled research is needed to determine whether green tea and sulindac might inhibit the growth of certain cancers in humans.

Alcohol
Drinking large quantities of alcoholic beverages over a long period may block the breakdown of sulindac, resulting in higher than normal blood levels of the drug.[9] Consequently, side effects and tissue damage caused by sulindac might occur unless an adjustment is made in the amount of drug taken each day.

SUMATRIPTAN

Common names: Imigran, Imitrex

Sumatriptan is a member of the selective serotonin receptor agonist family of drugs used to treat, but not prevent, migraine headaches. Sumatriptan is available in injection, nasal spray, and oral tablet forms.

Summary of Interactions for Sumatriptan
In some cases, an herb or supplement may appear in more than one category, which may seem contradictory. For clarification, read the full article for details about the summarized interactions.

⊘ Avoid: Adverse interaction	5-Hydroxytryptophan (5-HTP)* L-tryptophan*
Depletion or interference	None known
Side effect reduction/prevention	None known
Supportive interaction	None known
Reduced drug absorption/bioavailability	None known

Interactions with Dietary Supplements
5-hydroxytryptophan (5-HTP) and L-tryptophan
Sumatriptan works by stimulating serotonin receptors in the brain. 5-HTP and L-tryptophan are converted to serotonin in the brain, and taking them with sumatriptan could increase sumatriptan-induced side effects. However, no interactions have yet been reported with sumatriptan and 5-HTP or L-tryptophan.

Interactions with Foods and Other Compounds
Food
Sumatriptan tablets may begin to work faster when taken with fluid on an empty stomach at the first sign of migraine.[1, 2]

SYNALAR C

Contains the following ingredients:
Clioquinol
Fluocinolone

SYNALAR N

Contains the following ingredients:
Fluocinolone
Neomycin (page 187)

TACRINE

Common names: Cognex

Tacrine is used to treat Alzheimer's disease and is in a class of drugs known as acetylcholinesterase inhibitors.

Summary of Interactions for Tacrine
In some cases, an herb or supplement may appear in more than one category, which may seem contradictory. For clarification, read the full article for details about the summarized interactions.

✓ May be Beneficial: Side effect reduction/prevention	Milk thistle Vitamin C*
⊘ Avoid: Adverse interaction	Huperzine A*
Depletion or interference	None known
Supportive interaction	None known
Reduced drug absorption/bioavailability	None known

Interactions with Dietary Supplements
Vitamin C
Tacrine can cause reversible liver damage in some people who take the drug. Test tube studies have shown that vitamin C blocks the formation of cell-damaging substances produced when tacrine is broken down by the body.[1] Controlled studies are needed to determine whether supplemental vitamin C might prevent liver damage in people taking tacrine.

Interactions with Herbs
Huperzine A
Further studies are needed to determine the long-term safety of huperizine A. Until more is known about its

actions in the body, it is best to avoid using it together with tacrine, which also prevents the breakdown of acetylcholine.

Milk thistle (Silybum marianum)
Tacrine often causes elevations of a liver enzyme in the blood that indicates potential liver damage. One double-blind trial showed that taking 420 mg each day of silymarin, a compound found in milk thistle, together with tacrine did not prevent liver enzyme elevation. However, silymarin did reduce the number of people who developed more severe enzyme elevations. In addition, silymarin reduced adverse stomach and intestinal side effects that are common in individuals taking tacrine.[2] Therefore, supplementing with milk thistle or silymarin may be considered as a possible way to reduce the adverse effects of tacrine.

Interactions with Foods and Other Compounds
Food
Controlled studies show that the absorption of tacrine is significantly reduced when taken with food.[3] Consequently, tacrine should be taken an hour before or two hours after a meal unless stomach or intestinal upset occurs.

Smoking
Smoking cigarettes increases the elimination of tacrine from the body.[4] This may be a problem for people who either start or stop smoking while taking the drug. Those who start smoking may experience a reduction in the beneficial effects of tacrine, while those who stop smoking might experience more side effects.

TADALAFIL

Common names: Cialis

Tadalafil is used to treat erectile dysfunction. There are currently no reported nutrient or herb interactions involving tadalafil.

TAMOXIFEN

Common names: Apo-Tamox, Emblon, Fentamox, Gen-Tamoxifen, Nolvadex, Novo-Tamoxifen, Oestrifen, Tamofen, Tamone

Tamoxifen is an antiestrogen drug primarily used to treat women with breast cancer or possibly to help pre-

vent breast cancer in women at high risk. It is also used to treat mastalgia (painful breasts) and gynecomastia (abnormal breast enlargement in males).

Summary of Interactions for Tamoxifen
In some cases, an herb or supplement may appear in more than one category, which may seem contradictory. For clarification, read the full article for details about the summarized interactions.

✓ May be Beneficial: Supportive interaction	Gamma linolenic acid (GLA) Melatonin* Tocotrienols*
⊘ Avoid: Adverse interaction	Citrus flavonoids (tangeretin)
Depletion or interference	None known
Side effect reduction/prevention	None known
Reduced drug absorption/bioavailability	None known

Interactions with Dietary Supplements
Citrus flavonoids
Preliminary research in animals found that the citrus flavonoid tangeretin (found primarily in the peel of citrus fruits) interferes with the ability of tamoxifen to inhibit tumor growth.[1] Although the evidence is far from conclusive, people taking tamoxifen should probably avoid citrus bioflavonoid supplements, as well as beverages and foods to which citrus peel oils have been added.

Gamma-linolenic acid
Gamma-linolenic acid (GLA), found in evening primrose and borage oils, may enhance the therapeutic effects of tamoxifen. A small group of breast cancer patients took 2.8 g of oral GLA per day in addition to tamoxifen, in a preliminary trial.[2] Another group of breast cancer patients took tamoxifen alone. Those taking the GLA-tamoxifen combination appeared to have a better clinical response than did those taking tamoxifen alone. However, the results of this preliminary research are far from conclusive and need to be confirmed in a larger, more definitive trial.

Melatonin
In preliminary research, large amounts of melatonin were used successfully in combination with tamoxifen in a few people with breast cancer for whom tamoxifen had previously failed.[3] The amounts used in this study should be taken only under the supervision of a doctor.

Tocotrienols

Tocotrienols are compounds similar to vitamin E that are found in palm oil. Test tube studies have shown that tocotrienols enhance the effects of tamoxifen.[4] Controlled studies are needed to determine whether supplementing with tocotrienols might enhance the anticancer effects of tamoxifen.

TAMSULOSIN

Common names: Flomax

Tamsulosin is used to treat symptoms associated with benign prostatic hyperplasia (BPH). It is in a class of drugs known as alpha 1A-adrenoceptor antagonists.

Summary of Interactions for Tamsulosin

In some cases, an herb or supplement may appear in more than one category, which may seem contradictory. For clarification, read the full article for details about the summarized interactions.

Depletion or interference	None known
Side effect reduction/prevention	None known
Supportive interaction	None known
Reduced drug absorption/bioavailability	None known
Adverse interaction	None known

Interactions with Foods and Other Compounds
Food

Taking tamsulosin on an empty stomach significantly increases the amount of drug available in the blood.[1] Consequently, tamsulosin should be taken one hour before or two hours after a meal.

TARKA

Contains the following ingredients:
Trandolapril
Verapamil (page 280)

TAVIST-D

Contains the following ingredients:
Clemastine (page 69)
Phenylpropanolamine (page 218)

TEMPO TABLETS

Contains the following ingredients:
Aluminum hydroxide (page 10)
Calcium carbonate
Magnesium hydroxide (page 166)
Simethicone (page 239)

TENBEN

Contains the following ingredients:
Atenolol (page 28)
Bendroflumethiazide

TENCHLOR

Contains the following ingredients:
Atenolol (page 28)
Chlorthalidone

TENIF

Contains the following ingredients:
Atenolol (page 28)
Nifedipine (page 189)

TENORET 50

Contains the following ingredients:
Atenolol (page 28)
Chlorthalidone

TENORETIC

Contains the following ingredients:
Atenolol (page 28)
Chlorthalidone

TERAZOSIN

Common names: Alti-Terazosin, Apo-Terazosin, Hytrin BPH, Hytrin, Novo-Terazosin, Nu-Terazosin

Terazosin is a member of the alpha blocker family of drugs used to lower blood pressure in people with hypertension. Terazosin is also used to treat some instances of heart failure and symptoms of benign prostatic hyperplasia (BPH).

Summary of Interactions for Terazosin

In some cases, an herb or supplement may appear in more than one category, which may seem contradictory. For clarification, read the full article for details about the summarized interactions.

Depletion or interference	None known
Side effect reduction/prevention	None known
Supportive interaction	None known
Reduced drug absorption/bioavailability	None known
Adverse interaction	None known

TERBINAFINE

Common names: Lamisil

Terbinafine is an antifungal drug used to treat onychomycosis (fungal infection) of the toenails and fingernails.

Summary of Interactions for Terbinafine

In some cases, an herb or supplement may appear in more than one category, which may seem contradictory. For clarification, read the full article for details about the summarized interactions.

Depletion or interference	None known
Side effect reduction/prevention	None known
Supportive interaction	None known
Reduced drug absorption/bioavailability	None known
Adverse interaction	None known

Interactions with Foods and Other Compounds

Food

Food increases absorption of terbinafine.[1] People taking terbinafine should take it at the same time every day, always with or always without food.

TERCONAZOLE

Common names: Terazol

Terconazole is an antifungal drug used topically to treat vulvovaginal yeast infections.

Summary of Interactions for Terconazole

In some cases, an herb or supplement may appear in more than one category, which may seem contradictory. For clarification, read the full article for details about the summarized interactions.

Depletion or interference	None known
Side effect reduction/prevention	None known
Supportive interaction	None known
Reduced drug absorption/bioavailability	None known
Adverse interaction	None known

TERRA-CORTRIL

Contains the following ingredients:
  Hydrocortisone
  Oxytetracycline

TERRA-CORTRIL NYSTATIN

Contains the following ingredients:
  Hydrocortisone
  Nystatin (page 195)
  Oxytetracycline

TETRACYCLINE

Common names: Achromycin, Actisite, Apo-Tetra, Economycin, Novo-Tetra, Nu-Tetra, Sumycin, Tetrachel, Topicycline

Combination drugs: Deteclo, Helidac

Tetracycline is a member of the **tetracycline family** (page 255) of **antibiotics** (page 19). Tetracycline is used to treat a wide variety of infections and severe acne.

Summary of Interactions for Tetracycline

In some cases, an herb or supplement may appear in more than one category, which may seem contradictory. For clarification, read the full article for details about the summarized interactions.

✓ May be Beneficial: Depletion or interference	Folic acid Potassium Vitamin B₁₂ Vitamin B₂ Vitamin B₆ Vitamin C Vitamin K*
✓ May be Beneficial: Side effect reduction/prevention	*Bifidobacterium longum* *Lactobacillus acidophilus* *Lactobacillus casei* Probiotics* *Saccharomyces boulardii* *Saccharomyces cerevisiae* Vitamin K*
✓ May be Beneficial: Supportive interaction	Probiotics* *Saccharomyces boulardii* Vitamin B₃ (Niacinamide only, for bullous pemphigoid and dermatitis herpetiformis) Vitamin C*
⃠ Avoid: Reduced drug absorption/bioavailability	Minerals (Aluminum, Calcium, Iron, Magnesium, Zinc)
⃠ Avoid: Adverse interaction	Berberine-containing herbs such as Goldenseal, Barberry, and Oregon grape

Interactions with Dietary Supplements

Minerals

Many minerals can decrease the absorption of tetracycline, thus reducing its effectiveness. These minerals include aluminum (in **antacids** [page 18]), calcium (in antacids, dairy products, and supplements), magnesium (in antacids and supplements), iron (in food and supplements), zinc (in food and supplements), and others.

Probiotics

A common side effect of antibiotics is diarrhea, which may be caused by the elimination of beneficial bacteria normally found in the colon. Controlled studies have shown that taking probiotic microorganisms—such as *Lactobacillus casei*, *Lactobacillus acidophilus*, *Bifidobacterium longum*, or *Saccharomyces boulardii*—helps prevent antibiotic-induced diarrhea.[1]

The diarrhea experienced by some people who take antibiotics also might be due to an overgrowth of the bacterium *Clostridium difficile*, which causes a disease known as pseudomembranous colitis. Controlled studies have shown that supplementation with harmless yeast—such as *Saccharomyces boulardii*[2] or *Saccharomyces cerevisiae* (baker's or brewer's yeast)[3]—helps prevent recurrence of this infection. In one study, taking 500 mg of *Saccharomyces boulardii* twice daily enhanced the effectiveness of the antibiotic vancomycin in preventing recurrent clostridium infection.[4] Therefore, people taking antibiotics who later develop diarrhea might benefit from supplementing with saccharomyces organisms.

Treatment with antibiotics also commonly leads to an overgrowth of yeast *(Candida albicans)* in the vagina (candida vaginitis) and the intestines (sometimes referred to as "dysbiosis"). Controlled studies have shown that *Lactobacillus acidophilus* might prevent candida vaginitis.[5]

Vitamins

Tetracycline can interfere with the activity of folic acid, potassium, and vitamin B₂, vitamin B₆, vitamin B₁₂, vitamin C, and vitamin K.[6] This is generally not a problem when taking tetracycline for two weeks or less. People taking tetracycline for longer than two weeks should ask their doctor about vitamin and mineral supplementation. Taking 500 mg vitamin C simultaneously with tetracycline was shown to increase blood levels of tetracycline in one study.[7] The importance of this interaction is unknown.

Taking large amounts of niacinamide, a form of vitamin B₃, can suppress inflammation in the body. According to numerous preliminary reports, niacinamide, given in combination with tetracycline or **minocycline** (page 179), may be effective against bullous pemphigoid, a benign, autoimmune blistering disease of the skin.[8, 9, 10, 11, 12, 13, 14] Preliminary evidence also suggests a similar beneficial interaction may exist between tetracycline and niacinamide in the treatment of dermatitis herpetiformis.[15, 16]

Vitamin K
Several cases of excessive bleeding have been reported in people who take antibiotics.[17, 18, 19, 20] This side effect may be the result of reduced vitamin K activity and/or reduced vitamin K production by bacteria in the colon. One study showed that people who had taken broad-spectrum antibiotics had lower liver concentrations of vitamin K_2 (menaquinone), though vitamin K_1 (phylloquinone) levels remained normal.[21] Several antibiotics appear to exert a strong effect on vitamin K activity, while others may not have any effect. Therefore, one should refer to a specific antibiotic for information on whether it interacts with vitamin K. Doctors of natural medicine sometimes recommend vitamin K supplementation to people taking antibiotics. Additional research is needed to determine whether the amount of vitamin K_1 found in some multivitamins is sufficient to prevent antibiotic-induced bleeding. Moreover, most multivitamins do not contain vitamin K.

Interactions with Herbs
Berberine-containing herbs
Berberine, a chemical extracted from goldenseal *(Hydrastis canadensis)*, barberry *(Berberis vulgaris)*, and Oregon grape *(Berberis aquifolium)*, has been shown to have antibacterial activity. One double-blind study found that giving 100 mg of berberine at the same time as 500 mg of tetracycline four times daily led to a reduction of the efficacy of tetracycline in people with cholera.[22] Berberine may have decreased the absorption of tetracycline in this study. Another double-blind trial did not find that berberine interfered with tetracycline in cholera patients.[23] Until more studies are completed to clarify this issue, berberine-containing herbs should not be taken simultaneously with tetracycline.

Interactions with Foods and Other Compounds
Food
Tetracycline should be taken on an empty stomach, one hour before or two hours after any other food, drugs, or supplements, with a full glass of water.[24]

TETRACYCLINES

Common names: Declomycin, Demeclocycline, Ledermycin, Lymecycline, Oxymycin, Oxytetracycline, Oxytetramix, Terramycin

Combination drugs: Deteclo, Deteclo

Tetracyclines are a family of **antibiotics** (page 19) used to treat a broad spectrum of bacterial infections occurring in many areas of the body. Each drug within the family prevents the growth of specific bacteria; therefore, healthcare practitioners prescribe tetracyclines based on the individual's current needs.

There are interactions that are common to **antibacterial drugs** (page 19), interactions common to tetracyclines in general, and interactions involving specific tetracyclines. Interactions that are common to all tetracyclines are described below. For interactions involving specific tetracycline, refer to the highlighted drugs listed below.
- Demeclocycline (Declomycin)
- **Doxycycline** (page 101) (Monodox, Periostat, Vibramycin, Vibra-Tabs)
- **Minocycline** (page 179) (Dynacin, Minocin, Vectrin)
- Oxytetracycline (Terramycin)
- **Tetracycline** (page 253) (Sumycin, Tetracyn)

Summary of Interactions for Tetracyclines
In some cases, an herb or supplement may appear in more than one category, which may seem contradictory. For clarification, read the full article for details about the summarized interactions.

✓	May be Beneficial: Depletion or interference	Vitamin K*
✓	May be Beneficial: Side effect reduction/prevention	*Bifidobacterium longum** *Lactobacillus acidophilus** *Lactobacillus casei** Probiotics* *Saccharomyces boulardii** *Saccharomyces cerevisiae** Vitamin K*
✓	May be Beneficial: Supportive interaction	*Saccharomyces boulardii**

Tetracyclines

🚫 Avoid: Reduced drug absorption/ bioavailability	Aluminum Calcium Dairy products Food Iron Magnesium **Sodium bicarbonate** (page 240) Zinc
Adverse interaction	None known

Interactions common to many, if not all, Tetracycline preparations are described in this article. Interactions reported for only one or several drugs in this class may not be listed in this article. Some drugs listed in this article are linked to articles specific to that respective drug; please refer to those individual drug articles. The information in this article may not necessarily apply to drugs in this class for which no separate article exists. If you are taking a Tetracycline preparation for which no separate article exists, talk with your doctor or pharmacist.

Interactions with Dietary Supplements
Minerals

Taking mineral supplements or **antacids** (page 18) that contain aluminum, calcium, iron, magnesium, or zinc at the same time as tetracyclines inhibits the absorption of the drug.[1] Therefore, individuals should take tetracyclines at least two hours before or after products containing minerals.

Probiotics

A common side effect of antibiotics is diarrhea, which may be caused by the elimination of beneficial bacteria normally found in the colon. Controlled studies have shown that taking probiotic microorganisms—such as *Lactobacillus casei*, *Lactobacillus acidophilus*, *Bifidobacterium longum*, or *Saccharomyces boulardii*—helps prevent antibiotic-induced diarrhea.[2]

The diarrhea experienced by some people who take antibiotics also might be due to an overgrowth of the bacterium *Clostridium difficile*, which causes a disease known as pseudomembranous colitis. Controlled studies have shown that supplementation with harmless yeast—such as *Saccharomyces boulardii*[3] or *Saccharomyces cerevisiae* (baker's or brewer's yeast)[4]—helps prevent recurrence of this infection. In one study, taking 500 mg of *Saccharomyces boulardii* twice daily enhanced the effectiveness of the antibiotic vancomycin in preventing recurrent clostridium infection.[5] Therefore, people taking antibiotics who later develop diarrhea might benefit from supplementing with saccharomyces organisms.

Treatment with antibiotics also commonly leads to an overgrowth of yeast (*Candida albicans*) in the vagina (candida vaginitis) and the intestines (sometimes referred to as "dysbiosis"). Controlled studies have shown that *Lactobacillus acidophilus* might prevent candida vaginitis.[6]

Vitamin K

Several cases of excessive bleeding have been reported in people who take antibiotics.[7, 8, 9, 10] This side effect may be the result of reduced vitamin K activity and/or reduced vitamin K production by bacteria in the colon. One study showed that people who had taken broad-spectrum antibiotics had lower liver concentrations of vitamin K_2 (menaquinone), though vitamin K_1 (phylloquinone) levels remained normal.[11] Several antibiotics appear to exert a strong effect on vitamin K activity, while others may not have any effect. Therefore, one should refer to a specific antibiotic for information on whether it interacts with vitamin K. Doctors of natural medicine sometimes recommend vitamin K supplementation to people taking antibiotics. Additional research is needed to determine whether the amount of vitamin K_1 found in some multivitamins is sufficient to prevent antibiotic-induced bleeding. Moreover, most multivitamins do not contain vitamin K.

Interactions with Foods and Other Compounds
Food

The absorption of **tetracycline** (page 253), demeclocycline, and oxytetracycline is reduced when taken with a meal or with dairy products, such as milk, yogurt, and cheese.[12] Therefore, these drugs should be taken an hour before or two hours after eating a meal or dairy products. However, food and diary products do not reduce the absorption of **doxycycline** (page 101) and **minocycline** (page 179).[13]

Sodium bicarbonate (page 240)

Taking tetracyclines with sodium bicarbonate might inhibit the absorption and/or the excretion of the drug.[14] Therefore, to avoid alterations in clinical effect, tetracyclines should be taken an hour before or two hours after products containing sodium bicarbonate.

THEOPHYLLINE/ AMINOPHYLLINE

Common names: Amnivent 225 SR, Apo-Theo LA, Lasma, Norphyllin SR, Novo-Theophyl SR, Nuelin SA, Nuelin, Phyllocontin, Slo-

Bid, Slo-Phyllin, Theo-24, Theo-Bid, Theo-Dur, Theo-SR, Theochron SR, Theocron, Theolair, Theophylline Ethylenediamine, Truphylline, Uni-Dur, Uniphyllin Continuous, Uniphyl

Combination drug: Primatene Dual Action

Theophylline and aminophylline are bronchodilator drugs (i.e., drugs that open the lung passages) used to treat people with asthma. Aminophylline is a modified form of theophylline. Theophylline and aminophylline are used systemically (carried in the blood stream through the body) and have side effects throughout the body. Other drugs, which are administered by inhalation, are more commonly used to treat asthma, because they go directly to the lungs.

Summary of Interactions

In some cases, an herb or supplement may appear in more than one category, which may seem contradictory. For clarification, read the full article for details about the summarized interactions.

✓ May be Beneficial: Depletion or interference	Magnesium Potassium Vitamin B$_6$
⊘ Avoid: Reduced drug absorption/ bioavailability	St. John's wort* Tannin-containing herbs such as green tea, black tea, uva ursi, black walnut, red raspberry, oak, and witch hazel
⊘ Avoid: Adverse interaction	**Caffeine** (page 44) Pepper*
ⓘ Check: Other	Soy*
Side effect reduction/prevention	None known
Supportive interaction	None known

Interactions with Dietary Supplements

Potassium and magnesium

Preliminary evidence indicates that theophylline can promote potassium and magnesium deficiency.[1, 2] Some doctors have noted a tendency for persons on theophylline to become deficient in these minerals. Therefore, supplementing with these minerals may be necessary during theophylline therapy. Consult with a doctor to make this determination.

Vitamin B$_6$

Theophyline has been associated with depressed serum vitamin B$_6$ levels in children with asthma[3] and adults with chronic obstructive pulmonary disease.[4] In a short-term study of healthy adults, theophylline reduced serum vitamin B$_6$ levels and supplementation with vitamin B$_6$ (10 mg per day) normalized vitamin B$_6$ levels.[5] Some doctors believe that it makes sense for people taking this drug to accompany it with 10 mg of vitamin B$_6$ per day.

Soy

In a study of healthy volunteers given theophylline, ingesting daidzein (one of the major isoflavones in soy) in the amount of 200 mg twice a day for ten days inhibited the metabolism of theophylline, resulted in higher concentrations of the drug.[6] The amount of daidzein used in this study was greater than what would be found in a normal portion of soy foods; it is not known whether consuming average amounts of soy would have a similar effect.

Interactions with Herbs

Pepper (Piper nigrum, Piper longum)

Piperine is a chemical found in black peppers. A human study found that single doses of piperine could increase blood levels of theophylline.[7] Hypothetically, such an elevation could lead to increased theophylline side effects or dose reductions without loss of drug efficacy. However, further study is required before such conclusions are made. People should not change the amount of theophylline taken without consulting their physician.

Tannin-containing herbs

Herbs high in tannins can impair the absorption of theophylline.[8] High-tannin herbs include green tea, black tea, uva ursi (*Arctostaphylos uva-ursi*), black walnut (*Juglans nigra*), red raspberry (*Rubus idaeus*), oak (*Quercus* spp.), and witch hazel (*Hamamelis virginiana*).

St. John's wort (Hypericum perforatum)

One case study of a 42-year old asthmatic woman reported that taking 300 mg per day of St. John's wort extract led to a significant decrease in blood levels of theophylline.[9] Following discontinuation of St. John's wort, the patient's blood levels of theophylline returned to an acceptable therapeutic level. This may have occurred because certain chemicals found in St. John's wort activate liver enzymes that are involved in the elimination of some drugs.[10, 11] Until more is known, people taking theophylline should avoid St. John's wort.

Interactions with Foods and Other Compounds

Food

Low-carbohydrate, high-protein diets, charbroiled beef, and large amounts of cruciferous vegetables (broccoli, Brussels sprouts, cabbage, and cauliflower) can reduce theophylline activity.[12, 13] High-carbohydrate, low-protein diets can increase theophylline activity and side effects.[14] Sustained-release forms of theophylline should be taken on an empty stomach and should not be crushed or chewed.[15] Liquid and non-sustained release theophylline products are best taken on an empty stomach, but they may be taken with food if stomach upset occurs.[16] People with questions about theophylline and food should ask their prescribing doctor or pharmacist.

Caffeine (page 44)

Large amounts of caffeine (a substance that is related to theophylline) may increase the activity and side effects of theophylline.[17]Coffee, tea, colas, chocolate, guaraná, and some supplement products contain caffeine. Limiting intake of caffeine-containing beverages and products to small amounts will avoid this interaction.

Soy

In a study of healthy volunteers given theophylline, ingesting daidzein (one of the major isoflavones in soy) in the amount of 200 mg twice a day for ten days inhibited the metabolism of theophylline, resulted in higher concentrations of the drug.[18] The amount of daidzein used in this study was greater than what would be found in a normal portion of soy foods; it is not known whether consuming average amounts of soy would have a similar effect.

THERAFLU

Contains the following ingredients:
Acetaminophen (page 3)
Chlorpheniramine (page 59)
Pseudoephedrine

THIAZIDE DIURETICS

Common names: Apo-Chlorthalidone, Apo-Hydro, Aprinox, Bendrofluazide, Bendroflumethiazide, Benzthiazide, Berkozide, Chlorothiazide, Chlorphthalidone, Chlortalidone, Chlorthalidone, Cyclopenthiazide, Dihydrochlorothiazide, Diucardin, Diurexan, Diuril, Enduron, Esidrix, Exna, HCTZ, Hydrochlorothiazide, Hydro DIURIL, Hydroflumethiazide, Hydromox, HydroSaluric, Hygroton, Indapamide, Lozol, Metenix 5, Methyclothiazide, Metolazone, Mykrox, Naqua, Naturetin, Navidrex, Neo-Bendromax, Neo-

NaClex, Nephril, Opumide, Oretic, Polythiazide, Quinethazone, Renese, Saluric, Trichlormethiazide, Xipamide, Zaroxolyn

Combination drugs: Accuretic, Acezide, Aldactazide, Aldoclor, Aldoril, Apresazide, AtenixCo, Capto-Co, Captozide, Carace Plus, Co-Betaloc SA, Co-Betaloc, Co-Tendione, Co-Zidocapt, CoAprovel, Combipres, Cozaar-Comp, Dyazide, Hyzaar, Inderide, Innozide, Kalten, Lopressor HCT, Maxzide, Moducren, Moduretic, Monozide, Prinzide, Secradex, Tenchlor, Tenoret 50, Tenoretic, Timolide, Totaretic, Vaseretic, Zestoretic, Ziac

Thiazide diuretics are a family of drugs that remove water from the body. They are referred to as potassium-depleting because they cause the body to lose potassium as well as water. Potassium-depleting diuretics also cause the body to lose magnesium. Thiazide diuretics are used to lower blood pressure in people with high blood pressure. **Diuretics** (page 94) are also used to reduce water accumulation caused by other diseases.

Thiazide diuretics are also combined with other drugs to treat various conditions.

The information in this article pertains to thiazide diuretics in general. The interactions reported here may not apply to all the Also Indexed As terms. Talk to your doctor or pharmacist if you are taking any of these drugs.

Summary of Interactions for Thiazide Diuretics

In some cases, an herb or supplement may appear in more than one category, which may seem contradictory. For clarification, read the full article for details about the summarized interactions.

✓ May be Beneficial: Depletion or interference	Folic acid * Magnesium Potassium Zinc
🚫 Avoid: Adverse interaction	Alder Buckthorn* Buchu Buckthorn* Cleavers Dandelion Digitalis Ginkgo biloba* Gravel root Horsetail Juniper Licorice Uva ursi
ⓘ Check: Other	Calcium Sodium Vitamin D
Side effect reduction/prevention	None known
Supportive interaction	None known
Reduced drug absorption/bioavailability	None known

Interactions with Dietary Supplements

Calcium

Thiazide diuretics decrease calcium loss in the urine due to actions on the kidneys.[1] As a result, it may be less important for some people taking thiazide diuretics to supplement calcium than it is for other people.

Folic acid

One study showed that people taking diuretics for more than six months had dramatically lower blood levels of folic acid and higher levels of homocysteine compared with individuals not taking diuretics.[2] Homocysteine, a toxic amino acid by-product, has been associated with atherosclerosis. Until further information is available, people taking diuretics for longer than six months should probably supplement with folic acid.

Magnesium and potassium

Potassium-depleting diuretics, including thiazide diuretics, cause the body to lose potassium; they may also cause cellular magnesium depletion,[3] although this deficiency may not be reflected by a low blood level of magnesium.[4] Magnesium loss induced by potassium-depleting diuretics can cause additional potassium loss. Until more is known, it has been suggested that people taking potassium-depleting diuretics, including thiazide diuretics, should supplement both potassium and magnesium.[5]

People taking thiazide diuretics should be monitored by their prescribing doctor, who will prescribe potassium supplements if needed. Such supplementation is particularly critical before surgery in patients with a history of heart disease. In a preliminary study, people with low blood levels of potassium (in part related to diuretic use) had a higher incidence of serious problems resulting from surgery (including death) compared with those having normal potassium levels.[6] A double-blind trial showed that thiazide diuretic use led to a reduction in blood levels of potassium in some participants. Those experiencing decreased potassium levels were also more likely to experience cardiovascular events, such as heart attacks, stroke, heart failure, aneurysm, and sudden cardiac death.[7] Fruit is high in potassium, and increasing fruit intake (especially bananas) is another way of supplementing potassium.

Magnesium supplementation for people taking thiazide diuretics is typically 300–600 mg per day, though higher amounts (over 800 mg per day) have been reported in a controlled study to reduce side effects of thiazides.[8] Combining supplementation of both potassium and magnesium has been reported to correct abnormally low blood levels of potassium and also to protect against excessive loss of magnesium.[9]

Vitamin D

The reduction in urinary calcium loss resulting from treatment with thiazide diuretics is due primarily to changes in kidney function and may also be due, in part, to changes in vitamin D metabolism.[10] However, there is no evidence to suggest that people taking diuretics have different requirements for vitamin D.

Zinc

Thiazide diuretics can increase urinary zinc loss.[11]

Sodium

Diuretics, including thiazide diuretics, cause increased loss of sodium in the urine. By removing sodium from the body, diuretics also cause water to leave the body. This reduction of body water is the purpose of taking diuretics. Therefore, there is usually no reason to replace lost sodium, although strict limitation of salt intake in combination with the actions of diuretics can sometimes cause excessive sodium depletion. On the other hand, people who restrict sodium intake, and in the process reduce blood pressure, may need to have their dose of diuretics lowered.

Interactions with Herbs

Herbs that have a diuretic effect should be avoided when taking diuretic medications, as they may enhance the effect of these drugs and lead to possible cardiovascular side effects. These herbs include dandelion, uva ursi, juniper, buchu, cleavers, horsetail, and gravel root.[12]

Alder buckthorn, buckthorn (Rhamnus catartica, Rhamnus frangula, Frangula alnus)

Use buckthorn or alder buckthorn for more than ten days consecutively may cause a loss of electrolytes (especially the mineral potassium). Medications that also cause potassium loss, such as some diuretics, should be used with caution when taking buckthorn or alder buckthorn.[13]

Digitalis (Digitalis purpurea)

Digitalis refers to a family of plants commonly called foxglove, which contains digitalis glycosides, chemicals with actions and toxicities similar to the prescription drug **digoxin** (page 90). Thiazide diuretics can increase the risk of digitalis-induced heart disturbances.[14] Thiazide diuretics and digitalis-containing products should be used only under the direct supervision of a doctor trained in their use.

Ginkgo biloba

One case was reported in which ginkgo use was associated with high blood pressure in a person treated with a thiazide diuretic.[15] Ginkgo was not proven to be the cause of this reaction.

Licorice (Glycyrrhiza glabra)

Licorice may increase the side effects of potassium-depleting diuretics, including thiazide diuretics.[16] Thiazide diuretics and licorice should be used together only under careful medical supervision. At the time of this writing, no evidence was found of interactions between deglycyrrhizinated licorice (DGL) and any diuretic was found in the medical literature.

Interactions with Foods and Other Compounds
Food
Thiazide diuretics may be taken with food to avoid stomach upset.[17]

THIORIDAZINE

Common names: Apo-Thioridazine, Mellaril, Melleril, Rideril

Thioridazine is used to treat symptoms associated with psychosis; depression with worry and restlessness in adults; irritability, worry, and fear in elderly; and severe behavioral problems in children, including fighting and hyperactivity. It is classified as a phenothiazine neuroleptic.

Summary of Interactions for Thioridazine

In some cases, an herb or supplement may appear in more than one category, which may seem contradictory. For clarification, read the full article for details about the summarized interactions.

✓ May be Beneficial: Depletion or interference	Vitamin A
✓ May be Beneficial: Side effect reduction/prevention	Coenzyme Q10 Potassium*
✓ May be Beneficial: Supportive interaction	Niacin*
⊘ Avoid: Adverse interaction	Bacopa **Lithium** (page 157)*
ⓘ Check: Other	Vitamin C*
Reduced drug absorption/bioavailability	None known

Interactions with Dietary Supplements
Vitamin A
A review of people taking thioridazine showed that they had higher blood levels of vitamin A than did individu-

als not using the drug.[1] More research is necessary to determine whether taking vitamin A supplements with thioridazine might cause dangerously high vitamin A levels. Until more is known, people taking thioridazine should exercise caution with vitamin A supplementation and be alert for side effects such as bone pain, headaches, dry scaly skin, and hair loss.

Potassium
Some people taking thioridazine experience changes in the electrical activity of the heart, which sometimes improve with potassium supplementation.[2] More research is needed to determine if people taking thioridazine might prevent heart problems by supplementing with potassium.

Niacin (nicotinic acid)
In a controlled study, individuals taking thioridazine for psychosis cooperated better and withdrew less from other people when niacin, 300–1,500 mg each day, was added.[3] Whether people who are taking thioridazine for other mental health problems might benefit from niacin supplementation is unknown.

Coenzyme Q10
Phenothiazine drugs like thioridazine can cause changes in heart activity in some people, which might be prevented with coenzyme Q10 supplementation.[4] Therefore, some doctors and pharmacists may recommend coenzyme Q10 supplements to individuals taking thioridazine.

Lithium (page 157)
Lithium is a mineral that may be present in some supplements and is also used in large amounts to treat mood disorders such as bipolar disorder (manic depression). One study reviewed four cases in which individuals stabilized on lithium medication developed side effects such as delirium, seizures, and abnormal electrical activity in the brain when thioridazine was added.[5] Further research is needed to determine whether similar side effects might occur in individuals taking thioridazine and supplemental lithium.

Vitamin C
Taking phenothiazine drugs can stop menstruation in some women. A 45-year-old woman taking thioridazine started menstruating once she began supplementing with 6 grams of vitamin C daily.[6] Controlled studies are needed to determine whether women taking thioridazine, who are experiencing menstrual changes, might benefit from supplemental vitamin C. Vitamin C might also enhance the effectiveness of neuroleptic drugs, such as thioridazine, in the treatment of schizo-

phrenia. One uncontrolled study showed that 10 of 13 individuals experienced a reduction in disorganized thoughts, hallucinations, and suspicious thoughts when 8 grams of vitamin C was added to their daily drug therapy.[7] Controlled studies are needed to determine whether people taking thioridazine for schizophrenia might benefit from vitamin C supplementation.

Interactions with Herbs

Bacopa

An animal study found that the effects of chlorpromazine, a drug similar to (perphenazine, prochlorperazine, thioridazine), were enhanced when a bacopa extract was given along with it.[8] Until more is known, people taking medications from this family of drugs (called phenothiazines) should not take bacopa.

Interactions with Foods and Other Compounds

Alcohol

Drinking alcoholic beverages while taking thioridazine may enhance the actions of alcohol, such as drowsiness, dizziness, and lack of concentration,[9] and should be avoided. Two individuals withdrawing from chronic alcohol consumption experienced serious changes in heart function when they were given thioridazine;[10] therefore, the drug should be used with caution in people who are attempting to quit drinking.

THYROID HORMONES

Common names: Animal Levothyroxine/Liothyronine, Animal Thyroid, Armour Thyroid, Cytomel, Desiccated Thyroid, Eltroxin, Euthroid, L-Tri-iodothyronine, Levo-T, Levotec, Levothroid, Levothyroxine, Levothyroxine (Synthetic), Levoxyl, Liothyronine, Liothyronine (Synthetic), Liotrix, Proloid, Synthroid, Tertroxin, Thyar, Thyroglobulin, Thyrolar, Thyroxine, Tri-iodothyronine, Triostat, Unithroid

Thyroid medications are synthetic or animal-derived hormones used to treat people with hypothyroidism (low thyroid function), goiter, and Hashimoto's disease.

The information in this article pertains to thyroid hormones in general. The interactions reported here may not apply to all the Also Indexed As terms. Talk to your doctor or pharmacist if you are taking any of these drugs.

Summary of Interactions for Thyroid Hormones

In some cases, an herb or supplement may appear in more than one category, which may seem contradictory. For clarification, read the full article for details about the summarized interactions.

✓ May be Beneficial: Depletion or interference		Calcium
⊘ Avoid: Reduced drug absorption/ bioavailability		Calcium Soy
⊘ Avoid: Adverse interaction		Bugleweed* Lemon balm*
ⓘ Check: Other		Iron
Side effect reduction/prevention		None known
Supportive interaction		None known

Interactions with Dietary Supplements

Calcium

Thyroid hormones have been reported to increase urinary loss of calcium.[1] However, recent research suggests that, under most circumstances, taking thyroid hormones may not be associated with reduced bone density.[2, 3] Calcium supplementation for people taking long-term thyroid medication has not yet been proven to be either helpful or necessary.

Simultaneous ingestion of some calcium formulations with levothyroxine has been reported to reduce the effectiveness of levothyroxine.[4] For example, 1,200 mg per day of calcium as calcium carbonate, taken along with levothyroxine, significantly reduced absorption of the thyroid hormone.[5] Levothyroxine activity will not be blocked if it is taken in the morning and calcium carbonate is taken after lunch and dinner. Separating these medications by at least four hours is recommended.

Iron

Iron deficiency has been reported to impair the body's ability to make its own thyroid hormones,[6] which could increase the need for thyroid medication. In a preliminary trial, iron supplementation given to iron-deficient women with low blood levels of thyroid hormones, partially normalized these levels.[7] Diagnosing iron deficiency requires the help of a doctor. The body's ability to make its own thyroid hormones is also reduced during low-calorie dieting. Iron supplementation (27 mg per day) was reported in a controlled study to help maintain normal thyroid hormone levels in obese patients despite a very low-calorie diet.[8]

However, iron supplements may decrease absorption of thyroid hormone medications.[9, 10] People taking thyroid hormone medications should talk with their doctor before taking iron-containing products.

Soy

Ingestion of soy products simultaneously with thyroid hormones appears to reduce the absorption of the hormones. To be safe, people taking thyroid medication should not consume soy products within three hours of taking their medication. In addition, infants with congenital hypothyroidism given thyroid medication must not be given increased or reduced amounts of soy-based formula without consulting a pediatrician or pediatric endocrinologist.[11]

Interactions with Herbs

Bugleweed *(Lycopus virginicus, Lycopus europaeus)* and lemon balm *(Melissa officinalis)* may interfere with the action of thyroid hormones and should not be used during treatment with thyroid hormones.[12]

Interactions with Foods and Other Compounds
Food
Taking levothyroxine with food may decrease its absorption.[13] Levothyroxine absorption is increased when taken on an empty stomach.[14] High-fiber diets have been shown to decrease levothyroxine absorption.[15] Thyroid hormones should be taken an hour before eating, at the same time very day.[16]

TICLOPIDINE

Common names: Apo-Ticlopidine, Betimol, Nu-Ticlopidine, Ticlid

Ticlopidine is a platelet inhibiting drug. It is used to prevent stroke and to treat intermittent claudication and other conditions.

Summary of Interactions for Ticlopidine

In some cases, an herb or supplement may appear in more than one category, which may seem contradictory. For clarification, read the full article for details about the summarized interactions.

⊘ Avoid: Adverse interaction	Asian ginseng* Dan shen Devil's claw* Dong quai* Fenugreek* Garlic* *Ginkgo biloba* Horse chestnut* Quinine* Red clover* Salicylate-containing herbs* such as meadowsweet,
	poplar, willow, and wintergreen Sweet clover* Sweet woodruff*
ⓘ Check: Other	Eleuthero Ginger
Depletion or interference	None known
Side effect reduction/prevention	None known
Supportive interaction	None known
Reduced drug absorption/bioavailability	None known

Interactions with Herbs
Asian ginseng (Panax ginseng)
Ginseng was associated with a decrease in **warfarin** (page 281) activity in a case study.[1] This report suggests that ginseng may affect parameters of bleeding. Therefore, people taking ticlopidine should consult with a physician knowledgeable about botanical medicines before taking Asian ginseng or eleuthero/Siberian ginseng *(Eleutherococcus senticosus)*.

Dan shen (Salvia miltiorrhiza)
Dan shen, a Chinese herb, was associated with increased **warfarin** (page 281) activity in two cases.[2, 3] Although warfarin acts differently from ticlopidine, both affect parameters of bleeding. Until more is known, people taking ticlopidine should use dan shen only under close medical supervision. Sage *(Salvia officinalis)*, a plant relative of dan shen found in the West, has not been not associated with interactions involving warfarin.

Devil's claw (Harpagophytum procumbens)
Devil's claw was associated with purpura (bleeding under the skin) in a patient treated with **warfarin** (page 281).[4] As with dan shen, until more is known, people taking ticlopidine should avoid taking devil's claw concurrently.

Garlic (Allium sativum)
Garlic has been shown to help prevent atherosclerosis (hardening of the arteries), perhaps by reducing the ability of platelets to stick together.[5] Interfering with the action of platelets results in an increase in the tendency toward bleeding[6] and in theory could dangerously enhance the effect of ticlopidine. Standardized extracts of garlic have been associated with bleeding in people only on rare occasions.[7] People taking ticlopidine should consult with a doctor before taking prod-

ucts containing standardized extracts of garlic or eating more than one clove of garlic daily.

Ginger (Zingiber officinale)
Ginger has been shown to reduce platelet stickiness in test tubes. Although there appear to be no reports of interactions with platelet inhibiting drugs, people should talk with a healthcare professional if they are taking a platelet inhibitor and wish to use ginger.[8]

Ginkgo biloba
Ginkgo extracts may reduce the ability of platelets to stick together, possibly increasing the tendency toward bleeding.[9] In a rat study, a high intake of ginkgo increased the action of ticlopidine in a way that could prove dangerous if the same effect occurred in people.[10] Standardized extracts of ginkgo have been associated with two cases of spontaneous bleeding, although the ginkgo extracts were not definitively shown to be the cause of the problem.[11, 12] People taking ticlopidine should use ginkgo extracts only under the supervision of a doctor.

Herbs containing coumarin-derivatives
Although there are no specific studies demonstrating interactions with platelet inhibitors, the following herbs contain coumarin-like substances that may cause bleeding and therefore interact with ticlopidine. These herbs include dong quai, fenugreek, horse chestnut, red clover, sweet clover, and sweet woodruff.

Quinine *(page 227) (Cinchona sp.)*
Quinine, a chemical found in cinchona bark and available as a drug product, has been reported to increase **warfarin** (page 281) activity.[13] Although warfarin and ticlopidine are both considered "blood thinners," they have significantly different actions. Therefore, it remains unclear whether the reported interaction between quinine and warfarin would occur between ticlopidine and quinine.

Salicylate-containing herbs
Like ticlopidine, salicylates interfere with the action of platelets. Various herbs, including meadowsweet *(Filipendula ulmaria)*, poplar *(Populus tremuloides)*, willow *(Salix alba)*, and wintergreen *(Gaultheria procumbens)* contain salicylates. Though similar to **aspirin** (page 26), plant salicylates have been shown to have different actions in test tube studies.[14] Furthermore, salicylates are poorly absorbed and likely do not build up to levels sufficient to cause negative interactions that aspirin might cause.[15] No reports have been published of

negative interactions between salicylate-containing plants and aspirin or aspirin-containing drugs.[16] Therefore concerns about combining salicylate-containing herbs and any drug remain theoretical, and the risk of causing bleeding problems may be low.

Interactions with Foods and Other Compounds
Food
Ticlopidine should be taken with food to minimize gastrointestinal upset.[17]

TIMODINE

Contains the following ingredients:
  Benzalkonium chloride
  Dimeticone 350
  Hydrocortisone
  Nystatin (page 195)

TIMOLIDE

Contains the following ingredients:
  Hydrochlorothiazide
  Timolol (page 263)

TIMOLOL

Common names: Apo-Timol, Apo-Timop, Betim, Blocadren, Gen-Timolol, Glau-opt, Novo-Timol, Nu-Timolol, PMS-Timolol, Tim-Ak, Timoptic, Timoptol

Combination drugs: Cosopt, Moducren, Prestim, Timolide

Timolol is a beta-blocker drug used to lower blood pressure in people with hypertension, treat people after heart attacks, and prevent migraine headaches. Timolol is available alone and in a combination product used to lower blood pressure. Timolol is also available in eye drop and eye gel preparations used to lower high internal eye pressure due to glaucoma and other conditions.

Summary of Interactions for Timolol
In some cases, an herb or supplement may appear in more than one category, which may seem contradictory. For clarification, read the full article for details about the summarized interactions.

✓	May be Beneficial: Side effect reduction/prevention	Coenzyme Q$_{10}$
	Depletion or interference	None known
	Supportive interaction	None known
	Reduced drug absorption/bioavailability	None known
	Adverse interaction	None known

Interactions with Dietary Supplements

Coenzyme Q$_{10}$

In a group of 16 glaucoma patients treated with a timolol eye preparation, six weeks of oral coenzyme Q$_{10}$ (90 mg per day) was reported to reduce timolol-induced cardiovascular side effects without affecting intraocular pressure treatment.[1]

Potassium

Some beta-adrenergic blockers (called "nonselective" beta blockers) decrease the uptake of potassium from the blood into the cells,[2] leading to excess potassium in the blood, a potentially dangerous condition known as hyperkalemia.[3] People taking beta-blockers should therefore avoid taking potassium supplements, or eating large quantities of fruit (e.g., bananas), unless directed to do so by their doctor.

Interactions with Herbs

Pleurisy root

As pleurisy root and other plants in the *Aesclepius* genus contain cardiac glycosides, it is best to avoid use of pleurisy root with heart medications such as beta-blockers.[4]

Interactions with Foods and Other Compounds

Food

Timolol may be taken with or without food.[5]

Alcohol

Timolol may cause drowsiness, dizziness, lightheadedness, or blurred vision.[6] Alcohol may intensify these effects and increase the risk of accidental injury. To prevent problems, people taking timolol should avoid alcohol.

TOBRADEX

Contains the following ingredients:
   Dexamethasone
   Tobramycin (page 264)

TOBRAMYCIN

Common names: AKTob, Nebcin, Scheinpharm Tobramycin, TOBI, Tobrex

Combination drug: Tobradex

Tobramycin is an "aminoglycoside" **antibiotic** (page 19) used to treat infections caused by many different bacteria. Tobramycin is usually administered by intravenous (i.v.) infusion, intramuscular (i.m.) injection, or inhalation. Tobramycin is available in special preparations to treat eye infections, alone and in a combination product.

Summary of Interactions for Tobramycin

In some cases, an herb or supplement may appear in more than one category, which may seem contradictory. For clarification, read the full article for details about the summarized interactions.

✓	May be Beneficial: Depletion or interference	Calcium* Magnesium* Potassium* Vitamin K
✓	May be Beneficial: Side effect reduction/prevention	*Bifidobacterium longum** *Lactobacillus acidophilus** *Lactobacillus casei** *Saccharomyces boulardii** *Saccharomyces cerevisiae** Vitamin K
✓	May be Beneficial: Supportive interaction	*Saccharomyces boulardii**
	Reduced drug absorption/bioavailability	None known
	Adverse interaction	None known

Interactions with Dietary Supplements

Minerals

Calcium, magnesium, and potassium depletion requiring prolonged replacement were reported in a child with tetany who had just completed a three-week course of i.v. tobramycin.[1] The authors suggest this may have been due to kidney damage related to the drug. Seventeen patients with cancer developed calcium, magnesium, and potassium depletion after treatment with aminoglycoside antibiotics, including tobramycin.[2] The authors suggested a possible potentiating action of tobramycin-induced mineral depletion by **chemotherapy** (page 54) drugs, especially **doxorubicin** (page 100) (Adriamycin).

Until more is known, people receiving i.v. tobramycin should ask their doctor about monitoring calcium, magnesium, and potassium levels and the possibility of mineral replacement.

Probiotics

A common side effect of antibiotics is diarrhea, which may be caused by the elimination of beneficial bacteria normally found in the colon. Controlled studies have shown that taking probiotic microorganisms—such as *Lactobacillus casei, Lactobacillus acidophilus, Bifidobacterium longum,* or *Saccharomyces boulardii*—helps prevent antibiotic-induced diarrhea.[3]

The diarrhea experienced by some people who take antibiotics also might be due to an overgrowth of the bacterium *Clostridium difficile,* which causes a disease known as pseudomembranous colitis. Controlled studies have shown that supplementation with harmless yeast—such as *Saccharomyces boulardii*[4] or *Saccharomyces cerevisiae* (baker's or brewer's yeast)[5]—helps prevent recurrence of this infection. In one study, taking 500 mg of *Saccharomyces boulardii* twice daily enhanced the effectiveness of the antibiotic vancomycin in preventing recurrent clostridium infection.[6] Therefore, people taking antibiotics who later develop diarrhea might benefit from supplementing with saccharomyces organisms.

Treatment with antibiotics also commonly leads to an overgrowth of yeast *(Candida albicans)* in the vagina (candida vaginitis) and the intestines (sometimes referred to as "dysbiosis"). Controlled studies have shown that *Lactobacillus acidophilus* might prevent candida vaginitis.[7]

Vitamin K

Several cases of excessive bleeding have been reported in people who take antibiotics.[8, 9, 10, 11] This side effect may be the result of reduced vitamin K activity and/or reduced vitamin K production by bacteria in the colon. One study showed that people who had taken broad-spectrum antibiotics had lower liver concentrations of vitamin K_2 (menaquinone), though vitamin K_1 (phylloquinone) levels remained normal.[12] Several antibiotics appear to exert a strong effect on vitamin K activity, while others may not have any effect. Therefore, one should refer to a specific antibiotic for information on whether it interacts with vitamin K.

Doctors of natural medicine sometimes recommend vitamin K supplementation to people taking antibiotics. Additional research is needed to determine whether the amount of vitamin K_1 found in some multivitamins is sufficient to prevent antibiotic-induced bleeding. Moreover, most multivitamins do not contain vitamin K.

As with many **antibiotics** (page 19), tobramycin can deplete vitamin K.[13, 14] It makes sense for people taking tobramycin to supplement vitamin K to protect against drug-induced deficiency. Doctors sometimes suggest a daily intake between several hundred micrograms and one milligram.

TOLTERODINE

Common names: Detrol, Diflorasone Topical

Tolterodine is used to treat people with overactive bladders who have symptoms such as frequent urination, urgency, or loss of urinary control. It is a type of drug called a competitive muscarinic receptor antagonist.

Summary of Interactions for Tolterodine

In some cases, an herb or supplement may appear in more than one category, which may seem contradictory. For clarification, read the full article for details about the summarized interactions.

Depletion or interference	None known
Side effect reduction/prevention	None known
Supportive interaction	None known
Reduced drug absorption/bioavailability	None known
Adverse interaction	None known

TOPICAL CORTICOSTEROIDS

Common names: Aclometasone Topical, Aclovate Topical, Aeroseb-Dex Topical, Alclometasone, Aristocort Topical, Beclomethasone, Betacap, Betamethasone Topical, Betnovate-RD, Betnovate, Bettamousse, Clobetasol, Clobetasol Topical, Clobetasone, Clocortolone Pivalate Topical, Cloderm Topical, Cortaid Topical, Cortef Topical, Cortizone Topical, Cortone Topical, Cutivate, Cutivate Topical, Decadron Topical, Decaspray Topical, Deramcort, Derma-Smoothe/FS Topical, Dermovate, Desoximetasone Topical, Desoxymethasone, Dexamethasone Topical, Diflucortolone, Dioderm, Diprolene Topical, Diprosone, Efcortelan, Elocon, Elocon Topical, Eumovate, Florone Topical, Fludroxycortide, Fluocinolone, Fluocinolone Topical, Fluocinonide, Fluocortolone, Fluonid Topical, Flurandrenolone, Fluticasone Topical, FS Shampoo, Haelan, Halciderm Topical, Halcinonide, Hc45, Hydrocortisone Topical, Hytone Topical, Kenalog Topical, Lanacort, Locoid Crelo, Locoid, Locoid Topical, Luxiq Topical, Maxiflor Topical, Maxivate Topical, Metosyn, Mildison, Modrasone, Mometasone Topical, Nerisone Forte, Nerisone, Pandel Topical, Proctocort Topical, Propaderm, Psorcon Topical, Stiedex, Synalar, Synelar Topical, Synemol Topical, Temovate Topical, Topicort Topical, Triamcinolone, Triamcinolone Topical, Ultralanum Plain, Westcort Topical, Zenoxone

Combination drugs: Alphaderm, Betnovate-C, Betnovate-N, Calmurid HC, Canesten HC, Daktacort, Dermovate-NN, Diprosalic, Econacort, Eurax HC, Eurax-Hydrocortisone, FuciBET, Fucidin H, Gregoderm, Locoid C, Lotriderm, Mycolog II, Nystaform-HC, Quinocort, Synalar C, Synalar N, Terra-Cortril Nystatin, Terra-Cortril, Timodine, Vioform-Hydrocortisone

Corticosteroids are applied to the skin to treat mild to severe inflammation and itching resulting from conditions such as insect bites, allergic reactions, diaper rash, eczema, and psoriasis. They are combined with **antibiotics** (page 19) to treat ear infections, eye infections, and skin infections caused by bacteria. They are also combined with antifungal agents to treat fungal and yeast infections of the ear and skin.

The information in this article pertains to topical corticosteroids in general. The interactions reported here may not apply to all the Also Indexed As terms. Talk to your doctor or pharmacist if you are taking any of these drugs.

Summary of Interactions for Topical Corticosteroids

In some cases, an herb or supplement may appear in more than one category, which may seem contradictory. For clarification, read the full article for details about the summarized interactions.

✓ May be Beneficial: Supportive interaction	Biotin* (clobetasol) Licorice Zinc* (clobetasol)
ⓘ Check: Other	Aloe
Depletion or interference	None known
Side effect reduction/prevention	None known
Reduced drug absorption/bioavailability	None known
Adverse interaction	None known

Interactions with Dietary Supplements
Zinc and biotin
Children with alopecia areata who supplemented 100 mg of zinc and 20 mg biotin each day, combined with topical clobetasol, showed more improvement compared to children who took oral corticosteroid drugs.[1] Controlled research is needed to determine whether adding oral zinc and biotin to topical clobetasol therapy is more effective than clobetasol alone. However, until more information is available, caregivers should consider that children with alopecia who are currently taking oral corticosteroids might benefit from switching to supplements of zinc and biotin along with topical clobetasol.

Interactions with Herbs
Aloe (Aloe vera)
In animal research, applying aloe gel topically along with a topical corticosteroid enhanced the hormone's anti-inflammatory activity in the skin.[2] No human research has investigated this effect.

Licorice (Glycyrrhiza glabra)
When applied to the skin, glycyrrhetinic acid (a chemical found in licorice) increases the activity of hydrocortisone.[3] This effect might allow for less hydrocortisone to be used when combined with glycyrrhetinic acid, but further study is needed to test this possibility.[4]

TOTARETIC

Contains the following ingredients:
Atenolol (page 28)
Chlorthalidone

TRAMADOL

Common names: Dromadol SR, Tramake Insts, Tramake, Ultram, Zamadol SR, Zamadol, Zydol SR, Zydol XL, Zydol

Tramadol is a drug, unrelated to **nonsteroidal anti-inflammatory drugs** (page 193) (NSAIDs) or opiates, used to relieve moderate to moderately severe pain.

Summary of Interactions for Tramadol

In some cases, an herb or supplement may appear in more than one category, which may seem contradictory.

For clarification, read the full article for details about the summarized interactions.

⃠ Avoid: Adverse interaction	5-Hydroxytryptophan (5-HTP)* L-tryptophan*
Depletion or interference	None known
Side effect reduction/prevention	None known
Supportive interaction	None known
Reduced drug absorption/bioavailability	None known

Interactions with Dietary Supplements
5-Hydroxytryptophan (5-HTP) and L-tryptophan
Tramadol, which blocks serotonin reuptake in the brain, has been associated with two cases of serotonin syndrome.[1, 2] 5-HTP and L-tryptophan are converted to serotonin in the brain. While no interactions have yet been reported with tramadol and 5-HTP or L-tryptophan, taking 5-HTP or L-tryptophan with tramadol may increase the risk of tramadol-induced side effects, including serotonin syndrome.

Interactions with Foods and Other Compounds
Food
Tramadol may be taken with or without food.[3]

Alcohol
Tramadol may impair mental ability and physical coordination.[4] Alcohol may intensify these effects and increase the risk of accidental injury. People taking tramadol are cautioned to avoid alcohol.

TRASIDREX

Contains the following ingredients:
    Bendroflumethiazide
    Oxprenolol

TRAZODONE

Common names: Alti-Trazodone, Apo-Trazodone, Desyrel, Molipaxin, Novo-Trazodone, Nu-Trazodone, PMS-Trazodone, Trazorel

Trazodone is a weak serotonin reuptake inhibitor drug with other effects on brain neurotransmitters. It is used to treat people with depression. It is also used to treat people during cocaine withdrawal.

Summary of Interactions for Trazodone
In some cases, an herb or supplement may appear in more than one category, which may seem contradictory. For clarification, read the full article for details about the summarized interactions.

⃠ Avoid: Adverse interaction	*Ginkgo biloba** *St. John's wort**
ⓘ Check: Other	Digitalis
Depletion or interference	None known
Side effect reduction/prevention	None known
Supportive interaction	None known
Reduced drug absorption/bioavailability	None known

Interactions with Herbs
Digitalis (Digitalis lanata, Digitalis purpurea)
Digitalis refers to a family of plants commonly called foxglove that contain digitalis glycosides, chemicals with actions and toxicities similar to the prescription drug **digoxin** (page 90).

Trazodone was associated with increased serum digoxin levels in one case report.[1] No interactions between trazodone and digitalis have been reported. Until more is known, trazodone and digitalis-containing products should be used only under the direct supervision of a doctor trained in their use.

Ginkgo biloba
There is one case report of an elderly patient with Alzheimer's disease going into a coma while concurrently using trazodone and ginkgo.[2] Until more is known, ginkgo should not be combined with trazodone except under supervision of a doctor.

St. John's wort (Hypericum perforatum)
One report described a case of serotonin syndrome in a patient who took St. John's wort and trazodone.[3] The patient reportedly experienced mental confusion, muscle twitching, sweating, flushing, and ataxia. Until more is known, St. John's wort should not be combined with trazodone except under expert clinical supervision.

Interactions with Foods and Other Compounds
Food
Trazodone should be taken with food.[4]

Alcohol
Trazodone may cause drowsiness or dizziness.[5] Alcohol may compound these effects and increase the risk of accidental injury. To prevent problems, people taking trazodone should avoid alcohol.

TRETINOIN

Common names: All-Trans-Retinoic Acid, ATRA, Atragen, Avita, Rejuva-A, Renova, Retin-A, Retinova, Retisol-A, StieVA-A, Vesanoid, Vitamin A Acid, Vitinoin

Tretinoin is a slightly altered version of vitamin A. Topical tretinoin is available in cream, gel, and liquid forms to treat acne, other skin conditions, and some forms of skin cancer. Tretinoin is also available in oral capsules used to induce remission in people with acute promyelocytic leukemia.

Summary of Interactions for Tretinoin

In some cases, an herb or supplement may appear in more than one category, which may seem contradictory. For clarification, read the full article for details about the summarized interactions.

⊘ Avoid: Adverse interaction	Vitamin A*
Depletion or interference	None known
Side effect reduction/prevention	None known
Supportive interaction	None known
Reduced drug absorption/bioavailability	None known

Interactions with Dietary Supplements
Vitamin A
Large amounts of vitamin A can cause side effects, and oral tretinoin can cause similar side effects. Combining vitamin A with oral tretinoin is likely to increase the risk of side effects. People taking oral tretinoin should probably not take more than 10,000 IU of supplemental vitamin A per day.

Interactions with Foods and Other Compounds
Food
Food enhances absorption of retinoid drugs.[1] Tretinoin capsules (Vesanoid) should be taken with food.

TRI-ADCORTYL

Contains the following ingredients:
Gramicidin
Neomycin (page 187)
Nystatin (page 195)
Triamcinolone

TRIAMINIC-12

Contains the following ingredients:
  Chlorpheniramine (page 59)
  Phenylpropanolamine (page 218)

TRIAMTERENE

Common names: Dyrenium, Dytac

Combination drugs: Dyazide, Maxzide

Triamterene is a potassium-sparing **diuretic** (page 94) (i.e., it inhibits the urinary excretion of potassium). Diuretics increase urinary water loss from the body and are used to treat high blood pressure, congestive heart failure, and some kidney or liver conditions. Triamterene is available as a single agent and in combination products.

Summary of Interactions for Triamterene

In some cases, an herb or supplement may appear in more than one category, which may seem contradictory. For clarification, read the full article for details about the summarized interactions.

✓ May be Beneficial: Depletion or interference	Calcium* Folic acid*
✓ May be Beneficial: Side effect reduction/prevention	Folic acid
⊘ Avoid: Adverse interaction	Buchu Cleavers Dandelion Gravel root Horsetail Juniper Magnesium Potassium Uva ursi
ⓘ Check: Other	Sodium
Supportive interaction	None known
Reduced drug absorption/bioavailability	None known

Interactions with Dietary Supplements
Calcium
A review of the research literature indicates that triamterene may increase calcium loss.[1] The importance of this information is unclear.

Folic acid

Triamterene is a weak folic acid antagonist that has been associated with folic acid-deficiency anemia in people already at risk for folic acid deficiency.[2] However, people treated long term with triamterene, without additional risk for folic acid deficiency, were found to have normal folic acid levels and no signs of folic acid deficiency.[3] The use of multivitamin supplements containing folic acid appears to diminish the occurrence of birth defects associated with triamterene. According to one study,[4] pregnant women who took folic acid–containing multivitamin supplements in addition to their prescription drugs had fewer babies with heart defects and deformities of the upper lip and mouth.

One study showed that people taking diuretics for more than six months had dramatically lower blood levels of folic acid and higher levels of homocysteine compared with individuals not taking diuretics.[5] Homocysteine, a toxic amino acid by-product, has been associated with atherosclerosis. Until further information is available, people taking diuretics for longer than six months should probably supplement with folic acid.

Magnesium

Preliminary research in animals suggests that triamterene may inhibit the urinary excretion of magnesium.[6] It is unknown if this same effect would occur in humans. Persons taking more than 300 mg of magnesium per day and triamterene should consult with a doctor as this combination may lead to potentially dangerous increases in the level of magnesium in the body. The combination of triamterene and hydrochlorothiazide would likely eliminate this problem, as hydrochlorothiazide may deplete magnesium.

Potassium

As a potassium-sparing drug, triamterene reduces urinary loss of potassium, which can lead to elevated potassium levels.[7] People taking triamterene should avoid potassium supplements, potassium-containing salt substitutes (Morton Salt Substitute, No Salt, Lite Salt, and others) and even high-potassium foods (primarily fruit). Doctors should monitor potassium blood levels in patients taking triamterene to prevent problems associated with elevated potassium levels.

Sodium

Diuretics (page 94), including triamterene, cause increased loss of sodium in the urine. By removing sodium from the body, diuretics also cause water to leave the body. This reduction of body water is the purpose of taking diuretics. Therefore, there is usually no reason to replace lost sodium, although strict limitation of salt intake in combination with the actions of diuretics can sometimes cause excessive sodium depletion. On the other hand, people who restrict sodium intake and in the process reduce blood pressure may need to have their dose of diuretics lowered. People taking triamterene should talk with their prescribing doctor before severely restricting salt.

Interactions with Herbs

Diuretic herbs

Herbs that have a diuretic effect should be avoided when taking diuretic medications, as they may enhance the effect of these drugs and lead to possible cardiovascular side effects. These herbs include dandelion, uva ursi, juniper, buchu, cleavers, horsetail, and gravel root.[8]

Interactions with Foods and Other Compounds

Food

Triamterene is best taken after meals to avoid stomach upset.[9]

TRIAPIN

Contains the following ingredients:
Felodipine (page 113)
Ramipril (page 229)

TRIAVIL, ETRAFON

Contains the following ingredients:
Amitriptyline
Perphenazine (page 213)

TRIAZOLAM

Common names: Anafranil, Halcion

Triazolam is used for the short-term treatment of insomnia, and is in a family of drugs known as **benzodiazepines** (page 36).

Summary of Interactions for Triazolam

In some cases, an herb or supplement may appear in more than one category, which may seem contradictory.

Triazolam

For clarification, read the full article for details about the summarized interactions.

✓ May be Beneficial: Supportive interaction	Melatonin Vinpocetine*
🚫 Avoid: Adverse interaction	Alcohol Grapefruit juice
Depletion or interference	None known
Side effect reduction/prevention	None known
Reduced drug absorption/bioavailability	None known

Interactions with Dietary Supplements
Melatonin
A preliminary study showed that taking melatonin and triazolam together produces better quality of sleep than occurs when the drug is taken alone. The results also indicated that less triazolam is needed when melatonin and triazolam are taken together, which might reduce side effects such as morning grogginess.[1] Additional research is needed to determine whether individuals taking triazolam should also take melatonin.

Vinpocetine
In a preliminary trial, an extract of periwinkle called vinpocetine was shown to produce minor improvements in short-term memory among people taking flunitrazepam, a benzodiazepine.[2] Further study is needed to determine if vinpocetine would be a helpful adjunct to use of benzodiazepines, or triazolam specifically.

Interactions with Foods and Other Compounds
Grapefruit juice
Drinking grapefruit juice with triazolam dramatically increases the amount of drug absorbed and the amount of time it stays in the body.[3] Though the clinical significance of this interaction is unknown, some people may experience increased side effects, such as morning grogginess, dizziness, and poor coordination. Therefore, people taking triazolam should probably avoid drinking grapefruit juice or eating grapefruit for the duration of therapy.

Alcohol
Drinking alcoholic beverages while taking triazolam may enhance side effects such as drowsiness, confusion, and dizziness.[4] Consequently, people taking triazolam should avoid drinking alcohol, especially when they must stay alert.

TRICYCLIC ANTIDEPRESSANTS

Common names: Adapin, Alti-Desipramine, Alti-Doxepin, Amitriptyline, Amoxapine, Apo-Amitriptyline, Apo-Desipramine, Apo-Doxepin, Apo-Imipramine, Asendin, Clomipramine, Desipramine, Domical, Doxepin, Elavil, Imipramine, Janimine, Lentizol, Ludiomil, Maprotiline, Norpramin, Nortriptyline, Novo-Desipramine, Novo-Doxepin, Nu-Desipramine, Pamelor, Pertofrane, PMS-Desipramine, Protriptyline, Sinequan, Surmontil, Tofranil, Trimipramine Maleate, Tryptizol, Vivactil, Zonalon

Combination drug: Triavil, Etrafon

Tricyclic antidepressants are used to treat people with depression and less commonly to treat other illnesses.

Summary of Interactions for Tricyclic Antidepressants
In some cases, an herb or supplement may appear in more than one category, which may seem contradictory. For clarification, read the full article for details about the summarized interactions.

✓ May be Beneficial: Depletion or interference	CoQ$_{10}$*
✓ May be Beneficial: Supportive interaction	L-tryptophan* Niacinamide SAMe Vitamin B-complex Vitamin B$_1$ Vitamin B$_{12}$ Vitamin B$_2$ Vitamin B$_3$ Vitamin B$_5$ Vitamin B$_6$
🚫 Avoid: Reduced drug absorption/bioavailability	Tea*
🚫 Avoid: Adverse interaction	St. John's wort*
Side effect reduction/prevention	None known

Interactions with Dietary Supplements
B vitamins
Giving 10 mg per day each of vitamins B$_1$, B$_2$, and B$_6$ to elderly, depressed persons already on tricyclic antidepressants improved their depression and ability to think more than placebo did.[1] The subjects in this study were institutionalized, so it is unclear if these results apply to persons living at home.

L-tryptophan and vitamin B₃

L-tryptophan and vitamin B$_3$
Combination of 6 grams per day L-tryptophan and 1,500 mg per day niacinamide (a form of vitamin B$_3$) with imipramine has shown to be more effective than imipramine alone for people with bipolar disorder.[2] These levels did not improve the effects of imipramine in people with depression. Lower amounts (4 grams per day of L-tryptophan and 1,000 mg per day of niacinamide) did show some tendency to enhance the effect of imipramine.

The importance of the amount of L-tryptophan was confirmed in other studies, suggesting that if too much L-tryptophan (6 grams per day) is used, it is not beneficial, while levels around 4 grams per day may make tricyclic antidepressants work better.[3, 4]

Coenzyme Q$_{10}$
A number of tricyclic antidepressants have been shown to inhibit enzymes that require coenzyme Q$_{10}$ (CoQ$_{10}$), a nutrient that is needed for normal heart function.[5] It is therefore possible that CoQ$_{10}$ deficiency may be a contributing factor to the cardiac side effects that sometimes occur with tricyclic antidepressants. Some practitioners advise patients taking tricyclic antidepressants to supplement with 30–100 mg of CoQ$_{10}$ per day.

SAMe (S-adenosy-L-methionine)
SAMe may improve the clinical response to imipramine (Tofranil). In a double-blind trial, depressive symptoms decreased earlier in the people who received SAMe injections (200 mg per day) in combination with imipramine than in those who received imipramine with placebo injections.[6] Oral supplementation with SAMe has demonstrated antidepressant activity, independent of its combination with imipramine.[7]

Interactions with Herbs

St. John's wort (Hypericum perforatum)
Preliminary research has suggested that St. John's wort may reduce blood levels of the tricyclic antidepressant amitriptyline.[8] This may have occurred because certain chemicals found in St. John's wort activate liver enzymes that are involved in the elimination of some drugs.[9, 10] Until more is known, people taking tricyclic antidepressants should avoid St. John's wort.

Tea (Camellia sinensis)
Brewed black tea has been reported to cause precipitation of amitriptyline and imipramine in a test tube.[11] If this reaction occurred in the body, it could decrease absorption of these drugs. Until more is known, it makes sense to separate ingestion of tea and tricyclic antidepressants by at least two hours.

Interactions with Foods and Other Compounds

Alcohol
Tricyclic antidepressants can cause drowsiness and dizziness.[12] Alcohol may intensify these actions, increasing the risk for accidental injury. People taking tricyclic antidepressants should avoid alcohol.

TRIDESTRA

Contains the following ingredients:
   Estradiol (page 108)
   Medroxyprogesterone (page 167)

TRIMETHOPRIM

Common names: Monotrim, Proloprim, Trimogal, Trimopan, Trimpex, Triprimix

Trimethoprim is an **antibacterial** (page 19) drug used to treat people with urinary tract infections. The combination drug product **trimethoprim/sulfamethoxazole (TMP/SMX)** (page 273) is used to treat a wide variety of bacterial infections and some infections due to parasites.

Summary of Interactions for Trimethoprim
In some cases, an herb or supplement may appear in more than one category, which may seem contradictory. For clarification, read the full article for details about the summarized interactions.

✓ May be Beneficial: Depletion or interference	Calcium* Folic acid* Magnesium* Vitamin B$_{12}$* Vitamin B$_6$* Vitamin K*
✓ May be Beneficial: Side effect reduction/prevention	*Bifidobacterium longum* Folic acid *Lactobacillus acidophilus* *Lactobacillus casei* *Saccharomyces boulardii* *Saccharomyces cerevisiae* Vitamin K*
✓ May be Beneficial: Supportive interaction	*Saccharomyces boulardii*
⊘ Avoid: Adverse interaction	Potassium
Reduced drug absorption/bioavailability	None known

Interactions with Dietary Supplements

Calcium, magnesium, vitamin B₁₂

Sulfonamides, including **sulfamethoxazole** (page 245), can decrease absorption of calcium, magnesium, and vitamin B₁₂.[1] This is generally not a problem when taking sulfamethoxazole for two weeks or less. People taking sulfamethoxazole for longer than two weeks should ask their doctor about nutrient monitoring and supplementation.

> **Note:** Since sulfamethoxazole is often prescribed in combination with trimethoprim (e.g., Bactrim or Septra), it may be easy to associate this interaction with trimethoprim. However, this interaction is not known to occur with trimethoprim alone.

Folic acid, vitamin B₆, vitamin K

Sulfonamides, including **sulfamethoxazole** (page 245), can interfere with the activity of folic acid, vitamin B₆, and vitamin K.[2] This is generally not a problem when taking sulfamethoxazole for two weeks or less. People taking sulfamethoxazole for longer than two weeks should ask their doctor about nutrient monitoring and supplementation.

> **Note:** Since sulfamethoxazole is often prescribed in combination with trimethoprim (e.g., Bactrim or Septra), it may be easy to associate this interaction with trimethoprim. However, this interaction is not known to occur with trimethoprim alone.

The use of multivitamin supplements containing folic acid diminishes the occurrence of birth defects associated with trimethoprim. According to one study,[3] pregnant women who took folic acid–containing multivitamin supplements in addition to their prescription drugs had fewer babies with heart defects and deformities of the upper lip and mouth.

TMP/SMX (page 273) has been rarely associated with folic acid-deficiency anemia.[4] This action may be due to trimethoprim-induced folic acid depletion.[5] Trimethoprim and TMP/SMX should be used with caution in patients with folic acid deficiency, for which blood tests are available. Folic acid replacement does not interfere with the antibacterial activity of trimethoprim[6] or TMP/SMX.[7]

Potassium

TMP/SMX has been reported to elevate blood potassium and other constituents of blood (creatine and BUN).[8, 9] In particular, people with impaired kidney function should be closely monitored by their prescribing doctor for these changes. People taking trimethoprim or TMP/SMX should talk with the prescribing doctor before taking any potassium supplements or potassium-containing products, such as No Salt, Salt Substitute, Lite Salt, and even high-potassium foods (primarily fruit).

Probiotics

A common side effect of antibiotics is diarrhea, which may be caused by the elimination of beneficial bacteria normally found in the colon. Controlled studies have shown that taking probiotic microorganisms—such as *Lactobacillus casei, Lactobacillus acidophilus, Bifidobacterium longum,* or *Saccharomyces boulardii*—helps prevent antibiotic-induced diarrhea.[10]

The diarrhea experienced by some people who take antibiotics also might be due to an overgrowth of the bacterium *Clostridium difficile,* which causes a disease known as pseudomembranous colitis. Controlled studies have shown that supplementation with harmless yeast—such as *Saccharomyces boulardii*[11] or *Saccharomyces cerevisiae* (baker's or brewer's yeast)[12]—helps prevent recurrence of this infection. In one study, taking 500 mg of *Saccharomyces boulardii* twice daily enhanced the effectiveness of the antibiotic vancomycin in preventing recurrent clostridium infection.[13] Therefore, people taking antibiotics who later develop diarrhea might benefit from supplementing with saccharomyces organisms.

Treatment with antibiotics also commonly leads to an overgrowth of yeast *(Candida albicans)* in the vagina (candida vaginitis) and the intestines (sometimes referred to as "dysbiosis"). Controlled studies have shown that *Lactobacillus acidophilus* might prevent candida vaginitis.[14]

Vitamin K

Several cases of excessive bleeding have been reported in people who take antibiotics.[15, 16, 17, 18] This side effect may be the result of reduced vitamin K activity and/or reduced vitamin K production by bacteria in the colon. One study showed that people who had taken broad-spectrum antibiotics had lower liver concentrations of vitamin K₂ (menaquinone), though vitamin K₁ (phylloquinone) levels remained normal.[19] Several antibiotics appear to exert a strong effect on vitamin K activity, while others may not have any effect. Therefore, one should refer to a specific antibiotic for information on whether it interacts with vitamin K. Doctors of natural medicine sometimes recommend vitamin K supplementation to people taking antibiotics. Additional research is needed to determine whether the amount of vitamin K_1 found in some multivitamins is sufficient to prevent antibiotic-induced bleeding. Moreover, most multivitamins do not contain vitamin K.

TRIMETHOPRIM/ SULFAMETHOXAZOLE

Common names: Apo-Sulfatrim, Bactrim Roche, Bactrim, Chemotrim, Co-Trimoxazole, Comixco, Cotrim, Fectrim Forte, Fectrim, Novo-Trimel, Nu-Cotrimox, Septra, Septrin, SMX/TMP, TMP/SMX, Trimethoprim/Sulphamethoxazole, Uroplus

The antibiotic combination of **trimethoprim** (page 271) and **sulfamethoxazole** (page 245) (TMP/SMX) is used to treat a wide variety of bacterial infections and some infections due to parasites. Bactrim, Cotrim, and Septra are brand names for products containing identical amounts of TMP/SMX. Bactrim DS and Septra DS contain twice as much TMP and SMX as Bactrim and Septra.

Summary of Interactions for Trimethoprim/Sulfamethoxazole

In some cases, an herb or supplement may appear in more than one category, which may seem contradictory. For clarification, read the full article for details about the summarized interactions.

✓ May be Beneficial: Depletion or interference	Folic acid* Vitamin K*
✓ May be Beneficial: Side effect reduction/prevention	Bifidobacterium longum* Lactobacillus acidophilus* Lactobacillus casei* Saccharomyces boulardii* Saccharomyces cerevisiae* Vitamin K*
✓ May be Beneficial: Supportive interaction	Saccharomyces boulardii*
⊘ Avoid: Adverse interaction	PABA* Potassium
Reduced drug absorption/bioavailability	None known

Interactions with Dietary Supplements
Folic acid
TMP/SMX has, on rare occasions, been associated with anemia due to folic acid deficiency.[1] This effect may be

due to trimethoprim.[2] TMP/SMX should be used with caution in patients with folic acid deficiency, for which a blood test is available. Folic acid replacement does not interfere with the antibacterial activity of TMP/SMX.[3] People with AIDS-related pneumonia given TMP/SMX had a worse survival rate when folinic acid, an activated form of folic acid, was added.[4]

PABA (para-aminobenzoic acid)
PABA may interfere with the action of sulfamethoxazole. It should not be taken together with trimethoprim/sulfamethoxazole.

Potassium
TMP/SMX has been reported to increase blood potassium to levels above the normal range in some patients, particularly those with impaired kidney function.[5] People who have been prescribed TMP/SMX should ask their doctor whether they should avoid potassium supplements, potassium-containing salt substitutes (No Salt, Morton Salt Substitute, and others), and high-potassium foods (primarily fruit).

Probiotics
A common side effect of antibiotics is diarrhea, which may be caused by the elimination of beneficial bacteria normally found in the colon. Controlled studies have shown that taking probiotic microorganisms—such as *Lactobacillus casei*, *Lactobacillus acidophilus*, *Bifidobacterium longum*, or *Saccharomyces boulardii*—helps prevent antibiotic-induced diarrhea.[6]

The diarrhea experienced by some people who take antibiotics also might be due to an overgrowth of the bacterium *Clostridium difficile*, which causes a disease known as pseudomembranous colitis. Controlled studies have shown that supplementation with harmless yeast—such as *Saccharomyces boulardii*[7] or *Saccharomyces cerevisiae* (baker's or brewer's yeast)[8]—helps prevent recurrence of this infection. In one study, taking 500 mg of *Saccharomyces boulardii* twice daily enhanced the effectiveness of the antibiotic vancomycin in preventing recurrent clostridium infection.[9] Therefore, people taking antibiotics who later develop diarrhea might benefit from supplementing with saccharomyces organisms.

Treatment with antibiotics also commonly leads to an overgrowth of yeast (*Candida albicans*) in the vagina (candida vaginitis) and the intestines (sometimes referred to as "dysbiosis"). Controlled studies have shown that *Lactobacillus acidophilus* might prevent candida vaginitis.[10]

Vitamin K

Several cases of excessive bleeding have been reported in people who take antibiotics.[11, 12, 13, 14] This side effect may be the result of reduced vitamin K activity and/or reduced vitamin K production by bacteria in the colon. One study showed that people who had taken broad-spectrum antibiotics had lower liver concentrations of vitamin K_2 (menaquinone), though vitamin K_1 (phylloquinone) levels remained normal.[15] Several antibiotics appear to exert a strong effect on vitamin K activity, while others may not have any effect. Therefore, one should refer to a specific antibiotic for information on whether it interacts with vitamin K. Doctors of natural medicine sometimes recommend vitamin K supplementation to people taking antibiotics. Additional research is needed to determine whether the amount of vitamin K_1 found in some multivitamins is sufficient to prevent antibiotic-induced bleeding. Moreover, most multivitamins do not contain vitamin K.

TRIMOVATE

Contains the following ingredients:
  Clobetasone
  Neomycin (page 187)
  Nystatin (page 195)

TRIOTANN-S PEDIATRIC

This drug is a combination of two antihistamines, pyrilamine and **chlorpheniramine** (page 59), and a decongestant, phenylephrine. Triotann-S is used to treat symptoms associated with the common cold and hay fever, such as runny nose, itchy eyes, and sneezing.

Summary of Interactions for Triotann-S Pediatric

In some cases, an herb or supplement may appear in more than one category, which may seem contradictory. For clarification, read the full article for details about the summarized interactions.

✓ May be Beneficial: Depletion or interference	*Polygonum multiflorum**
✓ May be Beneficial: Supportive interaction	*Panax ginseng**
⊘ Avoid: Adverse interaction	Henbane*
Side effect reduction/prevention	None known
Reduced drug absorption/bioavailability	None known

Interactions with Herbs
Korean or Chinese ginseng (Panax ginseng)
Laboratory studies have shown that compounds found in *Panax ginseng* enhance the ability of phenylephrine to constrict blood vessels.[1] Controlled studies are necessary to determine whether taking *Panax ginseng* at the same time as phenylephrine will enhance the beneficial effects of the drug.

Polygonum multiflorum
Many drugs used in the treatment of high blood pressure cause relaxation or dilation of blood vessels. Laboratory studies show that emodin, a compound in *Polygonum multiflorum,* also relaxes blood vessels. However, animal studies reveal that phenylephrine blocks the action of emodin.[2] Controlled studies are needed to determine whether *Polygonum multiflorum* helps people with high blood pressure and whether phenylephrine blocks its beneficial effects.

Henbane (Hyoscyamus niger)
Antihistamines, including chlorpheniramine, can cause "anticholinergic" side effects such as dryness of mouth and heart palpitations. Henbane also has anticholinergic activity and side effects. Therefore, use of henbane with chlorpheniramine could increase the risk of anticholinergic side effects,[3] though apparently no interactions have yet been reported. Henbane should not be taken except by prescription from a physician trained in its use, as it is extremely toxic.

Interactions with Foods and Other Compounds
Alcohol
Drinking alcoholic beverages together with antihistamines can enhance side effects such as drowsiness and dizziness.[4] Consequently, people who are taking pyrilamine and chlorpheniramine should avoid alcohol, especially when staying alert is necessary.

TRISEQUENS

Contains the following ingredients:
  Estradiol (page 108)
  Norethisterone

TRISEQUENS FORTE

Contains the following ingredients:
  Estradiol (page 108)
  Norethisterone

TUSSIONEX

Contains the following ingredients:
  Chlorpheniramine (page 59)
  Hydrocodone (page 137)

TYLENOL ALLERGY SINUS

Contains the following ingredients:
  Acetaminophen (page 3)
  Diphenhydramine (page 93)
  Pseudoephedrine

TYLENOL WITH CODEINE

Contains the following ingredients:
  Acetaminophen (page 3)
  Codeine (page 75)

TYLENOL COLD

Contains the following ingredients:
  Acetaminophen (page 3)
  Chlorpheniramine (page 59)
  Dextromethorphan (page 87)
  Pseudoephedrine

TYLENOL FLU NIGHTTIME MAXIMUM STRENGTH POWDER

Contains the following ingredients:
  Acetaminophen (page 3)
  Diphenhydramine (page 93)
  Pseudoephedrine

TYLENOL MULTI-SYMPTOM HOT MEDICATION

Contains the following ingredients:
  Acetaminophen (page 3)
  Chlorpheniramine (page 59)
  Dextromethorphan (page 87)
  Pseudoephedrine

TYLENOL PM

Contains the following ingredients:
  Acetaminophen (page 3)
  Diphenhydramine (page 93)

TYLENOL SINUS

Contains the following ingredients:
  Acetaminophen (page 3)
  Pseudoephedrine

VALACYCLOVIR

Common names: Valtrex

Valacyclovir is an antiviral drug used to treat herpes zoster, or shingles, as well as recurrent episodes of genital herpes.

Summary of Interactions for Valcyclovir

In some cases, an herb or supplement may appear in more than one category, which may seem contradictory. For clarification, read the full article for details about the summarized interactions.

Depletion or interference	None known
Side effect reduction/prevention	None known
Supportive interaction	None known
Reduced drug absorption/bioavailability	None known
Adverse interaction	None known

VALPROIC ACID

Common names: Alti-Valproic, Apo-Valproic, Convulex, Depakene Syrup, Depakene, Depakote, Deproic, Divalproex Sodium, Epilim, Epival, Gen-Valproic, Novo-Valproic, Orlept, PMS-Valproic Acid, Sodium Valproate, Sondate 200 EC (sodium valproate)

Valproic acid, divalproex sodium, and sodium valproate are closely related drugs used to control (prevent) seizures in people with epilepsy.

Summary of Interactions for Valproic Acid

In some cases, an herb or supplement may appear in more than one category, which may seem contradictory.

Valproic Acid

For clarification, read the full article for details about the summarized interactions.

✓ May be Beneficial: Depletion or interference	Biotin*
	Calcium*
	Copper*
	Folic acid*
	L-carnitine*
	Vitamin A*
	Vitamin B₁₂*
	Vitamin B₆*
	Vitamin D*
	Vitamin K*
✓ May be Beneficial: Side effect reduction/prevention	Folic acid*
	L-carnitine*
	Vitamin B₁₂*
	Vitamin D*
	Vitamin K*
✓ May be Beneficial: Supportive interaction	Folic acid*
⊘ Avoid: Adverse interaction	Folic acid*
ⓘ Check: Other	Antioxidants (Selenium, Vitamin E)
	Zinc
Reduced drug absorption/bioavailability	None known

Interactions with Dietary Supplements

Antioxidants

On the basis of the biochemical actions of valproic acid, it has been suggested that people taking valproic acid should make sure they have adequate intakes of vitamin E and selenium.[1] The importance of supplementation with either nutrient has not yet been tested, however.

Biotin

Several controlled studies have shown that long-term anticonvulsant treatment decreases blood levels of biotin.[2, 3, 4, 5] In children, a deficiency of biotin can lead to withdrawn behavior and a delay in mental development. Adults with low biotin levels might experience a loss of appetite, feelings of discomfort or uneasiness, mental depression, or hallucinations. To avoid side effects, individuals taking anticonvulsants should supplement with biotin either alone or as part of a multivitamin.

Calcium

Individuals on long-term multiple anticonvulsant therapy may develop below-normal blood levels of calcium, which may be related to drug-induced vitamin D deficiency.[6] Two infants born to women taking

high doses of phenytoin and **phenobarbital** (page 215) while pregnant developed jitteriness and tetany (a syndrome characterized by muscle twitches), cramps, and spasms that can be caused by calcium deficiency during the first two weeks of life.[7] Controlled research is needed to determine whether pregnant women who are taking anticonvulsant medications should supplement with additional amounts of calcium and vitamin D.

Carnitine

Valproic acid causes depletion of carnitine in children,[8] and blood carnitine levels are often low in people taking valproic acid for long periods of time. While there have been several case reports of valproic acid-related carnitine deficiency causing abdominal pain in children, there is controversy about the need for carnitine supplements in children taking valproic acid.[9, 10, 11]

Complete disappearance of severe valproic acid-induced abdominal pain was achieved in one child with intractable epilepsy immediately following the introduction of 300 mg per day of L-carnitine.[12] Carnitine supplementation (50 mg per 2.2 pounds of body weight) has protected children from valproic acid-induced increases in blood ammonia levels in some research,[13] though other published work has questioned whether the depletion of carnitine and the increase in blood ammonia levels (both caused by valproic acid) are actually related to each other.[14] This last report found that the depletion of carnitine was significantly more severe when epileptics were taking valproic acid together with other anti-seizure medications. A double-blind, crossover study found that carnitine supplementation (100 mg per 2.2 pounds of body weight) was no more effective than placebo in improving the sense of well-being in children treated with valproic acid.[15] To date, the question of whether carnitine supplementation is beneficial for people taking valproic acid remains unresolved.[16] However, a panel of pediatric neurologists and experts on L-carnitine supplementation strongly recommended oral L-carnitine supplementation for all infants and children taking valproic acid, as well as for adults with carnitine deficiency syndromes, people with valproic acid-induced liver and kidney toxicity, people on kidney dialysis, and premature infants on total parenteral nutrition (intravenous feeding). The panel recommended an amount of 100 mg per 2.2 pounds of body weight per day, up to a maximum of 2 grams per day.[17]

Copper and zinc

In various studies of children treated with valproic acid for epilepsy compared with control groups, serum zinc levels remained normal[18, 19] or decreased,[20] serum copper levels remained normal[21, 22] or decreased,[23] and red blood cell zinc levels were decreased.[24] The importance of these changes and how frequently they occur remain unclear.

Folic acid

Several studies have shown that multiple anticonvulsant therapy reduces blood levels of folic acid and dramatically increases homocysteine levels.[25, 26, 27] Homocysteine, a potential marker for folic acid deficiency, is a compound used experimentally to induce seizures and is associated with atherosclerosis.

One preliminary study showed that pregnant women who use anticonvulsant drugs without folic acid supplementation have an increased risk of having a child with birth defects, such as heart defects, cleft lip and palate, neural tube defects, and skeletal abnormalities. However, supplementation with folic acid greatly reduces the risk.[28] Consequently, some healthcare practitioners recommend that women taking multiple anticonvulsant drugs supplement with 5 mg of folic acid daily, for three months prior to conception and during the first trimester, to prevent folic acid deficiency-induced birth defects.[29] Other practitioners suggest that 1 mg or less of folic acid each day is sufficient to prevent deficiency during pregnancy.[30]

One well-controlled study showed that adding folic acid to multiple anticonvulsant therapy resulted in reduced seizure frequency.[31] In addition, three infants with seizures who were unresponsive to medication experienced immediate relief following supplementation with the active form of folic acid.[32]

Despite the apparent beneficial effects, some studies have indicated that as little as 0.8 mg of folic acid taken daily can increase the frequency and/or severity of seizures.[33, 34, 35, 36] However, a recent controlled study showed that both healthy and epileptic women taking less than 1 mg of folic acid per day had no increased risk for seizures.[37] Until more is known about the risks and benefits of folic acid, individuals taking multiple anticonvulsant drugs should consult with their healthcare practitioner before supplementing with folic acid. In addition, pregnant women or women who might become pregnant while taking anticonvulsant drugs should discuss folic acid supplementation with their practitioner.

Vitamin A

Anticonvulsant drugs can occasionally cause birth defects when taken by pregnant women, and their toxicity might be related to low blood levels of vitamin A. One controlled study showed that taking multiple anticonvulsant drugs results in dramatic changes in the way the body utilizes vitamin A.[38] Further controlled research is needed to determine whether supplemental vitamin A might prevent birth defects in children born to women on multiple anticonvulsant therapy. Other research suggests that ingestion of large amounts of vitamin A may promote the development of birth defects, although the studies are conflicting.

Vitamin B6

Preliminary research has linked anticonvulsant therapy with possible depletion of vitamin B_6 in children.[39] One preliminary study found that a combination of 10–50 mg per 2.2 pounds of body weight of vitamin B_6 plus valproic acid was more effective than valproic acid or vitamin B_6 alone at treating children with recurrent seizures.[40] On the other hand, supplementation with large amounts of vitamin B_6 (80–200 mg per day) has been reported to reduce blood levels of some anticonvulsant drugs, which could theoretically trigger seizures. People taking anticonvulsant drugs should discuss with their doctor whether supplementing with vitamin B_6 is advisable.

Vitamin B12

Anemia is an uncommon side effect experienced by people taking anticonvulsant drugs. Though the cause may be folic acid deficiency in many cases, a deficiency of vitamin B_{12} may also be a factor in some cases. Deficiencies of folic acid and vitamin B_{12} can lead to nerve and mental problems. One study revealed that individuals on long-term anticonvulsant therapy had dramatically lower levels of vitamin B_{12} in their cerebrospinal fluid (the fluid that bathes the brain) when compared with people who were not taking seizure medications. Improvement in mental status and nerve function was observed in a majority of symptomatic individuals after taking 30 mcg of vitamin B_{12} daily for a few days.[41] Another study found that long-term anticonvulsant therapy had no effect on blood levels of vitamin B_{12}.[42] Despite these contradictory findings, people taking anticonvulsant drugs for several months or years might prevent nerve and mental problems by supplementing with vitamin B_{12}.

Vitamin D

Though research results vary, long-term use of anticonvulsant drugs appears to interfere with vitamin D activity, which might lead to softening of bones (osteomalacia). One study showed that blood levels of vitamin D in males taking anticonvulsants were lower than those found in men who were not taking seizure medication.[43] In a controlled study, bone strength improved in children taking anticonvulsant drugs who were supplemented with the activated form of vitamin D and 500 mg per day of calcium for nine months.[44] Some research suggests that differences in exposure to sunlight—which normally increases blood levels of vitamin D—might explain why some studies have failed to find a beneficial effect of vitamin D supplementation. In one controlled study, blood vitamin D levels in children taking anticonvulsants were dramatically lower in winter months than in summer months.[45] Another study of 450 people in Florida taking anticonvulsants found that few had drug-induced bone disease.[46] Consequently, people taking anticonvulsant drugs who do not receive adequate sunlight should supplement with 400 IU of vitamin D each day to help prevent osteomalacia.

Vitamin E
Two studies showed that individuals taking phenytoin and **phenobarbital** (page 215) had lower blood vitamin E levels than those who received no treatment for seizures.[47, 48] It is not known whether this same interaction occurs with valproic acid. Though the consequences of lower blood levels of vitamin E are unknown, people taking multiple anticonvulsant drugs should probably supplement with 100 to 200 IU of vitamin E daily to prevent a deficiency.

Vitamin K
Some studies have shown that babies born to women taking anticonvulsant drugs have low blood levels of vitamin K, which might cause bleeding in the infant.[49] Though some researchers recommend vitamin K supplementation prior to delivery,[50, 51] not all agree that supplementation for women taking anticonvulsant drugs is necessary.[52] Until more information is available, pregnant women or women who might become pregnant while taking anticonvulsant drugs should discuss vitamin K supplementation with their healthcare practitioner.

Interactions with Foods and Other Compounds
Food
Valproic acid, valproate, and divalproex may be taken with food to avoid/reduce stomach upset.[53] Capsules, tablets, and sprinkles containing these drugs should not be chewed, to avoid mouth and throat irritation.[54]

Alcohol
Valproic acid, valproate, and divalproex may all cause drowsiness and dizziness.[55] Alcohol may intensify these actions and increase the risk of accidental injury. People taking valproic acid, valproate, or divalproex should avoid alcohol.

VALSARTAN

Valsartan is an **angiotensin II receptor blocker** (page 17) used to treat high blood pressure.

Summary of Interactions for Valsartan
In some cases, an herb or supplement may appear in more than one category, which may seem contradictory. For clarification, read the full article for details about the summarized interactions.

Depletion or interference	None known
Side effect reduction/prevention	None known
Supportive interaction	None known
Reduced drug absorption/bioavailability	None known
Adverse interaction	None known

Interactions with Foods and Other Compounds
Food
Ingestion of food with valsartan may decrease the maximum blood level of the drug by 50%.[1] Therefore, valsartan should be taken an hour before or two hours after a meal.

VARDENAFIL

Common names: Levitra

Vardenafil is used to treat erectile dysfunction.

Summary of Interactions for Vardenafil
In some cases, an herb or supplement may appear in more than one category, which may seem contradictory. For clarification, read the full article for details about the summarized interactions.

⊘ Avoid: Reduced drug absorption/ bioavailability	Food
Depletion or interference	None known
Side effect reduction/prevention	None known
Supportive interaction	None known
Adverse interaction	None known

Interactions with Foods and Other Compounds
Food
A study comparing the effect of a high-fat meal and a moderate-fat meal on the absorption of vardenafil showed that taking the drug with a high-fat meal might result in a slight reduction in effectiveness and a delayed onset of action up to one hour.[1]

VASERETIC

Contains the following ingredients:
Enalapril (page 103)
Hydrochlorothiazide

VENLAFAXINE

Common names: Effexor

Venlafaxine is a drug used to treat depression. It is unrelated to other drugs used to treat depression.

Summary of Interactions for Venlafaxine
In some cases, an herb or supplement may appear in more than one category, which may seem contradictory. For clarification, read the full article for details about the summarized interactions.

⊘ Avoid: Adverse interaction	5-Hydroxytryptophan (5-HTP)* L-tryptophan* Sour date nut (Ziziphus jujube) St. John's wort*
ⓘ Check: Other	Sodium
Depletion or interference	None known
Side effect reduction/prevention	None known
Supportive interaction	None known
Reduced drug absorption/bioavailability	None known

Interactions with Dietary Supplements
5-hydroxytryptophan (5-HTP) and L-tryptophan
Venlafaxine, a potent serotonin reuptake inhibitor, has been associated with several cases of serotonin syndrome.[1, 2, 3, 4] 5-HTP and L-tryptophan are converted to serotonin in the brain, and taking them with venlafaxine may increase venlafaxine-induced side effects. While no interactions with venlafaxine and 5-HTP or L-tryptophan have been reported, until more is known, people taking venlafaxine are cautioned to avoid 5-HTP or L-tryptophan.

Sodium
One case was reported of a 79-year-old woman with depression treated with venlafaxine who experienced hyponatremia (abnormally low blood levels of sodium).[5] It remains unclear whether this interaction has any but rare ramifications.

Interactions with Herbs
Sour date nut (Ziziphus jujube)
There is one published report of a woman collapsing after taking venlafaxine in combination with the Chinese herbal remedy sour date nut (Ziziphus jujube),[6] although she tolerated venlafaxine by itself without side effects. People taking venlafaxine should not take sour date nut.

St. John's wort (Hypericum perforatum)
Although there have been no interactions reported in the medical literature, it is best to avoid using venlafaxine with St. John's wort unless you are under the supervision of a qualified healthcare professional.

Interactions with Foods and Other Compounds
Food
Venlafaxine is recommended to be taken with food.[7]

Alcohol
Venlafaxine may cause dizziness or drowsiness.[8] Alcohol may intensify these effects and increase the risk of accidental injury.[9] To prevent problems, people taking venlafaxine should avoid alcohol.

VENTIDE

Contains the following ingredient:
Salbutamol

Verapamil

VERAPAMIL

Common names: Alti-Verapamil, Apo-Verap, Berkatens, Calan, Chronovera, Cordilox, Covera-HS, Ethimil MR, Gen-Verapamil SR, Half Securon SR, Isoptin, Novo-Veramil, Nu-Verap, Securon, Univer, Verapress MR, Verelan, Vertab SR

Combination drug: Tarka

Verapamil is one of the calcium-channel blocker drugs used to treat angina pectoris, heart arrhythmias, and high blood pressure (hypertension).

Summary of Interactions for Verapamil

In some cases, an herb or supplement may appear in more than one category, which may seem contradictory. For clarification, read the full article for details about the summarized interactions.

✓ May be Beneficial: Side effect reduction/prevention	Calcium (for people with high blood pressure) Fiber Fluid
⊘ Avoid: Adverse interaction	Calcium (for people with high blood pressure) Pleurisy root* Vitamin D*
ⓘ Check: Other	Grapefruit juice
Depletion or interference	None known
Supportive interaction	None known
Reduced drug absorption/bioavailability	None known

Interactions with Dietary Supplements

Calcium

Calcium supplementation has been reported to reverse the blood pressure-lowering actions of this drug when used to treat arrhythmias.[1, 2] It remains unclear whether people taking verapamil for the purpose of lowering blood pressure should avoid calcium supplementation. These people should discuss the matter with the prescribing doctor.

On the other hand, people who take verapamil to treat other conditions, such as angina or heart arrhythmias, should discuss with their physicians the possibility of using low-level (as little as 27 mg per day) calcium supplementation, to reduce excessive blood pressure-lowering actions caused by verapamil in those who do not have high blood pressure.[3]

Vitamin D

Vitamin D may interfere with the effectiveness of verapamil.[4] People taking verapamil should ask their doctor before using vitamin D-containing supplements.

Fluid and fiber

Constipation is a common side effect of verapamil treatment.[5] Increasing fluid and fiber intake can ease constipation.

Interactions with Herbs

Pleurisy root

As pleurisy root and other plants in the *Aesclepius* genus contain cardiac glycosides, it is best to avoid use of pleurisy root with heart medications such as calcium-channel blockers.[6]

Interactions with Foods and Other Compounds

Grapefruit juice

Grapefruit juice may increase verapamil blood levels.[7] The importance of this interaction regarding verapamil effectiveness and side effects is unknown. Until more is known, it makes sense for people taking this drug to either avoid drinking grapefruit juice entirely or drink grapefruit juice only under the careful monitoring and supervision of the prescribing doctor. In theory, this last possibility might allow for a decrease in drug dose, but it could be dangerous in the absence of diligent monitoring. The same effects might be seen from eating grapefruit as from drinking its juice.

VICODIN

Contains the following ingredients:
Acetaminophen (page 3)
Hydrocodone (page 137)

VICOPROFEN

Contains the following ingredients:
Hydrocodone (page 137)
Ibuprofen (page 139)

VIOFORM-HYDROCORTISONE

Contains the following ingredients:
Clioquinol
Hydrocortisone

VISKALDIX

Contains the following ingredients:
Beclomethasone
Clopamide
Pindolol

WARFARIN

Common names: Coumadin, Marevan, Warfilone

Warfarin is an anticoagulant (slows blood clotting) used to prevent and treat people with venous thrombosis (blood clots in the veins) and pulmonary embolism (blood clots in the lungs). Warfarin is also used to treat or prevent dangerous blood clotting in people with atrial fibrillation (an irregularity in heartbeat) and, in some cases, to prevent stroke.

Summary of Interactions for Warfarin

In some cases, an herb or supplement may appear in more than one category, which may seem contradictory. For clarification, read the full article for details about the summarized interactions.

⊘ Avoid: Reduced drug absorption/ bioavailability	Coenzyme Q10 Green tea* Iron* Magnesium* St. John's wort* Vitamin C Zinc*
⊘ Avoid: Adverse interaction	American ginseng Asian ginseng* Cranberry Dan shen Devil's claw* Dong quai* Fenugreek* Garlic* Ginger* Ginkgo biloba* Horse chestnut* Lycium barbarum* Papain* Quilinggao* **Quinine** (page 227)* Red clover* Reishi
	Sweet clover* Sweet woodruff* Vitamin D* Vitamin K
ⓘ Check: Other	Alcohol Bromelain Eleuthero Olestra Protein Soy Vitamin C Vitamin E
Depletion or interference	None known
Side effect reduction/prevention	None known
Supportive interaction	None known

Interactions with Dietary Supplements

Bromelain

In theory, bromelain might enhance the action of anticoagulants. This theoretical concern has not been substantiated by human research, however.[1]

Coenzyme Q10

Coenzyme Q10 (CoQ10) is structurally similar to vitamin K and may affect blood coagulation.[2] Four case reports describe possible interference by CoQ10 with warfarin activity.[3, 4, 5] It remains unknown how common or rare this interaction is. Those taking warfarin should only take CoQ10 with the guidance of their doctor.

Minerals

Iron, magnesium, and zinc may bind with warfarin, potentially decreasing their absorption and activity.[6] People on warfarin therapy should take warfarin and iron/magnesium/zinc-containing products at least two hours apart.

Papain

Papain, an enzyme extract of papaya, was associated with increased warfarin activity in one patient.[7] Persons taking warfarin should avoid papain supplements until further information about this potential interaction becomes available.

Vitamin C

Although case reports have suggested that vitamin C might increase the activity of anticoagulants in a potentially dangerous way, this interaction has not been confirmed in research studies.[8] In fact, a possible interference by vitamin C with the effect of anticoagulants has also been reported.[9] A 52-year-old woman

Warfarin

maintained on 7.5 mg of warfarin per day had a short-ening of the blood clotting time which was not corrected by increasing warfarin up to 20 mg per day. Further questioning revealed she had begun taking an unspecified amount of vitamin C each morning. After stopping vitamin C, the blood clotting time returned to desired levels. Based on this and other case reports, people taking warfarin should consult with their physician before taking vitamin C supplements.

Vitamin D

In 1975, a single letter to the *Journal of the American Medical Association* suggested that vitamin D increases the activity of anticoagulants and that this interaction could prove dangerous.[10] However, there have been no other reports of such an interaction, even though tens of millions of people are taking multivitamins that contain vitamin D. Most doctors typically do not tell patients taking anticoagulant medications to avoid vitamin D.

Vitamin E

An isolated case was reported in 1974 of vitamin E (up to 1,200 IU per day) being associated with increased anticoagulation (blood thinning) in a patient treated with warfarin.[11] A study of 12 people undergoing warfarin therapy found that additional vitamin E (100 IU or 400 IU per day) did not induce a clinical bleeding state.[12] Moreover, a double-blind trial found that supplementation with vitamin E in amounts up to 1,200 IU per day had no effect on warfarin activity.[13] It now appears safe for people taking warfarin to supplement vitamin E despite information to the contrary often provided by doctors about this purported interaction. These warnings are based on the isolated case report from 1974.

Vitamin K

Warfarin slows blood clotting by interfering with vitamin K activity. Since vitamin K reverses the anticoagulant effects of warfarin,[14] people taking warfarin should avoid vitamin K-containing supplements unless specifically directed otherwise by their prescribing doctor. Some vegetables (broccoli, Brussels sprouts, kale, parsley, spinach, and others) are high in vitamin K. Eating large quantities[15] or making sudden changes in the amounts eaten of these vegetables can interfere with the effectiveness and safety of warfarin therapy. The greener the plant, the higher the vitamin K content.[16] Other significant dietary sources of vitamin K include soybean oil, olive oil, cottonseed oil, and canola oil.[17]

Vitamin K supplementation can be used, however, to counteract an overdose of warfarin.[18] Such treatment requires the supervision of a doctor.

Interactions with Herbs

Asian ginseng (Panax ginseng)
Asian ginseng was associated with a decrease in warfarin activity in a case report.[19] Persons taking warfarin should consult with a physician knowledgeable about botanical medicines if they are considering taking Asian ginseng or eleuthero/Siberian ginseng *(Eleutherococcus senticosus)*. A 1999 animal study did not reveal any significant interaction between warfarin and pure ginseng extract.[20]

In a study of healthy human volunteers, supplementing with American ginseng reduced warfarin's anticoagulant effect, apparently by stimulating the body to accelerate the metabolism of warfarin.[21] People taking warfarin should not take American ginseng, unless supervised by a doctor.

Cranberry
There have been at least five case reports suggesting that cranberry juice increases the activity of warfarin, possibly by inhibiting the breakdown of warfarin in the body.[22] Because of this potential interaction, people taking warfarin should avoid, or limit the intake of, cranberry juice. The U.K. Medicines Authority has advised people taking warfarin to avoid cranberry juice.

Dan shen (Salvia miltiorrhiza)
Dan shen, a Chinese herb, was associated with increased warfarin activity in several cases.[23, 24, 25, 26] Dan shen should only be used under close medical supervision by people taking warfarin. Sage *(Salvia officinalis)*, a plant relative of dan shen found in the West, is not associated with interactions involving warfarin.

Devil's claw (Harpagophytum procumbens)
Devil's claw was associated with purpura (bleeding under the skin) in a patient treated with warfarin.[27] However, key details in this case—including other medications taken and the amounts and duration of warfarin and devil's claw taken—were not reported, making it impossible to evaluate this reported interaction. Until more is known, people taking warfarin should avoid taking devil's claw.

Dong quai (Angelica sinensis)
A 46-year-old woman taking warfarin experienced increased strength of the anticoagulant properties of the

drug after starting to use dong quai for menopause.[28] The daily amount of dong quai was 1,130–2,260 mg per day. Her bleeding tendency returned to normal after discontinuing the dong quai. While little is known about the potential interaction of dong quai and warfarin, women should discuss the use of the herb with a healthcare professional if they are taking an anticoagulant drug and wish to use dong quai.

Feverfew (Tanacetum parthenium)
Although there are no documented cases of feverfew interacting with warfarin in humans, feverfew has been shown to interfere with certain aspects of blood clotting in test tube studies.[29, 30, 31]

Garlic (Allium sativum)
Garlic has been shown to help prevent atherosclerosis (hardening of the arteries), perhaps by reducing the ability of platelets to stick together.[32] This can result in an increase in the tendency toward bleeding.[33] Standardized extracts have, on rare occasions, been associated with bleeding in people.[34] Garlic extracts have also been associated with two human cases of increased warfarin activity.[35] The extracts were not definitively shown to be the cause of the problem. People taking warfarin should consult with a doctor before taking products containing standardized extracts of garlic or eating more than one clove of garlic daily.

Ginger (Zingiber officinale)
Ginger has been shown to reduce platelet stickiness in test tubes. Although there are no reports of interactions with anticoagulant drugs, people should consult a healthcare professional if they are taking an anticoagulant and wish to use ginger.[36]

Ginkgo biloba
Ginkgo extracts may reduce the ability of platelets to stick together, possibly increasing the tendency toward bleeding.[37] Standardized extracts of ginkgo have been associated with two cases of spontaneous bleeding, although the ginkgo extracts were not definitively shown to be the cause of the problem.[38, 39] There are two case reports of people taking warfarin in whom bleeding occurred after the addition of ginkgo.[40, 41] People taking warfarin should consult with a physician knowledgeable about botanical medicines if they are considering taking ginkgo.

Green tea (Camellia sinensis)
One man taking warfarin and one-half to one gallon of green tea per day developed signs based on laboratory testing suggesting his blood was too thick because the green tea was blocking the effect of warfarin.[42] Removal of the green tea caused normalization of his blood tests. Those taking green tea and warfarin together should have their blood monitored regularly to avert any problems and should consult with a doctor, healthcare practitioner and/or pharmacist before taking any medication.

Herbs containing coumarin derivatives
Although there are no specific studies demonstrating interactions with anticoagulants, the following herbs contain coumarin-like substances that may interact with warfarin and may cause bleeding.[43] These herbs include angelica root, arnica flower, anise, asafoetida, celery, chamomile, corn silk, fenugreek, horse chestnut, licorice root, lovage root, parsley, passion flower herb, quassia, red clover, rue, sweet clover, and sweet woodruff. Dong quai contains at least six coumarin derivatives, which may account for the interaction noted above. People should consult a healthcare professional if they are taking an anticoagulant and wish to use one of these herbs.

Lycium barbarum
There is one case report in which ingestion of a Chinese herbal tea made from *Lycium barbarum* appeared to interfere with the effect of warfarin.[44]

Quinine (page 227) (cinchona species)
Quinine, a chemical found in cinchona bark and available as a drug product, has been reported to increase warfarin activity.[45] People should read labels for quinine/cinchona content. People taking warfarin should avoid quinine-containing products.

Quilinggao
There is one published case report in which the Chinese herbal product quilinggao increased the action of warfarin and apparently contributed to a bleeding episode.[46] There are many different brands of quilinggao, and the composition varies between manufacturers. Individuals taking warfarin should not take quilinggao.

Reishi (Ganoderma lucidum)
As it may increase bleeding time, reishi is not recommended for those taking anticoagulant (blood-thinning) medications.[47]

St. John's wort (Hypericum perforatum)
According to a preliminary report, volunteers taking 900 mg per day of St. John's wort were given a single dose of an anticoagulant similar in action to warfarin.[48]

There was a significant drop in the amount of the drug measured in the blood. Seven case studies reported to the Medical Products Agency in Sweden also found a decrease in the anticoagulant activity of warfarin when St. John's wort was taken at the same time.[49] This may have occurred because certain chemicals found in St. John's wort activate liver enzymes that are involved in the elimination of some drugs.[50, 51] People taking warfarin should consult with their doctor before taking St. John's wort.

Interactions with Foods and Other Compounds

Alcohol

Alcohol use, especially long-term heavy drinking, can decrease the effectiveness of warfarin.[52] People taking warfarin are cautioned to avoid alcohol.

Food

Some vegetables (broccoli, Brussels sprouts, kale, parsley, spinach, and others) are high in vitamin K. Eating large quantities[53] or making sudden changes in the amounts eaten of these vegetables interferes with the effectiveness and safety of warfarin therapy. Eating charbroiled food may decrease warfarin activity,[54] while eating cooked onions may increase warfarin activity.[55] Soy foods have been reported both to increase[56] and to decrease[57] warfarin activity. The significance of these last three interactions remains unclear.

Preliminary evidence suggests that frequent consumption of mangoes may interfere with the effect of warfarin.[58]

There is one preliminary report in which a high-protein, low-carbohydrate diet appeared to interfere with the effect of warfarin in two people.[59] While additional research is needed to confirm that observation, people taking warfarin should consult their doctor before making large changes in the amount of protein they eat.

Olestra

The FDA-approved fat substitute, olestra, interferes with fat absorption, including the absorption of fat-soluble vitamins. Vitamin K, a fat-soluble vitamin, is added to olestra to offset this adverse effect.[60] Since vitamin K interferes with the activity of warfarin, eating snacks containing olestra may also interfere with the drug's activity. The impact of eating snacks containing olestra has not been evaluated in people taking warfarin. However, until more is known, it makes sense for people taking warfarin to avoid olestra-containing foods.[61]

WYGESIC

Contains the following ingredients:
Acetaminophen (page 3)
Propoxyphene (page 224)

ZAFIRLUKAST

Common names: Accolate

Zafirlukast is used in the prevention and treatment of mild to severe asthma, seasonal allergic asthma, exercise-induced asthma, and **aspirin** (page 26)-induced asthma. It belongs to a class of drugs called leukotriene-receptor antagonists (LTRA).

Summary of Interactions for Zafirlukast

In some cases, an herb or supplement may appear in more than one category, which may seem contradictory. For clarification, read the full article for details about the summarized interactions.

⊘ Avoid: Reduced drug absorption/ bioavailability	Food
⊘ Avoid: Adverse interaction	Willow*
Depletion or interference	None known
Side effect reduction/prevention	None known
Supportive interaction	None known

Interactions with Herbs

Willow (Salix alba)

Willow bark contains salicin, a substance similar to **aspirin** (page 26). Research has shown that aspirin significantly increases blood levels of zafirlukast,[1] which would increase the likelihood of side effects from zafirlukast. The same thing could theoretically happen if people took willow bark along with zafirlukast, although no studies have investigated this specific interaction. People may want to avoid combining willow bark with zafirlukast due to the possibility of increased side effects.

Interactions with Foods and Other Compounds

Food

The ingestion of food along with zafirlukast can reduce the overall absorption of the drug by about 40%.[2] Therefore, zafirlukast should be taken one hour before or two hours after a meal.

ZESTORETIC

Contains the following ingredients:
Hydrochlorothiazide
Lisinopril (page 156)

ZIAC

Contains the following ingredients:
Bisoprolol (page 41)
Hydrochlorothiazide

ZOLMITRIPTAN

Common names: Zomig

Zolmitriptan is used to treat acute attacks of migraine headache and is in a class of drugs known as serotonin antagonists. There are currently no reported nutrient or herb interactions involving zolmitriptan.

Summary of Interactions for Zolmitriptan

In some cases, an herb or supplement may appear in more than one category, which may seem contradictory. For clarification, read the full article for details about the summarized interactions.

⊘ Avoid: Adverse interaction	5-Hydroxytryp-tophan (5-HTP)* L-tryptophan*
Depletion or interference	None known
Side effect reduction/prevention	None known
Supportive interaction	None known
Reduced drug absorption/bioavailability	None known

Interactions with Dietary Supplements

5-hydroxytryptophan (5-HTP)
Zolmitriptan works by stimulating serotonin receptors in the brain. 5-HTP and L-tryptophan are converted to serotonin in the brain, and taking them with zolmitriptan could increase zolmitriptan-induced side effects. However, no interactions have yet been reported with zolmitriptan and 5-HTP or L-tryptophan.

ZOLPIDEM

Common names: Ambien, Stilnoct

Zolpidem a is hypnotic drug used for short-term treatment of people with insomnia.

Summary of Interactions for Zolpidem

In some cases, an herb or supplement may appear in more than one category, which may seem contradictory. For clarification, read the full article for details about the summarized interactions.

⊘ Avoid: Adverse interaction	5-Hydroxytryp-tophan (5-HTP)* L-tryptophan*
Depletion or interference	None known
Side effect reduction/prevention	None known
Supportive interaction	None known
Reduced drug absorption/bioavailability	None known

Interactions with Dietary Supplements

5-hydroxytryptophan (5-HTP) and L-tryptophan
Nine cases of zolpidem-induced hallucinations associated with serotonin reuptake inhibiting antidepressants have been reported, some lasting for several hours.[1] 5-HTP and L-tryptophan are converted to serotonin in the brain, and taking them with zolpidem may increase zolpidem-induced hallucinations, though no interactions have yet been reported with zolpidem and 5-HTP or L-tryptophan.

Interactions with Foods and Other Compounds

Food
Food may interfere with zolpidem absorption and slow the onset of sleep.[2] Zolpidem should be taken one hour before or two hours after food to avoid this interaction.

Alcohol
Zolpidem causes drowsiness. Alcohol may compound this effect and increase the risk of accidental injury.[3] To prevent problems, people taking zolpidem should avoid alcohol.

Zolpidem

Interactions by Herb or Vitamin

Herbs

Some interactions may increase the need for the herb (✓), other interactions may be negative (⊘) and indicate the herb should not be taken without first speaking with your physician or pharmacist. Others may require further explanation (ⓘ). Refer to the individual drug entry for specific details about an interaction. The following list only includes the generic or class name of a medicine—to find a specific brand name, use the index.

AHCC

At the time of writing, there were no well-known drug interactions with AHCC.

ALDER BUCKTHORN

Certain medicines interact with alder buckthorn:
Digoxin (page 90) ⓘ
Diuretics (page 94) ⊘
Loop Diuretics (page 159) ⊘
Oral Corticosteroids (page 200) ⓘ
Thiazide Diuretics (page 258) ⊘

ALFALFA

At the time of writing, there were no well-known drug interactions with alfalfa.

ALOE

Certain medicines interact with aloe:
Glyburide (page 132) ✓
Topical Corticosteroids (page 265) ⓘ

AMERICAN GINSENG

At the time of writing, there were no well-known drug interactions with American ginseng.

AMERICAN SCULLCAP

At the time of writing, there were no well-known drug interactions with American scullcap.

ANDROGRAPHIS

At the time of writing, there were no well-known drug interactions with andrographis.

ANISE

At the time of writing, there were no well-known drug interactions with anise.

ARTICHOKE

At the time of writing, there were no well-known drug interactions with artichoke.

ASHWAGANDHA

At the time of writing, there were no well-known drug interactions with ashwagandha.

ASIAN GINSENG

Certain medicines interact with Asian ginseng:
Influenza Virus Vaccine (page 142) ✓
Ticlopidine (page 262) ⊘
Triotann-S Pediatric (page 274) ✓
Warfarin (page 281) ⊘

ASTRAGALUS

At the time of writing, there were no well-known drug interactions with astragalus.

BACOPA

Certain medicines interact with bacopa:
   Perphenazine (page 213) ⊘
   Prochlorperazine (page 222) ⊘
   Thioridazine (page 260) ⊘

BARBERRY

Certain medicines interact with barberry:
   Doxycycline (page 101) ⓘ
   Tetracycline (page 253) ⊘

BASIL

At the time of writing, there were no well-known drug interactions with basil.

BILBERRY

At the time of writing, there were no well-known drug interactions with bilberry.

BITTER MELON

At the time of writing, there were no well-known drug interactions with bitter melon.

BITTER ORANGE

At the time of writing, there were no well-known drug interactions with bitter orange.

BLACK COHOSH

At the time of writing, there were no well-known drug interactions with black cohosh.

BLACK HOREHOUND

At the time of writing, there were no well-known drug interactions with black horehound.

BLACKBERRY

At the time of writing, there were no well-known drug interactions with blackberry.

BLADDERWRACK

At the time of writing, there were no well-known drug interactions with bladderwrack.

BLESSED THISTLE

At the time of writing, there were no well-known drug interactions with blessed thistle.

BLOODROOT

At the time of writing, there were no well-known drug interactions with bloodroot.

BLUE COHOSH

At the time of writing, there were no well-known drug interactions with blue cohosh.

BLUE FLAG

At the time of writing, there were no well-known drug interactions with blue flag.

BLUEBERRY

At the time of writing, there were no well-known drug interactions with blueberry.

BOLDO

At the time of writing, there were no well-known drug interactions with boldo.

BONESET

At the time of writing, there were no well-known drug interactions with boneset.

BOSWELLIA

At the time of writing, there were no well-known drug interactions with boswellia.

BUCHU

Certain medicines interact with buchu:
  Loop Diuretics (page 159) ⊘
  Spironolactone (page 243) ⊘
  Thiazide Diuretics (page 258) ⊘
  Triamterene (page 268) ⊘

BUCKTHORN

Certain medicines interact with buckthorn:
  Digoxin (page 90) ⓘ
  Diuretics (page 94) ⊘
  Loop Diuretics (page 159) ⊘
  Oral Corticosteroids (page 200) ⓘ
  Thiazide Diuretics (page 258) ⊘

BUGLEWEED

Certain medicines interact with bugleweed:
  Thyroid Hormones (page 261) ⊘

BUPLEURUM

Certain medicines interact with bupleurum:
  Interferon (page 144) ⊘

BURDOCK

At the time of writing, there were no well-known drug interactions with burdock.

BUTCHER'S BROOM

At the time of writing, there were no well-known drug interactions with butcher's broom.

CALENDULA

At the time of writing, there were no well-known drug interactions with calendula.

CARAWAY

At the time of writing, there were no well-known drug interactions with caraway.

CAROB

At the time of writing, there were no well-known drug interactions with carob.

CASCARA

Certain medicines interact with cascara:
  Digoxin (page 90) ⊘

CATNIP

At the time of writing, there were no well-known drug interactions with catnip.

CAT'S CLAW

At the time of writing, there were no well-known drug interactions with cat's claw.

CAYENNE

Certain medicines interact with cayenne:
  Aspirin (page 26) ✓

CENTAURY

At the time of writing, there were no well-known drug interactions with centaury.

CHAMOMILE

Certain medicines interact with chamomile:
  Chemotherapy (page 54) ✓
  Cisplatin (page 64) ✓
  Cyclophosphamide (page 79) ✓
  Docetaxel (page 95) ✓
  Fluorouracil (page 116) ✓
  Methotrexate (page 169) ✓
  Paclitaxel (page 205) ✓

CHAPARRAL

At the time of writing, there were no well-known drug interactions with chaparral.

CHICKWEED

At the time of writing, there were no well-known drug interactions with chickweed.

Chickweed

CHINESE SCULLCAP

Certain medicines interact with Chinese scullcap:
Cyclosporine (page 83) ⊘

CINNAMON

At the time of writing, there were no well-known drug interactions with cinnamon.

CLEAVERS

Certain medicines interact with cleavers:
Loop Diuretics (page 159) ⊘
Spironolactone (page 243) ⊘
Thiazide Diuretics (page 258) ⊘
Triamterene (page 268) ⊘

COLEUS

Certain medicines interact with coleus:
Albuterol (page 6) ✓
Aspirin (page 26) ⊘
Ephedrine and Pseudoephedrine (page 104) ✓
Epinephrine (page 105) ✓
Salmeterol (page 234) ✓

COLTSFOOT

At the time of writing, there were no well-known drug interactions with coltsfoot.

COMFREY

At the time of writing, there were no well-known drug interactions with comfrey.

CORDYCEPS

At the time of writing, there were no well-known drug interactions with cordyceps.

CORYDALIS

At the time of writing, there were no well-known drug interactions with corydalis.

CRANBERRY

Certain medicines interact with cranberry:
Lansoprazole (page 153) ✓
Omeprazole (page 197) ✓
Warfarin (page 281) ⊘

CRANESBILL

At the time of writing, there were no well-known drug interactions with cranesbill.

DAMIANA

At the time of writing, there were no well-known drug interactions with damiana.

DANDELION

Certain medicines interact with dandelion:
Ciprofloxacin (page 62) ⊘
Loop Diuretics (page 159) ⊘
Spironolactone (page 243) ⊘
Thiazide Diuretics (page 258) ⊘
Triamterene (page 268) ⊘

DEVIL'S CLAW

Certain medicines interact with devil's claw:
Ticlopidine (page 262) ⊘
Warfarin (page 281) ⊘

DONG QUAI

Certain medicines interact with dong quai:
Heparin (page 135) ⊘
Ticlopidine (page 262) ⊘
Warfarin (page 281) ⊘

ECHINACEA

Certain medicines interact with echinacea:
Chemotherapy (page 54) ⓘ
Cisplatin (page 64) ⓘ
Cyclophosphamide (page 79) ⓘ
Docetaxel (page 95) ⓘ
Econazole (page 103) ✓
Fluorouracil (page 116) ⓘ
Methotrexate (page 169) ⓘ
Paclitaxel (page 205) ⓘ

ELDERBERRY

At the time of writing, there were no well-known drug interactions with elderberry.

ELECAMPANE

At the time of writing, there were no well-known drug interactions with elecampane.

ELEUTHERO

Certain medicines interact with eleuthero:
Chemotherapy (page 54) ✓
Cisplatin (page 64) ✓
Cyclophosphamide (page 79) ✓
Digoxin (page 90) ⊘
Docetaxel (page 95) ✓
Fluorouracil (page 116) ✓
Influenza Virus Vaccine (page 142) ✓
Methotrexate (page 169) ✓
Paclitaxel (page 205) ✓
Ticlopidine (page 262) ⓘ
Warfarin (page 281) ⓘ

EUCALYPTUS

At the time of writing, there were no well-known drug interactions with eucalyptus.

EYEBRIGHT

At the time of writing, there were no well-known drug interactions with eyebright.

FALSE UNICORN

At the time of writing, there were no well-known drug interactions with false unicorn.

FENNEL

Certain medicines interact with fennel:
Ciprofloxacin (page 62) ⊘

FENUGREEK

Certain medicines interact with fenugreek:
Glipizide (page 131) ⊘
Heparin (page 135) ⊘
Insulin (page 144) ✓
Ticlopidine (page 262) ⊘
Warfarin (page 281) ⊘

FEVERFEW

At the time of writing, there were no well-known drug interactions with feverfew.

FO-TI

At the time of writing, there were no well-known drug interactions with fo-ti.

GARLIC

Certain medicines interact with garlic:
Chlorzoxazone (page 60) ⊘
Dipyridamole (page 94) ✓
Ticlopidine (page 262) ⊘
Warfarin (page 281) ⊘

GENTIAN

At the time of writing, there were no well-known drug interactions with gentian.

GINGER

Certain medicines interact with ginger:
Chemotherapy (page 54) ✓
Cisplatin (page 64) ✓
Cyclophosphamide (page 79) ✓
Docetaxel (page 95) ✓
Fluorouracil (page 116) ✓
General Anesthetics (page 129) ✓
Heparin (page 135) ⊘
Methotrexate (page 169) ✓
Nitrous Oxide (page 191) ✓
Paclitaxel (page 205) ✓
Ticlopidine (page 262) ⓘ
Warfarin (page 281) ⊘

Ginger

GINKGO BILOBA

Certain medicines interact with *Ginkgo biloba*:
Aspirin (page 26) ⊘
Citalopram (page 68) ✓
Cyclosporine (page 83) ✓
Fluoxetine (page 120) ✓
Fluvoxamine (page 122) ✓
Glimepiride (page 131) ⊘
Glipizide (page 131) ⊘
Glyburide (page 132) ⊘
Haloperidol (page 134) ✓
Heparin (page 135) ⊘
Metformin (page 168) ⊘
Paroxetine (page 208) ✓
Repaglinide (page 231) ⊘
Sertraline (page 237) ✓
Thiazide Diuretics (page 258) ⊘
Ticlopidine (page 262) ⊘
Trazodone (page 267) ⊘
Warfarin (page 281) ⊘

GOLDENSEAL

Certain medicines interact with goldenseal:
Doxycycline (page 101) ⓘ
Tetracycline (page 253) ⊘

GOTU KOLA

At the time of writing, there were no well-known drug interactions with gotu kola.

GREATER CELANDINE

At the time of writing, there were no well-known drug interactions with greater celandine.

GREEN TEA

Certain medicines interact with green tea:
Atropine (page 30) ⊘
Cardec DM (page 50) ⊘
Codeine (page 75) ⊘
Ephedrine and Pseudoephedrine (page 104) ⊘
Lomotil/Lonox (page 158) ⊘
Theophylline/Aminophylline (page 256) ⊘
Warfarin (page 281) ⊘

GUARANÁ

Certain medicines interact with guaraná:
Caffeine (page 44) ⓘ

GUGGUL

At the time of writing, there were no well-known drug interactions with guggul.

GYMNEMA

Certain medicines interact with gymnema:
Glipizide (page 131) ⊘
Glyburide (page 132) ⓘ
Insulin (page 144) ✓ ⊘

HAWTHORN

Certain medicines interact with hawthorn:
Digoxin (page 90) ⓘ

HOPS

At the time of writing, there were no well-known drug interactions with hops.

HOREHOUND

At the time of writing, there were no well-known drug interactions with horehound.

HORSE CHESTNUT

Certain medicines interact with horse chestnut:
Heparin (page 135) ⊘
Ticlopidine (page 262) ⊘
Warfarin (page 281) ⊘

HORSERADISH

At the time of writing, there were no well-known drug interactions with horseradish.

HORSETAIL

Certain medicines interact with horsetail:
Loop Diuretics (page 159) ⊘
Spironolactone (page 243) ⊘
Thiazide Diuretics (page 258) ⊘
Triamterene (page 268) ⊘

Ginkgo Biloba

HUPERZIA

Certain medicines interact with huperzia:
> **Donepezil** (page 99) ⃠
> **Tacrine** (page 250) ⃠

HYSSOP

At the time of writing, there were no well-known drug interactions with hyssop.

IPECAC

At the time of writing, there were no well-known drug interactions with ipecac.

IVY LEAF

At the time of writing, there were no well-known drug interactions with ivy leaf.

JUNIPER

Certain medicines interact with juniper:
> **Loop Diuretics** (page 159) ⃠
> **Spironolactone** (page 243) ⃠
> **Thiazide Diuretics** (page 258) ⃠
> **Triamterene** (page 268) ⃠

KAVA

Certain medicines interact with kava:
> **Alprazolam** (page 9) ⃠
> **Buspirone** (page 44) ⃠

KUDZU

At the time of writing, there were no well-known drug interactions with kudzu.

LAVENDER

At the time of writing, there were no well-known drug interactions with lavender.

LEMON BALM

Certain medicines interact with lemon balm:
> **Thyroid Hormones** (page 261) ⃠

LICORICE

Certain medicines interact with licorice:
> **Aspirin** (page 26) ✓
> **Digoxin** (page 90) ⃠
> **Etodolac** (page 111) ✓
> **Ibuprofen** (page 139) ✓
> **Interferon** (page 144) ✓
> **Isoniazid** (page 146) ✓
> **Loop Diuretics** (page 159) ⃠
> **Nabumetone** (page 184) ✓
> **Naproxen/Naproxen Sodium** (page 186) ✓
> **Oral Corticosteroids** (page 200) ⓘ
> **Oxaprozin** (page 203) ✓
> **Risperidone** (page 232) ⓘ
> **Thiazide Diuretics** (page 258) ⃠
> **Topical Corticosteroids** (page 265) ✓

LIGUSTRUM

At the time of writing, there were no well-known drug interactions with ligustrum.

LINDEN

At the time of writing, there were no well-known drug interactions with linden.

LOBELIA

Certain medicines interact with lobelia:
> **Nicotine Alternatives** (page 189) ⓘ

LOMATIUM

At the time of writing, there were no well-known drug interactions with lomatium.

MAITAKE

At the time of writing, there were no well-known drug interactions with maitake.

MALLOW

At the time of writing, there were no well-known drug interactions with mallow.

Mallow

MARSHMALLOW

At the time of writing, there were no well-known drug interactions with marshmallow.

MEADOWSWEET

Certain medicines interact with meadowsweet:
>   **Bismuth Subsalicylate** (page 40) ⊘
>   **Ticlopidine** (page 262) ⊘

MILK THISTLE

Certain medicines interact with milk thistle:
>   **Acetaminophen** (page 3) ✓
>   **Chemotherapy** (page 54) ✓
>   **Cisplatin** (page 64) ✓
>   **Clofibrate** (page 71) ✓
>   **Fluorouracil** (page 116) ✓
>   **General Anesthetics** (page 129) ✓
>   **Haloperidol** (page 134) ✓
>   **Lovastatin** (page 163) ✓
>   **Methotrexate** (page 169) ✓
>   **Metronidazole** (page 177) ①
>   **Nitrous Oxide** (page 191) ✓
>   **Paclitaxel** (page 205) ✓
>   **Pravastatin** (page 220) ✓
>   **Tacrine** (page 250) ✓

MISTLETOE

At the time of writing, there were no well-known drug interactions with mistletoe.

MOTHERWORT

At the time of writing, there were no well-known drug interactions with motherwort.

MULLEIN

At the time of writing, there were no well-known drug interactions with mullein.

MYRRH

At the time of writing, there were no well-known drug interactions with myrrh.

NETTLE

Certain medicines interact with nettle:
>   **Diclofenac** (page 87) ✓

NONI

At the time of writing, there were no well-known drug interactions with noni.

OAK

Certain medicines interact with oak:
>   **Atropine** (page 30) ⊘
>   **Cardec DM** (page 50) ⊘
>   **Codeine** (page 75) ⊘
>   **Ephedrine and Pseudoephedrine** (page 104) ⊘
>   **Lomotil/Lonox** (page 158) ⊘
>   **Theophylline/Aminophylline** (page 256) ⊘

OATS

At the time of writing, there were no well-known drug interactions with oats.

OLIVE LEAF

At the time of writing, there were no well-known drug interactions with olive leaf.

ONION

At the time of writing, there were no well-known drug interactions with onions.

OREGANO/WILD MARJORAM

At the time of writing, there were no well-known drug interactions with Oregano/Wild Marjoram.

OREGON GRAPE

Certain medicines interact with Oregon grape:
>   **Doxycycline** (page 101) ①
>   **Tetracycline** (page 253) ⊘

PASSION FLOWER

At the time of writing, there were no well-known drug interactions with passion flower.

PAU D'ARCO

At the time of writing, there were no well-known drug interactions with pau d'arco.

PENNYROYAL

At the time of writing, there were no well-known drug interactions with pennyroyal.

PEONY

At the time of writing, there were no well-known drug interactions with peony.

PEPPERMINT

At the time of writing, there were no well-known drug interactions with peppermint.

PERIWINKLE

At the time of writing, there were no well-known drug interactions with periwinkle.

PHYLLANTHUS

At the time of writing, there were no well-known drug interactions with phyllanthus.

PICRORHIZA

Certain medicines interact with picrorhiza:
Isoniazid (page 146) ✓

PLANTAIN

At the time of writing, there were no well-known drug interactions with plantain.

PLEURISY ROOT

Certain medicines interact with pleurisy root:
Acebutolol (page 3) ⃠
Amlodipine (page 13) ⃠
Atenolol (page 28) ⃠
Beta-Adrenergic Blockers (page 37) ⃠
Betaxolol (page 38) ⃠
Bisoprolol (page 41) ⃠
Calcium-Channel Blockers (page 46) ⃠

Digoxin (page 90) ⃠
Felodipine (page 113) ⃠
Labetalol (page 151) ⃠
Metoprolol (page 176) ✓ ⃠
Nadolol (page 185) ✓
Nifedipine (page 189) ⃠
Propranolol (page 224) ⃠
Sotalol (page 242) ⃠
Verapamil (page 280) ⃠

PRICKLY ASH

At the time of writing, there were no well-known drug interactions with prickly ash.

PSYLLIUM

Certain medicines interact with psyllium:
Lithium (page 157) ⓘ
Mesalamine (page 168) ✓
Orlistat (page 202) ✓

PUMPKIN

At the time of writing, there were no well-known drug interactions with pumpkin.

PYGEUM

At the time of writing, there were no well-known drug interactions with pygeum.

RED CLOVER

Certain medicines interact with red clover:
Estrogens (Combined) (page 109) ⃠
Heparin (page 135) ⃠
Ticlopidine (page 262) ⃠
Warfarin (page 281) ⃠

RED RASPBERRY

Certain medicines interact with red raspberry:
Atropine (page 30) ⃠
Cardec DM (page 50) ⃠
Codeine (page 75) ⃠
Ephedrine and Pseudoephedrine (page 104) ⃠
Lomotil/Lonox (page 158) ⃠
Theophylline/Aminophylline (page 256) ⃠

Red Raspberry

RED YEAST RICE

Certain medicines interact with red yeast rice:
> **Gemfibrozil** (page 127) ⊘
> **Lovastatin** (page 163) ⊘
> **Pravastatin** (page 220) ⊘

REISHI

Certain medicines interact with reishi:
> **Heparin** (page 135) ⊘
> **Warfarin** (page 281) ⊘

RHODIOLA

At the time of writing, there were no well-known drug interactions with Rhodiola.

ROOIBOS

At the time of writing, there were no well-known drug interactions with Rooibos.

ROSEMARY

At the time of writing, there were no well-known drug interactions with rosemary.

SAGE

At the time of writing, there were no well-known drug interactions with sage.

SANDALWOOD

At the time of writing, there were no well-known drug interactions with sandalwood.

SARSAPARILLA

Certain medicines interact with sarsaparilla:
> **Bismuth Subsalicylate** (page 40) ⊘
> **Digoxin** (page 90) ⊘

SASSAFRAS

At the time of writing, there were no well-known drug interactions with sassafras.

SAW PALMETTO

At the time of writing, there were no well-known drug interactions with saw palmetto.

SCHISANDRA

Certain medicines interact with schisandra:
> **Acetaminophen** (page 3) ⓘ

SENNA

Certain medicines interact with senna:
> **Digoxin** (page 90) ⊘

SHIITAKE

Certain medicines interact with shiitake:
> **Didanosine** (page 90) ✓

SLIPPERY ELM

At the time of writing, there were no well-known drug interactions with slippery elm.

ST. JOHN'S WORT

Certain medicines interact with St. John's wort:
> **Atazanavir** (page 28) ⊘
> **Benzodiazepines** (page 36) ⊘
> **Chemotherapy** (page 54) ⊘
> **Cyclosporine** (page 83) ⊘
> **Digoxin** (page 90) ⊘
> **Fexofenadine** (page 115) ⓘ
> **Fluoxetine** (page 120) ⊘
> **Fluvoxamine** (page 122) ⊘
> **Fosamprenavir** (page 125) ⊘
> **Indinavir** (page 141) ⊘
> **Nefazodone** (page 187) ⊘
> **Oral Contraceptives** (page 198) ⊘
> **Paroxetine** (page 208) ⊘
> **Phenelzine** (page 214) ⊘
> **Sertraline** (page 237) ⊘
> **Theophylline/Aminophylline** (page 256) ⊘
> **Trazodone** (page 267) ⊘
> **Tricyclic Antidepressants** (page 270) ⊘
> **Venlafaxine** (page 279) ⊘
> **Warfarin** (page 281) ⊘

STEVIA

At the time of writing, there were no well-known drug interactions with stevia.

SUMA

At the time of writing, there were no well-known drug interactions with suma.

SUNDEW

At the time of writing, there were no well-known drug interactions with sundew.

SWEET ANNIE

At the time of writing, there were no well-known drug interactions with sweet Annie.

TEA TREE

At the time of writing, there were no well-known drug interactions with tea tree.

THYME

At the time of writing, there were no well-known drug interactions with thyme.

TURMERIC

At the time of writing, there were no well-known drug interactions with turmeric.

TYLOPHORA

At the time of writing, there were no well-known drug interactions with tylophora.

USNEA

At the time of writing, there were no well-known drug interactions with usnea.

UVA URSI

Certain medicines interact with uva ursi:
- **Atropine** (page 30) ⊘
- **Cardec DM** (page 50) ⊘
- **Codeine** (page 75) ⊘
- **Ephedrine and Pseudoephedrine** (page 104) ⊘
- **Lomotil/Lonox** (page 158) ⊘
- **Loop Diuretics** (page 159) ⊘
- **Spironolactone** (page 243) ⊘
- **Theophylline/Aminophylline** (page 256) ⊘
- **Thiazide Diuretics** (page 258) ⊘
- **Triamterene** (page 268) ⊘

VALERIAN

At the time of writing, there were no well-known drug interactions with valerian.

VERVAIN

At the time of writing, there were no well-known drug interactions with vervain.

VITEX

At the time of writing, there were no well-known drug interactions with vitex.

WILD CHERRY

At the time of writing, there were no well-known drug interactions with wild cherry.

WILD INDIGO

At the time of writing, there were no well-known drug interactions with wild indigo.

WILD YAM

At the time of writing, there were no well-known drug interactions with wild yam.

WILLOW

Certain medicines interact with willow:
- **Bismuth Subsalicylate** (page 40) ⊘
- **Celecoxib** (page 51) ⊘
- **Diclofenac** (page 87) ⊘
- **Etodolac** (page 111) ⊘
- **Flurbiprofen** (page 121) ⊘
- **Ibuprofen** (page 139) ⊘
- **Indomethacin** (page 141) ⊘
- **Ketoprofen** (page 150) ⊘
- **Ketorolac** (page 150) ⊘
- **Live Influenza Virus** (page 158) ⊘
- **Metoclopramide** (page 175) ✓
- **Nabumetone** (page 184) ⊘
- **Nadolol** (page 185) ⊘
- **Naproxen/Naproxen Sodium** (page 186) ⊘
- **Nonsteroidal Anti-Inflammatory Drugs** (page 193) ⊘
- **Oxaprozin** (page 203) ⊘
- **Piroxicam** (page 219) ⓘ
- **Repaglinide** (page 231) ⊘
- **Salsalate** (page 235) ⊘
- **Sulindac** (page 249) ⊘
- **Ticlopidine** (page 262) ⊘
- **Zafirlukast** (page 284) ⊘

Willow

WITCH HAZEL

Certain medicines interact with witch hazel:
Atropine (page 30) ⊘
Cardec DM (page 50) ⊘
Codeine (page 75) ⊘
Ephedrine and Pseudoephedrine (page 104) ⊘
Lomotil/Lonox (page 158) ⊘
Theophylline/Aminophylline (page 256) ⊘

WOOD BETONY

At the time of writing, there were no well-known drug interactions with wood betony.

WORMWOOD

At the time of writing, there were no well-known drug interactions with wormwood.

YARROW

At the time of writing, there were no well-known drug interactions with yarrow.

YELLOW DOCK

At the time of writing, there were no well-known drug interactions with Yellow Dock.

YOHIMBE

Certain medicines interact with yohimbe:
Brimonidine (page 42) ⊘
Bupropion (page 43) ✓
Fluvoxamine (page 122) ✓

YUCCA

At the time of writing, there were no well-known drug interactions with yucca.

Witch Hazel

Vitamins

Some interactions may increase the need for the herb (✓), other interactions may be negative (⊘) and indicate the herb should not be taken without first speaking with your physician or pharmacist. Others may require further explanation (ⓘ). Refer to the individual drug entry for specific details about an interaction. The following list only includes the generic or class name of a medicine—to find a specific brand name, use the index.

5-HYDROXYTRYPTOPHAN

Certain medicines interact with 5-hydroxytryptophan:
Carbidopa (page 48) ⓘ
Carbidopa/Levodopa (page 49) ⓘ
Fluoxetine (page 120) ⊘
Fluvoxamine (page 122) ⊘
Paroxetine (page 208) ⊘
Selegiline (page 236) ✓
Sertraline (page 237) ⊘
Sibutramine (page 238) ⊘
Sumatriptan (page 250) ⊘
Tramadol (page 266) ⊘
Venlafaxine (page 279) ⊘
Zolmitriptan (page 285) ⊘
Zolpidem (page 285) ⊘

7-KETO

At the time of writing, there were no well-known drug interactions with 7-KETO.

ACETYL-L-CARNITINE

Certain medicines interact with acetyl-L-carnitine:
Didanosine (page 90) ✓

ADENOSINE MONOPHOSPHATE

At the time of writing, there were no well-known drug interactions with adenosine monophosphate.

ADRENAL EXTRACT

At the time of writing, there were no well-known drug interactions with adrenal extract.

ALANINE

At the time of writing, there were no well-known drug interactions with alanine.

ALPHA LIPOIC ACID

At the time of writing, there were no well-known drug interactions with alpha lipoic acid.

AMYLASE INHIBITORS

At the time of writing, there were no well-known drug interactions with amylase inhibitors.

ARGININE

At the time of writing, there were no well-known drug interactions with arginine.

BETA-CAROTENE

Certain medicines interact with beta-carotene:
Bile Acid Sequestrants (page 39) ✓
Chemotherapy (page 54) ✓
Cisplatin (page 64) ✓

Colchicine (page 76) ✓
Colestipol (page 76) ✓
Cyclophosphamide (page 79) ✓
Docetaxel (page 95) ✓
Fluorouracil (page 116) ✓
Lansoprazole (page 153) ✓
Methotrexate (page 169) ✓
Methyltestosterone (page 175) ✓
Mineral Oil (page 178) ✓
Neomycin (page 187) ✓
Orlistat (page 202) ✓
Paclitaxel (page 205) ✓
Quinidine (page 227) ✓

BETA-GLUCAN

At the time of writing, there were no well-known drug interactions with beta-glucan.

BETA-SITOSTEROL

At the time of writing, there were no well-known drug interactions with beta-sitosterol.

BETAINE (TRIMETHYLGLYCINE)

At the time of writing, there were no well-known drug interactions with betaine.

BETAINE HYDROCHLORIDE

At the time of writing, there were no well-known drug interactions with betaine hydrochloride.

BIOTIN

Certain medicines interact with biotin:
Anticonvulsants (page 21) ✓
Gabapentin (page 125) ✓
Glyburide (page 132) ⓘ
Insulin (page 144) ✓
Phenobarbital (page 215) ✓
Topical Corticosteroids (page 265) ✓
Valproic Acid (page 275) ✓

BLUE-GREEN ALGAE

At the time of writing, there were no well-known drug interactions with blue-green algae.

BORAGE OIL

At the time of writing, there were no well-known drug interactions with borage oil.

BORIC ACID

At the time of writing, there were no well-known drug interactions with boric acid.

BORON

At the time of writing, there were no well-known drug interactions with boron.

BOVINE COLOSTRUM

At the time of writing, there were no well-known drug interactions with bovine colostrum.

BRANCHED-CHAIN AMINO ACIDS

At the time of writing, there were no well-known drug interactions with branched-chain amino acids.

BREWER'S YEAST

Certain medicines interact with brewer's yeast:
Aminoglycoside Antibiotics (page 11) ✓
Amoxicillin (page 13) ✓
Ampicillin (page 15) ✓
Antibiotics (page 19) ✓
Azithromycin (page 31) ✓
Cephalosporins (page 52) ✓
Chlorhexidine (page 58) ✓
Ciprofloxacin (page 62) ✓
Clarithromycin (page 68) ✓
Clindamycin Oral (page 70) ✓
Clindamycin Topical (page 71) ✓
Dapsone (page 85) ✓
Dicloxacillin (page 88) ✓
Doxycycline (page 101) ✓
Erythromycin (page 106) ✓
Gentamicin (page 129) ✓
Levofloxacin (page 155) ✓
Loracarbef (page 161) ✓
Macrolides (page 164) ✓
Minocycline (page 179) ✓
Neomycin (page 187) ✓
Nitrofurantoin (page 190) ✓

Ofloxacin (page 195) ✓
Penicillin V (page 210) ✓
Penicillins (page 211) ✓
Quinolones (page 228) ✓
Sulfamethoxazole (page 245) ✓
Sulfasalazine (page 246) ✓
Sulfonamides (page 248) ✓
Tetracycline (page 253) ✓
Tetracyclines (page 255) ✓
Tobramycin (page 264) ✓
Trimethoprim (page 271) ✓
Trimethoprim/Sulfamethoxazole (page 273) ✓

BROMELAIN

Certain medicines interact with bromelain:
Amoxicillin (page 13) ✓
Erythromycin (page 106) ✓
Penicillamine (page 209) ✓
Penicillin V (page 210) ✓
Warfarin (page 281) ⓘ

CALCIUM

Certain medicines interact with calcium:
Albuterol (page 6) ✓
Alendronate (page 7) ⓘ
Aluminum Hydroxide (page 10) ✓
Anticonvulsants (page 21) ✓
Bile Acid Sequestrants (page 39) ✓
Caffeine (page 44) ✓
Calcitonin (page 45) ✓
Calcium Acetate (page 45) ⊘
Ciprofloxacin (page 62) ⊘
Cisplatin (page 64) ✓
Colestipol (page 76) ✓
Cycloserine (page 82) ✓
Diclofenac (page 87) ✓
Doxycycline (page 101) ⊘
Erythromycin (page 106) ⓘ
Estrogens (Combined) (page 109) ✓
Felodipine (page 113) ✓
Flurbiprofen (page 121) ✓
Gabapentin (page 125) ✓
Gemifloxacin (page 128) ⊘
Gentamicin (page 129) ✓
Hydroxychloroquine (page 137) ✓
Indapamide (page 140) ✓
Indomethacin (page 141) ✓
Inhaled Corticosteroids (page 143) ✓

Isoniazid (page 146) ✓
Lactase (page 152) ⓘ
Metformin (page 168) ✓
Mineral Oil (page 178) ✓
Minocycline (page 179) ✓ ⊘
Nadolol (page 185) ⊘
Neomycin (page 187) ✓
Ofloxacin (page 195) ⊘
Oral Contraceptives (page 198) ⓘ
Oral Corticosteroids (page 200) ✓
Phenobarbital (page 215) ✓
Quinolones (page 228) ⊘
Risedronate (page 232) ✓ ⊘
Sodium Fluoride (page 241) ⓘ
Sotalol (page 242) ⊘
Sucralfate (page 244) ✓
Sulfamethoxazole (page 245) ✓
Tetracycline (page 253) ⊘
Tetracyclines (page 255) ⊘
Thiazide Diuretics (page 258) ⓘ
Thyroid Hormones (page 261) ✓ ⊘
Tobramycin (page 264) ✓
Triamterene (page 268) ✓
Trimethoprim (page 271) ✓
Valproic Acid (page 275) ✓
Verapamil (page 280) ✓ ⊘

CALCIUM D-GLUCARATE

At the time of writing, there were no well-known drug interactions with calcium D-glucarate.

CARNOSINE

At the time of writing, there were no well-known drug interactions with carnosine.

CAROTENOIDS

Certain medicines interact with carotenoids:
Bile Acid Sequestrants (page 39) ✓
Colestipol (page 76) ✓

CARTILAGE AND COLLAGEN

At the time of writing, there were no well-known drug interactions with cartilage.

Cartilage and Collagen

CETYL MYRISTOLEATE

At the time of writing, there were no well-known drug interactions with cetyl myristoleate.

CHITOSAN

At the time of writing, there were no well-known drug interactions with chitosan.

CHLOROPHYLL

At the time of writing, there were no well-known drug interactions with chlorophyll.

CHONDROITIN SULFATE

At the time of writing, there were no well-known drug interactions with chondroitin sulfate.

CHROMIUM

Certain medicines interact with chromium:
Glyburide (page 132) ⊘
Insulin (page 144) ✓ ⊘
Oral Corticosteroids (page 200) ✓
Sertraline (page 237) ✓

COCONUT OIL

At the time of writing, there were no well-known drug interactions with coconut oil.

COENZYME Q₁₀

Certain medicines interact with coenzyme Q_{10}:
Atorvastatin (page 29) ✓
Doxorubicin (page 100) ✓
Fluvastatin (page 122) ✓
Gemfibrozil (page 127) ✓
Lovastatin (page 163) ✓
Perphenazine (page 213) ✓
Pravastatin (page 220) ✓
Propranolol (page 224) ✓
Simvastatin (page 239) ✓
Thioridazine (page 260) ✓
Timolol (page 263) ✓
Tricyclic Antidepressants (page 270) ✓
Warfarin (page 281) ⊘

COLLOIDAL SILVER

At the time of writing, there were no well-known drug interactions with colloidal silver.

CONJUGATED LINOLEIC ACID

At the time of writing, there were no well-known drug interactions with conjugated linoleic acid.

COPPER

Certain medicines interact with copper:
AZT (page 33) ✓
Ciprofloxacin (page 62) ⊘
Etodolac (page 111) ✓
Famotidine (page 112) ⓘ
Ibuprofen (page 139) ✓
Nabumetone (page 184) ✓
Naproxen/Naproxen Sodium (page 186) ✓
Nizatidine (page 192) ⓘ
Oral Contraceptives (page 198) ⓘ
Oxaprozin (page 203) ✓
Penicillamine (page 209) ⓘ
Valproic Acid (page 275) ✓

CREATINE MONOHYDRATE

At the time of writing, there were no well-known drug interactions with creatine monohydrate.

CYSTEINE

At the time of writing, there were no well-known drug interactions with cysteine.

D-MANNOSE

At the time of writing, there were no well-known drug interactions with D-mannose.

DEHYDROEPIANDROSTERONE (DHEA)

Certain medicines interact with dehydroepiandrosterone:
Amlodipine (page 13) ⓘ
Clonidine (page 72) ✓
Diltiazem (page 92) ⊘
Fluoxetine (page 120) ✓

Inhaled Corticosteroids (page 143) ✓
Insulin (page 144) ✓
Metformin (page 168) ⓘ
Methyltestosterone (page 175) ⓘ

DMAE

At the time of writing, there were no well-known drug interactions with DMAE.

DMSO

At the time of writing, there were no well-known drug interactions with DMSO.

DIGESTIVE ENZYMES

Certain medicines interact with digestive enzymes:
Warfarin (page 281) ⊘

DOCOSAHEXAENOIC ACID

At the time of writing, there were no well-known drug interactions with docosahexaenoic acid.

EVENING PRIMROSE OIL

Certain medicines interact with evening primrose oil:
Tamoxifen (page 251) ✓

FIBER

Certain medicines interact with fiber:
Lovastatin (page 163) ⊘
Propoxyphene (page 224) ⓘ
Verapamil (page 280) ✓

FISH OIL AND COD LIVER OIL (EPA AND DHA)

Certain medicines interact with fish oil and cod liver oil:
Cyclosporine (page 83) ✓
Pravastatin (page 220) ✓
Simvastatin (page 239) ✓

FLAVONOIDS

Certain medicines interact with flavonoids:
Acyclovir Oral (page 5) ✓

FLAXSEED AND FLAXSEED OIL

At the time of writing, there were no well-known drug interactions with flaxseed oil.

FLUORIDE

At the time of writing, there were no well-known drug interactions with fluoride.

FOLIC ACID

Certain medicines interact with folic acid:
Aluminum Hydroxide (page 10) ✓
Anticonvulsants (page 21) ✓ ⊘
Aspirin (page 26) ✓
Azathioprine (page 31) ✓
Bile Acid Sequestrants (page 39) ✓
Chemotherapy (page 54) ⊘
Colestipol (page 76) ✓
Cycloserine (page 82) ✓
Diuretics (page 94) ✓
Erythromycin (page 106) ⓘ
Famotidine (page 112) ⓘ
Fenofibrate (page 114) ✓
Fluoxetine (page 120) ✓
Gabapentin (page 125) ✓ ⊘
Indomethacin (page 141) ✓
Isoniazid (page 146) ✓
Lansoprazole (page 153) ✓
Lithium (page 157) ✓
Loop Diuretics (page 159) ✓
Magnesium Hydroxide (page 166) ✓
Medroxyprogesterone (page 167) ⓘ
Metformin (page 168) ✓
Methotrexate (page 169) ✓ ⊘
Neomycin (page 187) ✓
Nitrous Oxide (page 191) ✓
Nizatidine (page 192) ✓ ⓘ
Omeprazole (page 197) ✓
Oral Contraceptives (page 198) ✓
Phenobarbital (page 215) ✓ ⊘
Piroxicam (page 219) ⓘ
Ranitidine (page 230) ✓
Salsalate (page 235) ✓
Sodium Bicarbonate (page 240) ✓
Sulfamethoxazole (page 245) ✓
Sulfasalazine (page 246) ✓
Sulindac (page 249) ⓘ
Tetracycline (page 253) ✓

Thiazide Diuretics (page 258) ✓
Triamterene (page 268) ✓
Trimethoprim (page 271) ✓
Trimethoprim/Sulfamethoxazole (page 273) ✓
Valproic Acid (page 275) ✓ ⊘

FRUCTO-OLIGOSACCHARIDES (FOS) AND OTHER OLIGOSACCHARIDES

At the time of writing, there were no well-known drug interactions with fructo-oligosaccharides (FOS) and other oligosaccharides.

FUMARIC ACID

At the time of writing, there were no well-known drug interactions with fumaric acid.

GABA (GAMMA-AMINO BUTYRIC ACID)

At the time of writing, there were no well-known drug interactions with GABA.

GAMMA ORYZANOL

At the time of writing, there were no well-known drug interactions with gamma oryzanol.

GLUCOMANNAN

At the time of writing, there were no well-known drug interactions with glucomannan.

GLUCOSAMINE

At the time of writing, there were no well-known drug interactions with glucosamine.

GLUTAMIC ACID

At the time of writing, there were no well-known drug interactions with glutamic acid.

GLUTAMINE

Certain medicines interact with glutamine:
Chemotherapy (page 54) ✓
Cisplatin (page 64) ✓
Cyclophosphamide (page 79) ✓
Docetaxel (page 95) ✓

Fluorouracil (page 116) ✓
Methotrexate (page 169) ✓
Paclitaxel (page 205) ✓

GLUTATHIONE

Certain medicines interact with glutathione:
Cisplatin (page 64) ✓ ⓘ
Cyclophosphamide (page 79) ✓

GLYCINE

Certain medicines interact with glycine:
Clozapine (page 74) ⊘
Haloperidol (page 134) ✓
Olanzapine (page 196) ✓
Risperidone (page 232) ✓

GRAPEFRUIT SEED EXTRACT

At the time of writing, there were no well-known drug interactions with grapefruit seed extract.

GREEN-LIPPED MUSSEL

At the time of writing, there were no well-known drug interactions with green-lipped mussel.

HISTIDINE

At the time of writing, there were no well-known drug interactions with histidine.

HMB

At the time of writing, there were no well-known drug interactions with HMB.

HYDROXYCITRIC ACID

At the time of writing, there were no well-known drug interactions with hydroxycitric acid.

INDOLE-3-CARBINOL

At the time of writing, there were no well-known drug interactions with indole-3-carbinol.

INOSINE

At the time of writing, there were no well-known drug interactions with inosine.

INOSITOL

Certain medicines interact with inositol:
Lithium (page 157) ✓

IODINE

At the time of writing, there were no well-known drug interactions with iodine.

IP-6

At the time of writing, there were no well-known drug interactions with IP-6.

IPRIFLAVONE

Certain medicines interact with ipriflavone:
Estrogens (Combined) (page 109) ✓

IRON

Certain medicines interact with iron:
Angiotensin-Converting Enzyme (ACE) Inhibitors (page 17) ✓
Aspirin (page 26) ✓
Benazepril (page 34) ✓
Captopril (page 47) ✓
Carbidopa (page 48) ⊘
Carbidopa/Levodopa (page 49) ⊘
Chlorhexidine (page 58) ⊘
Cimetidine (page 61) ✓
Ciprofloxacin (page 62) ⊘
Deferoxamine (page 86) ⊘
Dipyridamole (page 94) ✓
Doxycycline (page 101) ⊘
Enalapril (page 103) ✓
Etodolac (page 111) ✓
Famotidine (page 112) ✓
Gemifloxacin (page 128) ⊘
Haloperidol (page 134) ✓
Hyoscyamine (page 138) ✓
Ibuprofen (page 139) ✓
Indomethacin (page 141) ⓘ
Levofloxacin (page 155) ⊘

Magnesium Hydroxide (page 166) ✓
Methyldopa (page 174) ⊘
Minocycline (page 179) ✓ ⊘
Moexipril (page 182) ✓
Nabumetone (page 184) ✓
Naproxen/Naproxen Sodium (page 186) ✓
Neomycin (page 187) ✓
Nizatidine (page 192) ✓
Ofloxacin (page 195) ⊘
Oral Contraceptives (page 198) ⓘ
Oxaprozin (page 203) ✓
Penicillamine (page 209) ⊘
Quinapril (page 226) ✓
Ramipril (page 229) ✓
Ranitidine (page 230) ✓
Risedronate (page 232) ⊘
Sodium Bicarbonate (page 240) ✓
Stanozolol (page 244) ✓
Sulfasalazine (page 246) ⊘
Tetracycline (page 253) ⊘
Tetracyclines (page 255) ⊘
Thyroid Hormones (page 261) ⓘ
Warfarin (page 281) ⊘

KELP

At the time of writing, there were no well-known drug interactions with kelp.

L-CARNITINE

Certain medicines interact with L-carnitine:
Allopurinol (page 8) ⓘ
Anticonvulsants (page 21) ✓
AZT (page 33) ✓
Chemotherapy (page 54) ✓
Doxorubicin (page 100) ✓
Gabapentin (page 125) ✓
Phenobarbital (page 215) ✓
Valproic Acid (page 275) ✓

L-TYROSINE

Certain medicines interact with L-tyrosine:
Mixed Amphetamines (page 181) ✓

LACTASE

At the time of writing, there were no well-known drug interactions with lactase.

Lactase

LECITHIN/PHOSPHATIDYL CHOLINE

At the time of writing, there were no well-known drug interactions with lecithin/phosphatidylcholine/choline.

LIPASE

At the time of writing, there were no well-known drug interactions with lipase.

LIVER EXTRACTS

At the time of writing, there were no well-known drug interactions with liver extracts.

LUTEIN

At the time of writing, there were no well-known drug interactions with lutein.

LYCOPENE

At the time of writing, there were no well-known drug interactions with lycopene.

LYSINE

At the time of writing, there were no well-known drug interactions with lysine.

MAGNESIUM

Certain medicines interact with magnesium:

Albuterol (page 6) ✓
Alendronate (page 7) ⓘ
Amiloride (page 11) ⊘
Amphotericin B (page 15) ✓
Azithromycin (page 31) ⓘ
Cimetidine (page 61) ⊘
Ciprofloxacin (page 62) ⊘
Cisplatin (page 64) ✓
Cycloserine (page 82) ✓
Cyclosporine (page 83) ✓
Digoxin (page 90) ✓
Docusate (page 99) ✓
Doxycycline (page 101) ⊘
Epinephrine (page 105) ⓘ
Erythromycin (page 106) ✓
Estrogens (Combined) (page 109) ⓘ
Famotidine (page 112) ⓘ

Felodipine (page 113) ✓
Fentanyl (page 115) ✓
Gemifloxacin (page 128) ⊘
Gentamicin (page 129) ✓
Glimepiride (page 131) ✓
Glipizide (page 131) ⓘ
Hydroxychloroquine (page 137) ⊘
Isoniazid (page 146) ✓
Levofloxacin (page 155) ⊘
Loop Diuretics (page 159) ✓
Medroxyprogesterone (page 167) ⓘ
Metformin (page 168) ⓘ
Minocycline (page 179) ✓ ⊘
Misoprostol (page 180) ⊘
Mixed Amphetamines (page 181) ✓ ⊘
Neomycin (page 187) ✓
Nitrofurantoin (page 190) ⊘
Nizatidine (page 192) ⓘ
Ofloxacin (page 195) ⊘
Oral Contraceptives (page 198) ✓
Oral Corticosteroids (page 200) ✓ ⊘
Quinidine (page 227) ✓
Quinolones (page 228) ⊘
Risedronate (page 232) ⊘
Sotalol (page 242) ✓
Spironolactone (page 243) ⊘
Sulfamethoxazole (page 245) ✓
Tetracycline (page 253) ⊘
Tetracyclines (page 255) ⊘
Theophylline/Aminophylline (page 256) ✓
Thiazide Diuretics (page 258) ✓
Tobramycin (page 264) ✓
Triamterene (page 268) ⊘
Trimethoprim (page 271) ✓
Warfarin (page 281) ⊘

MALIC ACID

At the time of writing, there were no well-known drug interactions with malic acid.

MANGANESE

Certain medicines interact with manganese:

Ciprofloxacin (page 62) ⊘
Oral Contraceptives (page 198) ⓘ

MEDIUM CHAIN TRIGLYCERIDES

At the time of writing, there were no well-known drug interactions with medium chain triglycerides.

MELATONIN

Certain medicines interact with melatonin:

Chemotherapy (page 54) ✓
Cisplatin (page 64) ✓
Cyclophosphamide (page 79) ✓
Docetaxel (page 95) ✓
Doxorubicin (page 100) ✓
Fluorouracil (page 116) ✓
Fluoxetine (page 120) ✓ ⓘ
Fluvoxamine (page 122) ⓘ
Methotrexate (page 169) ✓
Mirtazapine (page 180) ⓘ
Oral Corticosteroids (page 200) ✓
Paclitaxel (page 205) ✓
Tamoxifen (page 251) ✓
Triazolam (page 269) ✓

METHIONINE

At the time of writing, there were no well-known drug interactions with methionine.

METHOXYISOFLAVONE

At the time of writing, there were no well-known drug interactions with methoxyisoflavone.

METHYLSULFONYLMETHANE

At the time of writing, there were no well-known drug interactions with methylsulfonylmethane.

MOLYBDENUM

At the time of writing, there were no well-known drug interactions with molybdenum.

N-ACETYL CYSTEINE

Certain medicines interact with N-Acetyl Cysteine:

Acetaminophen (page 3) ✓
AZT (page 33) ⓘ
Chemotherapy (page 54) ✓
Cisplatin (page 64) ✓

Clozapine (page 74) ✓
Cyclophosphamide (page 79) ✓
Docetaxel (page 95) ✓
Doxorubicin (page 100) ⓘ
Fluorouracil (page 116) ✓
Flurbiprofen (page 121) ✓
Gentamicin (page 129) ✓
Interferon (page 144) ✓
Isosorbide Dinitrate (page 148) ✓
Isosorbide Mononitrate (page 148) ✓
Metoclopramide (page 175) ⊘
Nitroglycerin (page 191) ✓ ⊘
Oral Corticosteroids (page 200) ✓
Paclitaxel (page 205) ✓

N-ACETYL-GLUCOSAMINE

At the time of writing, there were no well-known drug interactions with N-acetyl-glucosamine.

NADH

At the time of writing, there were no well-known drug interactions with NADH.

OCTACOSANOL

At the time of writing, there were no well-known drug interactions with octacosanol.

ORNITHINE

At the time of writing, there were no well-known drug interactions with ornithine.

ORNITHINE ALPHA-KETOGLUTARATE

At the time of writing, there were no well-known drug interactions with ornithine alpha-ketoglutarate.

PABA

Certain medicines interact with PABA:

Dapsone (page 85) ✓
Methotrexate (page 169) ⊘
Sulfamethoxazole (page 245) ⊘
Sulfasalazine (page 246) ⊘
Trimethoprim/Sulfamethoxazole (page 273) ⊘

PABA

PANTOTHENIC ACID

Certain medicines interact with pantothenic acid:
  Tricyclic Antidepressants (page 270) ✓

PHENYLALANINE

At the time of writing, there were no well-known drug interactions with phenylalanine.

PHOSPHATIDYLSERINE

At the time of writing, there were no well-known drug interactions with phosphatidylserine.

PHOSPHORUS

Certain medicines interact with phosphorus:
  Albuterol (page 6) ✓
  Aluminum Hydroxide (page 10) ✓
  Cisplatin (page 64) ✓
  Mineral Oil (page 178) ✓
  Sucralfate (page 244) ✓

POLICOSANOL

At the time of writing, there were no well-known drug interactions with policosanol.

POLLEN

At the time of writing, there were no well-known drug interactions with pollen.

POTASSIUM

Certain medicines interact with potassium:
  Acebutolol (page 3) ⊘
  Albuterol (page 6) ✓
  Amiloride (page 11) ⊘
  Angiotensin-Converting Enzyme (ACE) Inhibitors (page 17) ⊘
  Atenolol (page 28) ⊘
  Benazepril (page 34) ⊘
  Beta-Adrenergic Blockers (page 37) ⊘
  Betaxolol (page 38) ⊘
  Bisacodyl (page 39) ✓
  Bisoprolol (page 41) ⊘
  Captopril (page 47) ⊘
  Celecoxib (page 51) ✓

Cisplatin (page 64) ✓
Colchicine (page 76) ✓
Digoxin (page 90) ✓ ⓘ
Docusate (page 99) ✓
Enalapril (page 103) ⊘
Epinephrine (page 104) ⓘ
Etodolac (page 111) ⓘ
Felodipine (page 113) ✓
Gentamicin (page 129) ✓
Haloperidol (page 134) ⓘ
Heparin (page 135) ⓘ
Ibuprofen (page 139) ⓘ
Indapamide (page 140) ✓
Indomethacin (page 141) ⊘
Ipecac (page 145) ✓
Ketorolac (page 150) ⊘
Labetalol (page 151) ⊘
Lisinopril (page 156) ⊘
Loop Diuretics (page 159) ✓
Losartan (page 162) ⓘ
Magnesium Hydroxide (page 166) ⓘ
Metoprolol (page 176) ✓ ⊘
Mineral Oil (page 178) ✓
Moexipril (page 182) ✓ ⊘
Nabumetone (page 184) ⓘ
Nadolol (page 185) ⊘
Naproxen/Naproxen Sodium (page 186) ⓘ
Neomycin (page 187) ✓
Oral Corticosteroids (page 200) ✓
Oxaprozin (page 203) ⓘ
Piroxicam (page 219) ⊘
Propranolol (page 224) ⊘
Quinapril (page 226) ⊘
Quinidine (page 227) ✓
Ramipril (page 229) ⊘
Salsalate (page 235) ✓
Senna (page 236) ⓘ
Sotalol (page 242) ⊘
Spironolactone (page 243) ⊘
Sulfamethoxazole (page 245) ⊘
Sulindac (page 249) ✓
Tetracycline (page 253) ✓
Theophylline/Aminophylline (page 256) ✓
Thiazide Diuretics (page 258) ✓
Thioridazine (page 260) ✓
Tobramycin (page 264) ✓
Triamterene (page 268) ⊘
Trimethoprim (page 271) ⊘
Trimethoprim/Sulfamethoxazole (page 273) ⊘

PREGNENOLONE

At the time of writing, there were no well-known drug interactions with pregnenolone.

PROANTHOCYANIDINS

At the time of writing, there were no well-known drug interactions with proanthocyanidins.

PROBIOTICS

Certain medicines interact with probiotics:
- **Aminoglycoside Antibiotics** (page 11) ✓
- **Amoxicillin** (page 13) ✓
- **Ampicillin** (page 15) ✓
- **Antibiotics** (page 19) ✓
- **Azithromycin** (page 31) ✓
- **Cephalosporins** (page 52) ✓
- **Chlorhexidine** (page 58) ✓
- **Ciprofloxacin** (page 62) ✓
- **Clarithromycin** (page 68) ✓
- **Clindamycin Oral** (page 70) ✓
- **Clindamycin Topical** (page 71) ✓
- **Dapsone** (page 85) ✓
- **Dicloxacillin** (page 88) ✓
- **Doxycycline** (page 101) ✓
- **Erythromycin** (page 106) ✓
- **Gentamicin** (page 129) ✓
- **Levofloxacin** (page 155) ✓
- **Loracarbef** (page 161) ✓
- **Macrolides** (page 164) ✓
- **Metronidazole** (page 177) ✓
- **Minocycline** (page 179) ✓
- **Neomycin** (page 187) ✓
- **Nitrofurantoin** (page 190) ✓
- **Ofloxacin** (page 195) ✓
- **Penicillin V** (page 210) ✓
- **Penicillins** (page 211) ✓
- **Quinolones** (page 228) ✓
- **Sulfamethoxazole** (page 245) ✓
- **Sulfasalazine** (page 246) ✓
- **Sulfonamides** (page 248) ✓
- **Tetracycline** (page 253) ✓
- **Tetracyclines** (page 255) ✓
- **Tobramycin** (page 264) ✓
- **Trimethoprim** (page 271) ✓
- **Trimethoprim/Sulfamethoxazole** (page 273) ✓

PROGESTERONE

At the time of writing, there were no well-known drug interactions with progesterone.

PROPOLIS

At the time of writing, there were no well-known drug interactions with propolis.

PYRUVATE

At the time of writing, there were no well-known drug interactions with pyruvate.

QUERCETIN

Certain medicines interact with quercetin:
- **Cyclosporine** (page 83) ⊘
- **Estradiol** (page 108) ⊘
- **Felodipine** (page 113) ⊘

RESVERATROL

At the time of writing, there were no well-known drug interactions with resveratrol.

RIBOSE

At the time of writing, there were no well-known drug interactions with ribose.

ROYAL JELLY

At the time of writing, there were no well-known drug interactions with royal jelly.

SAMe

Certain medicines interact with SAMe:
- **Tricyclic Antidepressants** (page 270) ✓

SELENIUM

Certain medicines interact with selenium:
- **Cisplatin** (page 64) ✓
- **Clozapine** (page 74) ✓
- **Oral Corticosteroids** (page 200) ✓
- **Valproic Acid** (page 275) ⓘ

Selenium

SILICA HYDRIDE

At the time of writing, there were no well-known drug interactions with silica hydride.

SILICON

At the time of writing, there were no well-known drug interactions with silicon.

SOY

Certain medicines interact with soy:
- **Estrogens (Combined)** (page 109) ⊘
- **Ipratropium Bromide** (page 146) ⓘ
- **Thyroid Hormones** (page 261) ⊘
- **Warfarin** (page 281) ⓘ

SPLEEN EXTRACTS

Certain medicines interact with spleen extracts:
- **Chemotherapy** (page 54) ✓
- **Cisplatin** (page 64) ✓
- **Cyclophosphamide** (page 79) ✓
- **Docetaxel** (page 95) ✓
- **Fluorouracil** (page 116) ✓
- **Methotrexate** (page 169) ✓
- **Paclitaxel** (page 205) ✓

STRONTIUM

At the time of writing, there were no well-known drug interactions with strontium.

SULFORAPHANE

At the time of writing, there were no well-known drug interactions with sulforaphane.

SULFUR

At the time of writing, there were no well-known drug interactions with sulfur.

TAURINE

Certain medicines interact with taurine:
- **Chemotherapy** (page 54) ✓
- **Cisplatin** (page 64) ✓
- **Fluorouracil** (page 116) ✓
- **Paclitaxel** (page 205) ✓

THYMUS EXTRACTS

Certain medicines interact with thymus extracts:
- **Chemotherapy** (page 54) ✓
- **Cisplatin** (page 64) ✓
- **Cyclophosphamide** (page 79) ✓
- **Docetaxel** (page 95) ✓
- **Fluorouracil** (page 116) ✓
- **Interferon** (page 144) ✓ ⊘
- **Paclitaxel** (page 205) ✓

THYROID EXTRACTS

At the time of writing, there were no well-known drug interactions with thyroid extracts.

TOCOTRIENOLS

Certain medicines interact with tocotrienols:
- **Tamoxifen** (page 251) ✓

VANADIUM

At the time of writing, there were no well-known drug interactions with vanadium.

VINPOCETINE

Certain medicines interact with vinpocetine:
- **Benzodiazepines** (page 36) ✓

VITAMIN A

Certain medicines interact with vitamin A:
- **Anticonvulsants** (page 21) ✓
- **Atorvastatin** (page 29) ⊘
- **Bile Acid Sequestrants** (page 39) ✓
- **Chemotherapy** (page 54) ⓘ
- **Cisplatin** (page 64) ⓘ
- **Colestipol** (page 76) ✓
- **Cyclophosphamide** (page 79) ✓ ⓘ
- **Docetaxel** (page 95) ⓘ
- **Fluorouracil** (page 116) ⓘ
- **Fluvastatin** (page 122) ⊘
- **Gabapentin** (page 125) ✓
- **Isotretinoin** (page 149) ⊘
- **Lovastatin** (page 163) ⓘ
- **Medroxyprogesterone** (page 167) ⓘ
- **Methotrexate** (page 169) ⓘ
- **Methyltestosterone** (page 175) ✓

Mineral Oil (page 178) ✓
Minocycline (page 179) ⊘
Neomycin (page 187) ✓
Oral Contraceptives (page 198) ⓘ
Oral Corticosteroids (page 200) ✓ ⓘ
Orlistat (page 202) ✓
Paclitaxel (page 205)
Phenobarbital (page 215) ✓
Pravastatin (page 220) ⓘ
Simvastatin (page 239) ⊘
Thioridazine (page 260) ✓
Tretinoin (page 268) ⊘
Valproic Acid (page 275) ✓

VITAMIN B₁

Certain medicines interact with vitamin B₁:
Loop Diuretics (page 159) ✓
Oral Contraceptives (page 198) ✓
Stavudine (page 244) ✓
Tricyclic Antidepressants (page 270) ✓

VITAMIN B₂

Certain medicines interact with vitamin B₂:
AZT (page 33) ✓
Didanosine (page 90) ✓
Doxorubicin (page 100) ✓
Oral Contraceptives (page 198) ✓
Tetracycline (page 253) ✓
Tricyclic Antidepressants (page 270) ✓

VITAMIN B₃

Certain medicines interact with vitamin B₃:
Atorvastatin (page 29) ⓘ
Benztropine (page 37) ✓
Carbidopa (page 48) ✓
Carbidopa/Levodopa (page 49) ✓
Cerivastatin (page 53) ⓘ
Fluvastatin (page 122) ⓘ
Gemfibrozil (page 127) ✓
Glimepiride (page 131) ⊘
Isoniazid (page 146) ✓
Lovastatin (page 163) ⓘ
Minocycline (page 179) ✓
Oral Contraceptives (page 198) ✓
Pravastatin (page 220) ⓘ
Repaglinide (page 231) ⓘ
Rosuvastatin (page 234) ✓ ⊘

Simvastatin (page 239) ⓘ
Tetracycline (page 253) ✓
Thioridazine (page 260) ✓
Tricyclic Antidepressants (page 270) ✓

VITAMIN B₆

Certain medicines interact with vitamin B₆:
Anticonvulsants (page 21) ✓
Carbidopa (page 48) ⓘ
Carbidopa/Levodopa (page 49) ⓘ
Cycloserine (page 82) ✓
Docetaxel (page 95) ✓
Erythromycin (page 106) ✓
Estrogens (Combined) (page 109) ✓
Fenofibrate (page 114) ✓
Fluorouracil (page 116) ✓
Folic Acid (page 123) ✓ ⊘
Gabapentin (page 125) ✓
Gentamicin (page 129) ⓘ
Hydralazine (page 136) ✓
Hydroxychloroquine (page 137) ✓
Isoniazid (page 146) ⓘ
Levodopa (page 154) ✓
Mixed Amphetamines (page 181) ✓
Neomycin (page 187) ✓
Oral Contraceptives (page 198) ✓
Oral Corticosteroids (page 200) ✓
Penicillamine (page 209) ✓
Phenelzine (page 214) ✓
Phenobarbital (page 215) ✓ ⊘
Risperidone (page 232) ✓
Sulfamethoxazole (page 245) ✓
Tetracycline (page 253) ✓
Theophylline/Aminophylline (page 256) ✓
Tricyclic Antidepressants (page 270) ✓
Trimethoprim (page 271) ✓
Valproic Acid (page 275) ✓

VITAMIN B₁₂

Certain medicines interact with vitamin B₁₂:
Anticonvulsants (page 21) ✓
Aspirin (page 26) ✓
AZT (page 33) ✓
Cimetidine (page 61) ✓
Clofibrate (page 71) ✓
Colchicine (page 76) ✓
Cycloserine (page 82) ✓
Erythromycin (page 106) ✓

Vitamin B₁₂

Famotidine (page 112) ✓
Fenofibrate (page 114) ✓
Gabapentin (page 125) ✓
Gentamicin (page 129) ✓
Isoniazid (page 146) ✓
Lansoprazole (page 153) ✓
Metformin (page 168) ✓
Methyldopa (page 174) ✓
Neomycin (page 187) ✓
Nitrous Oxide (page 191) ✓
Nizatidine (page 192) ✓
Omeprazole (page 197) ✓
Oral Contraceptives (page 198) ✓
Phenobarbital (page 215) ✓
Ranitidine (page 230) ✓
Sulfamethoxazole (page 245) ✓
Tetracycline (page 253) ✓
Tricyclic Antidepressants (page 270) ✓
Trimethoprim (page 271) ✓
Valproic Acid (page 275) ✓

VITAMIN C

Certain medicines interact with vitamin C:
Acetaminophen (page 3) ✓
Ampicillin (page 15) ✓
Aspirin (page 26) ✓
Carbidopa (page 48) ✓
Carbidopa/Levodopa (page 49) ✓
Cardec DM (page 50) ⓘ
Chemotherapy (page 54) ⓘ
Cisplatin (page 64) ⓘ
Clozapine (page 74) ✓
Cyclophosphamide (page 79) ✓ ⓘ
Dapsone (page 85) ✓
Docetaxel (page 95) ⓘ
Doxorubicin (page 100) ✓
Ephedrine and Pseudoephedrine (page 104) ⓘ
Epinephrine (page 105) ⓘ
Fenofibrate (page 114) ✓
Fluorouracil (page 116) ⓘ
Indomethacin (page 141) ✓
Isosorbide Mononitrate (page 148) ⓘ
Methotrexate (page 169) ⓘ
Minocycline (page 179) ✓
Mixed Amphetamines (page 181) ⊘
Nitroglycerin (page 191) ✓
Oral Contraceptives (page 198) ✓
Oral Corticosteroids (page 200) ⓘ
Paclitaxel (page 205) ⓘ

Perphenazine (page 213) ⓘ
Salsalate (page 235) ✓
Tacrine (page 250) ✓
Tetracycline (page 253) ✓
Thioridazine (page 260) ⓘ
Warfarin (page 281) ⊘ ⓘ

VITAMIN D

Certain medicines interact with vitamin D:
Allopurinol (page 8) ⓘ
Anticonvulsants (page 21) ✓
Bile Acid Sequestrants (page 39) ✓
Cimetidine (page 61) ✓
Colestipol (page 76) ✓
Estradiol (page 108) ⓘ
Estrogens (Combined) (page 109) ✓ ⊘
Flurbiprofen (page 121) ✓
Gabapentin (page 125) ✓
Heparin (page 135) ✓
Hydroxychloroquine (page 137) ✓
Indapamide (page 140) ✓
Isoniazid (page 146) ✓
Medroxyprogesterone (page 167) ⓘ
Mineral Oil (page 178) ✓
Neomycin (page 187) ✓
Oral Corticosteroids (page 200) ✓
Orlistat (page 202) ✓
Phenobarbital (page 215) ✓
Sodium Fluoride (page 241) ✓
Thiazide Diuretics (page 258) ⓘ
Valproic Acid (page 275) ✓
Verapamil (page 280) ⊘
Warfarin (page 281) ⊘

VITAMIN E

Certain medicines interact with vitamin E:
Amiodarone (page 12) ✓
Anthralin (page 18) ✓
Aspirin (page 26) ⊘
AZT (page 33) ⓘ
Benzamycin (page 35) ✓
Bile Acid Sequestrants (page 39) ✓
Chemotherapy (page 54) ✓
Cisplatin (page 64) ✓
Colestipol (page 76) ✓
Cyclophosphamide (page 79) ✓
Cyclosporine (page 83) ✓

Dapsone (page 85) ✓
Docetaxel (page 95) ✓
Doxorubicin (page 100) ✓
Fenofibrate (page 114) ✓
Fluorouracil (page 116) ✓
Gemfibrozil (page 127) ✓
Glyburide (page 132) ⓘ
Griseofulvin (page 133) ✓
Haloperidol (page 134) ✓
Insulin (page 144) ✓
Isoniazid (page 146) ✓
Isotretinoin (page 149) ✓
Lindane (page 156) ✓
Lovastatin (page 163) ⓘ
Mineral Oil (page 178) ✓
Orlistat (page 202) ✓
Paclitaxel (page 205) ✓
Pentoxifylline (page 212) ✓
Risperidone (page 232) ✓
Simvastatin (page 239) ⓘ
Sodium Fluoride (page 241) ✓
Valproic Acid (page 275) ⓘ
Warfarin (page 281) ⓘ

VITAMIN K

Certain medicines interact with vitamin K:
Aminoglycoside Antibiotics (page 11) ✓
Amoxicillin (page 13) ✓
Ampicillin (page 15) ✓
Antibiotics (page 19) ✓
Anticonvulsants (page 21) ✓
Azithromycin (page 31) ✓
Bile Acid Sequestrants (page 39) ✓
Cephalosporins (page 52) ✓
Chlorhexidine (page 58) ✓
Ciprofloxacin (page 62) ✓
Clarithromycin (page 68) ✓
Clindamycin Oral (page 70) ✓
Clindamycin Topical (page 71) ✓
Colestipol (page 76) ✓
Cycloserine (page 82) ✓
Dapsone (page 85) ✓
Dicloxacillin (page 88) ✓
Doxycycline (page 101) ✓
Erythromycin (page 106) ✓
Gabapentin (page 125) ✓
Gentamicin (page 129) ✓
Isoniazid (page 146) ✓
Levofloxacin (page 155) ✓

Loracarbef (page 161) ✓
Macrolides (page 164) ✓
Mineral Oil (page 178) ✓
Minocycline (page 179) ✓
Neomycin (page 187) ✓
Nitrofurantoin (page 190) ✓
Ofloxacin (page 195) ⓘ
Oral Corticosteroids (page 200) ⓘ
Penicillin V (page 210) ✓
Penicillins (page 211) ✓
Phenobarbital (page 215) ✓
Quinolones (page 228) ✓
Sulfamethoxazole (page 245) ✓
Sulfasalazine (page 246) ✓
Sulfonamides (page 248) ✓
Tetracycline (page 253) ✓
Tetracyclines (page 255) ✓
Tobramycin (page 264) ✓
Trimethoprim (page 271) ✓
Trimethoprim/Sulfamethoxazole (page 273) ✓
Valproic Acid (page 275) ✓
Warfarin (page 281) ⊘

WHEY PROTEIN

At the time of writing, there were no well-known drug interactions with whey protein.

XYLITOL

At the time of writing, there were no well-known drug interactions with xylitol.

ZINC

Certain medicines interact with zinc:
Aspirin (page 26) ✓
AZT (page 33) ✓
Benazepril (page 34) ✓
Benzamycin (page 35) ✓
Bile Acid Sequestrants (page 39) ✓
Calcium Acetate (page 45) ✓
Captopril (page 47) ✓
Chemotherapy (page 54) ✓
Chlorhexidine (page 58) ⓘ
Ciprofloxacin (page 62) ⊘
Cisplatin (page 64) ✓
Clindamycin Topical (page 71) ✓
Colestipol (page 76) ✓
Cyclophosphamide (page 79) ✓

Zinc

Zinc

Index

About Healthnotes

Healthnotes, Inc. (HNI) is the premier provider of reliable, easy-to-use health, food, and lifestyle information for Web sites and interactive touch-screen kiosks. Used by leading supermarkets, pharmacies, and health food stores in the United States, Canada, and the United Kingdom, Healthnotes Retail Solutions empower consumers to make educated decisions and drive product sales—online and in-store. HNI also generates Web applications that are licensed to e-commerce and health-related Internet sites worldwide. On the Web: www.healthnotes.com.

Overseen by Chief Medical Editor Alan R. Gaby, M.D., the Healthnotes interdisciplinary writing team includes experts from the fields of medicine, pharmacy, nursing, naturopathy, public health, and chiropractic. We regularly update our knowledgebase, annually reviewing thousands of articles published in more than 600 peer-reviewed medical journals to ensure that consumers receive fully referenced, up-to-date health information based on the latest scientific and medical research.

Alan R. Gaby, M.D., *Chief Medical Editor*

An expert in nutritional therapies, Chief Medical Editor Alan R. Gaby is a former professor at Bastyr University of Natural Health Sciences, where he served as the Endowed Professor of Nutrition. He is past president of the American Holistic Medical Association and gave expert testimony to the White House Commission on Complementary and Alternative Medicine on the cost-effectiveness of nutritional supplements. He has authored *Preventing and Reversing Osteoporosis* (Prima Lifestyles, 1995) and *B6: The Natural Healer* (Keats, 1987) and coauthored *The Patient's Book of Natural Healing* (Prima, 1999), *The Natural Pharmacy* (Three Rivers Press, 2006), and the *A–Z Guide to Drug-Herb-Vitamin Interactions* (Three Rivers Press, 2006). Dr. Gaby has conducted nutritional seminars for physicians and has collected over 30,000 scientific papers related to the field of nutritional and natural medicine.

Also Available from Healthnotes

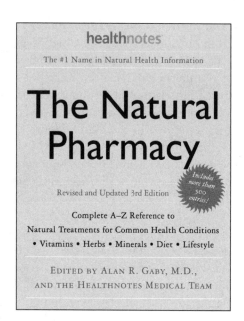

The Natural Pharmacy
0-307-33665-4
$24.95 paper (Canada: $34.95)

Written by some of the world's most respected natural health experts, *The Natural Pharmacy* offers timely, practical, fully integrated advice on treating troublesome conditions the natural way. Inside you will find complete coverage of the most common health concerns with useful treatments based on reliable, up-to-date research.

Healthnotes' trusted health, food, and lifestyle information is available throughout the United States and United Kingdom. Ask your local pharmacy, supermarket, or health food store if they offer Healthnotes in-store or online.

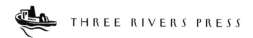 THREE RIVERS PRESS

Available from Three Rivers Press
wherever books are sold